"In her beautifully written book, *The Emergence of Analytic Oneness*: *Into the Heart of Psychoanalysis*, Ofra Eshel offers a radical change in the way we conceive of the analytic endeavor, a change that opens new possibilities for everyone engaged in the lifelong process of becoming a psychotherapist. She discusses and clinically illustrates what it is to be there with the patient so thoroughly that a new subjective entity and depth of experiencing emerges, an experiential process she calls 'withnessing.' The book is a tour de force of cutting-edge psychoanalytic theory and practice, which is particularly valuable in work with severely disturbed patients."

—**Thomas Ogden**, author of *Reclaiming Unlived Life* and *Creative Readings: Essays on Seminal Analytic Works*

"This is a very special book you will not want to miss. If you ever wanted to learn more about psychoanalysis and psychotherapy or experience fuller appreciation of how they work, this book serves as a fusion of Virgil and Beatrice as guides. Just as you think you can't go any further, more opens, wave after wave of psychic vision and reality. Depth psychology transforms as you read and your sense of being shifts with it. Psychoanalysis enters a new age, a further age. Whatever your viewpoint or practice, you will appreciate many new beginnings as windows of experience appear out of nowhere and beg you to open them."

—**Michael Eigen, PhD**, author of *The Challenge of Being Human* and *Contact with the Depths*

"This comprehensive work reflects Dr. Ofra Eshel's many years of clinical focus on the need for a deep sense of oneness with the patient, which she feels is a paradigm shift in psychoanalysis brought about by Winnicott's work and the late work of Bion. The book includes powerful clinical descriptions of psychoanalytic work with severe early loss and trauma, breakdowns of the emerging self, and 'Black Holes' in the interpersonal psychic space. *The Emergence of Analytic Oneness: Into the Heart of Psychoanalysis* stands out in its clear description of Bion's idea of at-one-ment with the patient, and the necessity of accompanying the patient into these painful depths. This scholarly book will speak to psychoanalysts and psychotherapists interested in learning about the early frontiers of the self, and Eshel's openness to these painful states of mind is an important guide to the kind of work necessary in psychoanalysis of the 21st century."

—**Annie Reiner**, author, *Bion And Being: Passion and the Creative Mind. Of Things Invisible to Mortal Sight: Celebrating the Work of James S. Grotstein* (editor), Los Angeles

The Emergence of Analytic Oneness

The Emergence of Analytic Oneness is a profound and penetrating exploration of a fundamental dimension of analytic presence and patient–analyst interconnectedness that offers new possibilities for extending the reach of psychoanalytic treatment and working with some of the most difficult treatment situations.

Eshel listens with a "hearing heart" and gives herself over to being within the patient's experiential world and the grip of the unfolding analytic process. She has gone with her patients into black holes, dissociation, deadness, sleepiness, petrifaction, silence, longings, the depths of perversion, and the enigmas of telepathic dreams, while experiencing the emergence of patient–analyst two-in-oneness, with its challenges and mysteries. Drawing on Winnicott's posthumous writings and Bion's late work, and going beyond recent analytic notions of intersubjectivity and witnessing to interconnectedness and "withnessing," Eshel offers her own understanding of at-one-ment or "being-in-oneness" with the patient's emotional reality as the only state of analytic being that can meet and transform core unthinkable breakdown and mental catastrophe. The critical question here is to what extent the analyst is willing and able to open the boundaries of his or her psyche to the patient, especially in difficult, unbearable and devastated-devastating states.

Eshel's clinical narratives are detailed, intense, theoretically grounded, and very moving. *The Emergence of Analytic Oneness* will be an invaluable guide for psychoanalysts, psychotherapists, and students in these fields who want to extend their reach into deeper levels of disturbance in the difficult clinical work they do.

Ofra Eshel is a faculty member, training and supervising analyst of the Israel Psychoanalytic Society and Institute, and member of the International Psychoanalytical Association (IPA); vice-president of the International Winnicott Association (IWA); founder and head of the postgraduate track "Independent Psychoanalysis: Radical Breakthroughs" at the advanced studies of the Program of Psychotherapy, Sackler Faculty of Medicine, Tel Aviv University. Her papers have been published in psychoanalytic journals and books and presented in national and international conferences all over the world. She is in private practice in Tel Aviv, Israel.

PSYCHOANALYSIS IN A NEW KEY BOOK SERIES

DONNEL STERN
Series Editor

When music is played in a new key, the melody does not change, but the notes that make up the composition do: change in the context of continuity, continuity that perseveres through change. Psychoanalysis in a New Key publishes books that share the aims psychoanalysts have always had, but that approach them differently. The books in the series are not expected to advance any particular theoretical agenda, although to this date most have been written by analysts from the Interpersonal and Relational orientations.

The most important contribution of a psychoanalytic book is the communication of something that nudges the reader's grasp of clinical theory and practice in an unexpected direction. Psychoanalysis in a New Key creates a deliberate focus on innovative and unsettling clinical thinking. Because that kind of thinking is encouraged by exploration of the sometimes surprising contributions to psychoanalysis of ideas and findings from other fields, Psychoanalysis in a New Key particularly encourages interdisciplinary studies. Books in the series have married psychoanalysis with dissociation, trauma theory, sociology, and criminology. The series is open to the consideration of studies examining the relationship between psychoanalysis and any other field—for instance, biology, literary and art criticism, philosophy, systems theory, anthropology, and political theory.

But innovation also takes place within the boundaries of psychoanalysis, and Psychoanalysis in a New Key therefore also presents work that reformulates thought and practice without leaving the precincts of the field. Books in the series focus, for example, on the significance of personal values in psychoanalytic practice, on the complex interrelationship between the analyst's clinical work and personal life, on the consequences for the clinical situation when patient and analyst are from different cultures, and on the need for psychoanalysts to accept the degree to which they knowingly satisfy their own wishes during treatment hours, often to the patient's detriment. A full list of all titles in this series is available at: www.routledge.com/series/LEAPNKBS

TITLES IN THIS SERIES INCLUDE:

Vol. 50 *The Emergence of Analytic Oneness: Into the Heart of Psychoanalysis* Ofra Eshel

Vol. 49 *Homosexuality, Transsexuality, Psychoanalysis and Traditional Judaism* Edited by Alan Slomowitz and Alison Feit

Vol. 48 *Psychodynamic Perspectives on Asylum Seekers and the Asylum-Seeking Process* Barbara K. Eisold

Vol. 47 *Bearing Witness to the Witness: A Psychoanalytic Perspective on Four Modes of Traumatic Testimony* Dana Amir

Vol. 46 *Travels with the Self: Interpreting Psychology as Cultural History* Philip Cushman

Vol. 45 *The Critique of Regression: A Psychoanalytic Model of Irreversible Lifespan Development* Gregory S. Rizzolo

The Emergence of Analytic Oneness

Into the Heart of Psychoanalysis

Ofra Eshel

Routledge
Taylor & Francis Group
LONDON AND NEW YORK

First published 2019
by Routledge
2 Park Square, Milton Park, Abingdon, Oxon OX14 4RN

and by Routledge
52 Vanderbilt Avenue, New York, NY 10017

Routledge is an imprint of the Taylor & Francis Group, an informa business

British Library Cataloguing in Publication Data
A catalogue record for this book is available from the British Library

Library of Congress Cataloging in Publication Data
A catalog record has been requested for this book

ISBN: 978-1-138-18633-0 (hbk)
ISBN: 978-1-138-18634-7 (pbk)
ISBN: 978-1-315-21253-1 (ebk)

Typeset in Times New Roman
by Swales & Willis Ltd, Exeter, Devon, UK

To the memory of my father, Jeruham, and to my husband Uzi, whose love and pride in me are always with me.

Contents

Acknowledgments

First and foremost, my thanks for this book go to Dr. Donnel Stern. He had first suggested that I write this book back in 2004, when he was the editor of *Contemporary Psychoanalysis*, which published two of my papers that year. It was then too early for me to write a book, but the seed was planted; and he continued to encourage me over the years until I felt that I could move on from writing articles to conceiving a book. I am, therefore, happy to publish the book in *Psychoanalysis in a New Key Book Series*, of which he is the editor.

I am profoundly indebted to my patients over the years, my true partners in unknown ways through unbearable and unthinkable psychic realities and experiences of dread, deadness, distress, despair, as well as yearning, devotion, faith and struggle. I hope I have been able to convey in this book how deep and formative the impact of these experiences has been on me. I learned *with* them the true meaning of delving into the heart of psychoanalysis.

I also wish to thank my many students, supervisees, and candidates over the years at the psychoanalytic training of the Israel Psychoanalytic Institute, and the Program of Psychoanalytic Psychotherapy for Advanced Psychotherapists at the Israel Psychoanalytic Society; at the Program of Psychotherapy, Sackler Faculty of Medicine, Tel Aviv University; at the Israel Winnicott Center; at "Mabatim," the department of psychology, Bar Ilan University; at my Wednesdays reading groups; and most recently—at the postgraduate track "Independent Psychoanalysis: Radical Breakthroughs" that I founded (2016) and chair at the advanced studies of the Program of Psychotherapy, Sackler Faculty of Medicine, Tel Aviv University. Together with them, we have had and still have the opportunity to learn, explore, think, discuss and exchange theoretical-clinical ideas and questions regarding more fundamental and experiential forms of analytic work, especially of Winnicott's thinking.

Many thanks to *Sihot—Dialogue, Israel Journal of Psychotherapy* for offering a welcoming space for the evolution of my writing for the last 23 years.

I am glad to have the opportunity to thank Yolanda Gampel and Raanan Kulka for supporting my own personal way of thinking and working analytically in the earlier years of my analytic work; the late James Grotstein for generously encouraging my analytic writing from the start; the members of my long-time peer reading group: Yossi Tamir, Nili Zaidman, Naama Keinan, Ilan Treves, and Ahuva Barkan, for our meetings over the last 25 years that have been a true learning and friendly experience; and Errica Moustaki for a longstanding, thought-provoking friendship, spanning Jerusalem, Tel Aviv, and London.

I would like to thank Ilan Amir and Amit Fachler for providing invaluable enriching material on telepathic dreams; Michal Heiman for introducing to me Cathy Caruth's writing on trauma; and Sharon Hass for sharing with me her special understanding of Dante—all these have greatly added to my understanding and writings.

I owe a special acknowledgment to Chava Cassel, Patricia Marra, and Lieske Bloom who have edited my writings in English over the years. It is difficult to write in a language that is not my inner tongue; therefore, the care and thought that they put into this editing have been much needed. Special acknowledgment also to Kristopher Spring for his help in acquiring the copyright permissions.

Finally, I am profoundly grateful to my husband Uzi for years of true love and deep t(w)ogetherness, and to our daughter Lee and son Matan, for their heart-warming presence in my life.

Copyright permissions

I wish to thank the following journals:

The *International Journal of Psychoanalysis* and John Wiley and Sons, Inc. for permission to use my following articles, here in revised form:

"Black Holes," deadness and existing analytically. International *Journal of Psychoanalysis*, 79:1115–1130, 1998. Copyright © Institute of Psychoanalysis, London, 1998.

Whose sleep is it, anyway? Or *Night Moves*. *International Journal of Psychoanalysis*, 82:545–562, 2001. Copyright © Institute of Psychoanalysis, London, 2001.

Pentheus rather than Oedipus: On perversion, survival and analytic "presencing." *International Journal of Psychoanalysis*, 86:1071–1097, 2005. Copyright © Institute of Psychoanalysis, London, 2005.

Where are you, my beloved? On absence, loss, and the enigma of telepathic dreams. *International Journal of Psychoanalysis*, 87:1603–1627, 2006. Copyright © Institute of Psychoanalysis, London, 2006.

The *Psychoanalytic Quarterly* and John Wiley and Sons, Inc. for permission to use my following articles, here in revised form:

Patient–analyst "withness": On analytic "presencing," passion, and compassion in states of breakdown, despair, and deadness. *Psychoanalytic Quarterly*, 82: 925–963, 2013.

From extension to revolutionary change in clinical psychoanalysis: The radical influence of Bion and Winnicott. *Psychoanalytic Quarterly*, 86:753–794, 2017.

Contemporary Psychoanalysis and Taylor and Francis, LLC for permission to use my following article:

The "voice" of breakdown: On facing the unbearable traumatic experience in psychoanalytic work. *Contemporary Psychoanalysis*, 52:76–110, 2016.

I also thank *Contemporary Psychoanalysis* and Taylor and Francis, LLC for permission to use clinical material from my papers:

Let it be and become me: Notes on containing, identification, and the possibility of being. *Contemporary Psychoanalysis*, 40:323–351, 2004. Copyright © *Contemporary Psychoanalysis*.

From the "Green Woman" to "Scheherazade": The becoming of a fundamentally new experience in psychoanalytic treatment. *Contemporary Psychoanalysis*, 40:527–556, 2004.

The *Psychoanalytic Review* for permission to use my following article:

A beam of "chimeric" darkness: Presence, interconnectedness and transformation in the psychoanalytic treatment of a patient convicted of sex offences. *Psychoanalytic Review*, 99:149–178, 2012. Reprinted with permission of Guilford Press, Inc.

Studies in Gender and Sexuality and Taylor & Francis Group, LLC for permission to use material from my article: Beyond sexuality, beyond perversion: The annihilated last scream. *Studies in Gender and Sexuality*, 18:154–166, 2017. This paper was also the winner of the 2017 Symonds Prize.

I am grateful for the permission to publish my article:

Into the depths of a "black hole" and deadness, in *Of Things Invisible to Mortal Sight: Celebrating the Work of James S. Grotstein*, edited by Annie Reiner (published by Karnac Books in 2017), and reprinted with kind permission of Taylor & Francis, LLC.

I am grateful for permission to use material from the following works:

Hernandez, Max. Winnicott's "Fear of Breakdown": On and Beyond Trauma. *diacritics* 28:4 (1998), 137–139. Copyright © 1999 The Johns Hopkins University Press. Reprinted with permission of Johns Hopkins University Press.

Derrida, J. (1988) Telepathy. N. Royle (trans.), *Oxford Literary Review*, 10:3–41. Reprinted with permission of Edinburgh University Press.

Guntrip, Harry. My experience of analysis with Fairbairn and Winnicott: (How complete a result does psychoanalytic therapy achieve?) Harry Guntrip's paper was first published in the *International Review of Psycho-Analysis* (1975, 2: 145–156). Copyright © Institute of Psycho-Analysis, London, 1996.

Excerpt from *Beyond Good & Evil: Prelude To A Philosophy Of The Future* by Friedrich Nietzsche, translated by Walter Kaufmann. Copyright © 1966 by Penguin Random House LLC. Used by permission of Random House, an imprint and division of Penguin Random House LLC. All rights reserved.

Excerpts from *Moments of Being: Autobiographical Writings* by Virginia Woolf, published by Chatto & Windus. Reproduced by permission of the Random House Group Ltd. (world). Copyright © 1976 by Quentin Bell and Angelica Garnett. Reprinted by permission of Houghton Mifflin Harcourt Publishing Company (United States).

From God's Christ Theory by Anne Carson, from *Glass, Irony, And God.* Copyright ©1995 by Anne Carson. Reprinted by permission of New Directions Publishing Corp.

And Death Shall Have No Dominion by Dylan Thomas, from *The Poems of Dylan Thomas*. Copyright ©1943 by New Directions Publishing Corp. Reprinted by permission of New Directions Publishing Corp. British Commonwealth rights by David Higham Associates Limited.

From Autotomy by Wislawa Szymborska, translated by Czeslaw Milosz. *Postwar Polish Poetry: An Anthology*, 1983. Republished with permission of University of California Press—Books; permission conveyed through Copyright Clearance Center, Inc.

From Poppies in October by Sylvia Plath. *The Collected Poems by Sylvia Plath.* Edited by Ted Hughes. Copyright © 1960, 1965, 1971, 1981, by the Estate of Sylvia Plath. Editorial material copyright © 1981 by Ted Hughes. Reprinted by permission of HarperCollins *Publishers*. World permission granted by Faber and Faber Ltd.

From East Coker and Little Gidding from *Collected Poems 1909–1962* by T. S. Eliot. Copyright 1936 by Houghton Mifflin Harcourt Publishing Company. Copyright © renewed 1964 by Thomas Stearns Eliot. Reprinted by permission of Houghton Mifflin Harcourt Publishing Company. All rights reserved. World permission granted by Faber and Faber Ltd.

From God full of mercy (1962) by Yehuda Amichai. Translated by B. & B. Harshav, *Shirim [Poems], 1948–1962*. Reprinted by kind permission of Hana Sokolov Amichai.

From *My Michael* by Amos Oz, translated from the Hebrew by Nicolas de Lange in collaboration with the author. Copyright © 1968, Amos Oz, by Am Oved Publishers Ltd, used by permission of the Wylie Agency (UK) Limited. English Translation copyright ©1972 by Chatto & Windus Ltd, and Alfred A. Knopf Inc. Reprinted by permission (United States and Canada) of Houghton Mifflin Harcourt Publishing Company. All rights reserved. Reproduced by permission (UK & Commonwealth) of The Random House Group Ltd. Copyright ©1972.

From Wait for me and I'll come back! by Konstantin Simonov (1941); translated by Avraham Shlonsky (1943). All rights reserved to author, Avraham Shlonsky and ACUM.

From What's love got to do with it? Words and Music by Terry Britten and Graham Lyle. Copyright © 1984 WB Music Corp and Songs of Kobalt Music Publishing. All rights reserved. Used by permission of Alfred Music.

From Suzanne, words and music by Leonard Cohen. Copyright (c) 1967, 1995 Sony/ATV Music Publishing LLC. Copyright Renewed. All Rights Administered by Sony/ATV Music Publishing LLC, 424 Church Street, Suite 1200, Nashville, TN 37219. International Copyright Secured All Rights Reserved. *Reprinted by Permission of Hal Leonard LLC.*

For Cover Image: 'A cosmic couple' (Star WR 124 and the nebula M1-67).Credit: ESA/Hubble & NASA. Acknowledgment: Judy Schmidt.

About the author

Ofra Eshel, PsyD, is senior faculty member, and training and supervising analyst at the Israel Psychoanalytic Society, and a fellow of the International Psychoanalytical Association (IPA). She is Vice-president of the International Winnicott Association (IWA); co-founder, former coordinator and faculty member of the Program of Psychoanalytic Psychotherapy for Advanced Psychotherapists at the Israel Psychoanalytic Society, and of the Israel Winnicott Center; and founder and head of the postgraduate track "Independent Psychoanalysis: Radical Breakthroughs" (2016) at the advanced studies of the Program of Psychotherapy, Sackler Faculty of Medicine, Tel Aviv University. She is book review editor of *Sihot—Dialogue, Israel Journal of Psychotherapy*.

Her papers have been published in psychoanalytic journals and books, and presented at national and international conferences allover the world. She also co-edited the book *Was It or Was It Not? When Shadows of Sexual Abuse Emerge in Psychoanalytic Treatment* (2017, in Hebrew). She received the Leonard J. Comess Fund grant at the New Center for Psychoanalysis (Los Angeles, 2011), the David Hammond grant at the Massachusetts Institute for Psychoanalysis (Boston, 2016), was a visiting scholar at the Psychoanalytic Institute of North California (San Francisco, 2013), visiting lecturer and supervisor at the Beijing Advanced International Training Program in Winnicott's Psychoanalysis (Beijing, China, 2018), and was awarded the 2013 Frances Tustin Memorial Prize and the 2017 Symonds Prize. She was featured in 2012 in *Globes* (Israel's financial newspaper and magazine) as sixteenth of the fifty most influential women in Israel. She is in private practice in Tel Aviv, Israel.

Introduction

On the emergence of analytic oneness—challenges and mysteries

This book explores and expands on ideas that have long been at the heart of my clinical work, perhaps from the very beginning of my therapeutic work with patients. Over the years, and particularly over the last 30 years of my analytic work, these ideas have crystallized and developed into my own way of psychoanalytic thinking and writing, which center on the essential function of the analyst/therapist's[1] presence and patient–analyst interconnectedness in the psychoanalytic treatment process—particularly with more disturbed patients and various difficult treatment situations. Along the way, enriching psychoanalytic theoretical and clinical influences—primarily Winnicott and Bion (especially late Bion), and also Green, Searles, Grotstein, Tustin, Bollas, Ogden, and Eigen—have provided me with deeply compelling ways of delving into the nature and meaning of these therapeutic experiences. Yet, the most profound and critical impact on my way of thinking and working has been and remains the lived experience with my patients—the vital "experiencing experience" through and within the psychoanalytic situation.

With time, I realized that a different clinical dimension had entered into my work and that I should follow its calling. This dimension is created by the analyst/therapist's "presencing" (being there) within the patient's experiential world and within the grip of the analytic process, and the ensuing deep patient–analyst interconnectedness. Patient and analyst thus forge an emergent new entity of interconnectedness or "withnessing" that goes beyond the confines of their separate subjectivities and the simple summation of the two—*a two-in-oneness*. I have also called this process "quantum interconnectedness" (from physicist David Bohm's [1980] phrase "the quantum interconnectedness of distant systems").

This fundamental dimension, with its profound ontological[2] implications, engenders markedly new possibilities in clinical experience, especially at deeper levels of disturbance. It has become an essential and integral part of the way I practice, think of, and envision psychoanalytic work. Thus, I went with my patients through "black holes," through feelings of deadness, sleepiness, dissociation, vanished last screams, petrifaction and silences, yearnings and longings, into the depths of perversion, and the enigma of telepathic dreams, while staying within the intense impact of the treatment situation and communing with it. I came to feel that analytic treatments have to reach *a moment of patient–analyst profound interconnectedness,* a moment of be(com)ing-at-one with the patient's experience, which is of critical transformative importance when being in touch with the patient's deeper levels of traumatic or core experiences.

Over the last decade, I further developed this dimension of patient–analyst interconnected being and experiencing, expanding it beyond recent analytic notions of intersubjectivity and witnessing, to a more radical patient–analyst "analytic oneness" and "transformations in Oneness." I venture to suggest that patient–analyst deep-level interconnectedness or "withnessing," which grows into *"at-one-ment"* with the patient's innermost experience, is the only state of analytic being that can meet and transform core breakdown and mental catastrophe. This idea draws on my understanding of Winnicott's (1974, 1965a, 1967a) posthumous writings and Bion's (1967a, 1970) late writing on at-one-ment or being-in-oneness with the patient's unthinkable and ultimately unknown psychic reality.

Using detailed clinical illustrations, accompanied by theoretical and clinical psychoanalytic material, the book describes the evolution of my theoretical-clinical psychoanalytic approach over the years, and the kind of knowledge, experience, and powerful effects that come into being when the analyst interconnects psychically with the patient in living through the process. Each of the chapters in the book grew out of an attempt to come to grips with a problem, a struggle, or a particularly poignant situation in my clinical experience. This involved pursuing the ontological (being) rather than the epistemological (interpretive) dimension of experience, and drawing on experiential-developmental modes of being, relating, and becoming in my analytic technique and therapeutic action. Thus, the book charts my endeavor to explore and grasp the true experiential scope and therapeutic significance of working within this fundamental dimension of analytic presence and interconnectedness, with the emergence of analytic oneness and its various, sometimes most radical, expressions. I have found that working analytically within this dimension deepens and extends the reach of analytic experience in ways that I had not thought possible.

In the last chapter of the book, I address the radical departure of Winnicott's and late Bion's theoretical-clinical ideas from traditional psychoanalytic work, introducing a revolutionary change in clinical psychoanalysis—a transition from "extension" to "scientific revolution," and "paradigm change or paradigm shift" (to use Thomas Kuhn's 1962 terminology). For me, these revolutionary ideas of late Bion and Winnicott are profoundly important, theoretically and practically, as they provide a formative matrix and a mode of transformation that relationships cannot offer at deep levels of disturbance. I believe that the ontological *experience of analytic oneness*, suspended, even if momentarily, from epistemological and relational discourse, becomes an experience and language of new possibility, especially within states of breakdown, devastation, core deadness, and emptiness. It is, in my view, the place wherein lies the very heart of psychoanalysis and, I would add, its wonder.

The trajectory of the chapters of this book follows the exploration and evolution, in some specific way, of the dimension of analytic presence, deep patient–analyst interconnectedness or "withnessing," and the emergence of analytic oneness as it occurs in the clinical situation.

Part I. Within the depths of being: experiences in a new dimension

In chapters 1 through 7, I describe the development of my theoretical-clinical approach over time, and how it expands beyond recent analytic notions of intersubjectivity and witnessing to more radical patient–analyst deep-level interconnectedness or "withnessing" that may grow into at-one-ment.

What does it mean to approach the heart of psychoanalytic work? Chapter 1—The heart. Or, what's *heart* got to do with it?—brings the "hearing heart" that King Solomon requested from God (I Kings 3:9) and Frances Tustin's emphasis on experiencing "the heart-break which is at the centre of human existence" into psychoanalytic treatment. The experiencing and "hearing heart"—the willingness to dare to open one's heart and soul to another human being—is at the core of the analyst's difficult struggle to give him/herself over to being within the troubled emotional experience of the patient's world, particularly when sensing, hearing and experiencing the "voice" of the patient's trauma or breakdown that cries out.

Chapter 2—Two-in-oneness: Transformations in "O"—introduces the two main pillars of the clinical thinking that I develop and explore in this book—the analyst's "presencing" (being-within), and the ensuing deep patient–analyst interconnectedness or "withnessing," in which the analyst's psyche is there to be used as an area of experiencing, processing, and transforming for the patient's expelled, unbearable experiences. Thus, it is not a one- or two-person psychology, but an emergent two-in-oneness that is fundamentally inseparable into its two participants—an analytic oneness that transcends the duality of patient and analyst, transference and countertransference. I highlight how this dimension of analytic work converges with and differs from other forms of profound interconnectedness (developed in recent years by Ogden, Botella and Botella, the Barangers and Ferro).

Chapter 3—Into the depths of a "black hole" and deadness—makes metaphorical use of the astrophysical "black hole" and the event horizon, applying them to an interpersonal phenomenon of individuals whose interpersonal and intersubjective psychic space is dominated by a central object that is experienced as a black hole. Thus, they are either gripped by its enormous, compelling pull, or are petrified in their interpersonal psychic space out of fear of being pulled over its edge. This black hole experience in the interpersonal psychic space is caused mainly by the impact of a psychically "dead" parent, particularly the impact of the psychically "dead mother" on her child (Green, 1986). The analysis that I present in this chapter, of a man who grew up with a "dead" mother, brings to the fore, experientially and theoretically, the pivotal role of the analyst's capacity to be there and remain alive, while experiencing and going through annihilation and death along with the patient—a years-long struggle that could not be completed without reaching a moment of "at-one-ment" with the patient's desperate and painful innermost experience.

Chapter 4—Whose sleep is it, anyway? Or, *Night Moves*—deals with the analyst's "sleep" during sessions, a puzzling, troubling, extreme experience, which has hardly been described in the psychoanalytic literature. Using a clinical illustration in which my recurring "sleep" during the sessions was approached as an open, central issue, I explore theoretically and clinically the analyst's sleep, first with a review and examination of the psychoanalytic literature on the subject and on related phenomena, and then by offering my own explanation of it, which emphasizes the analyst's being in the grip of a dissociative process and the ensuing state of deep experiential patient–analyst interconnectedness and impact on each other. This thinking addresses notions of "the uncanny," dissociation, and the mitigation of the patient's dissociative self-experience via the analyst's own vicarious dissociative experience.

In chapter 5—A beam of "chimeric" darkness: Presence, interconnectedness, and transformation in the psychoanalytic treatment of a patient convicted of sex offenses—the dimension created by the analytic presence and ensuing patient–analyst interconnectedness takes on an almost transplant-like, or immunological form of "chimeric" antibodies that do not trigger the immune reaction in the body, generally triggered by regular antibodies toward what they perceive as "foreign" elements. The chapter focuses on the "chimeric" element or quality of patient–analyst interconnectedness—the term "chimeric" chosen here for its wealth of mythological, genetic, biological, biomedicinal (chimeric proteins), and psychoanalytical associations—to highlight the complex quality of patient–analyst interconnectedness, especially in difficult, psychotic, psychically foreclosed, profoundly dissociated and perverse states. I include an extensive clinical account of the psychoanalytic treatment of a patient convicted of sex offenses to illustrate "presencing," interconnectedness, and the extent and intricate emotional meaning of the extreme chimerism that this kind of difficult treatment entailed.

Chapter 6—Where are you, my beloved? On absence, loss, and the enigma of telepathic dreams—focuses on the subject of dream telepathy (especially patients' telepathic dreams) and related phenomena in the psychoanalytic context, which has been a controversial, disturbing "foreign body" ever since it was introduced into psychoanalysis by Freud in 1921. Telepathy—suffering (or intense feeling) at a distance (Greek: *pathos* + *tele*)—is the transfer or communication of thoughts, impressions and information between two people without using the recognized sense organs. The chapter opens with a comprehensive historical review of the psychoanalytic literature on this controversial issue, beginning with Freud's years-long struggle over the possibility of thought-transference and dream telepathy. This is followed by a description of my own analytic encounters over the years with the telepathic dreams of five patients—dreams involving precise details of the time, place, sensory impressions, and experiential states that the analyst was in at that time, which the patients could not have known through ordinary sensory perception and communication. My ensuing explanation combines contributory factors of the patient, archaic communication, and the analyst. The mother of each of these patients in their early childhood was emotionally absent-within-absence of a significant figure in her own life, resulting in a fixation on a nonverbal, archaic mode of communication. The patients' telepathic dreams are formed to serve as a search engine to find the analyst when he or she is suddenly emotionally absent, and thus halt the process of abandonment and prevent a collapse into the despair of the early traumatization. Hence, the telepathic dream embodies an enigmatic "impossible" extreme of patient–analyst deep-level interconnectedness and unconscious communication in the analytic process.

Chapter 7—Pentheus rather than Oedipus: On perversion, survival, and analytic "presencing"—begins with a review of the main developments in psychoanalytic thinking on perversion, followed by my own understanding of perversion and its treatment, which is based on the psychoanalytic treatment of patients with severe sexual perversions. I use the term "autotomy" (borrowed from the field of biology) to describe perversion formation as an "autotomous," massive splitting defense in the service of psychic survival within violent, deeply traumatic, early childhood situations. Thus, a compulsively enacted "desire for ritualized trauma" ensues—a last-ditch attempt to prevent, by its corporeality and intensity, a collapse into dread, psychic deadness, and annihilation. The specific nature of the perverse scenario embodies the specific experiential core quality of the traumatic situation while, at the same time, controlling, sanitizing and disavowing it. Hence, the world of severe perversion is no longer oedipal, but rather the world of Pentheus, Euripides's most tragic hero—a world dominated by a mixture of a mother's madness, devourment, destruction, and rituals of desire. From this perspective, I emphasize the importance of the analyst's abiding "presencing" and interconnection with the perverse patient, thus being with-in and listening to the perversion beyond its pathology, for its survival function and the profound loneliness and despair it carries. This approach creates a new, alternative experiential-emotional reality within the patient's alienated world, eventually generating a change in the perverse essence. I provide several clinical vignettes that illustrate the genesis of my thinking on perversion.

Part II. The "voice" of breakdown

In chapters 8 through 10, I continue to describe how working within the dimension of analytic presence and patient–analyst deep interconnectedness or "withnessing" that grows into at-one-ment enables me to meet, reach, and transform the patient's most unknown, unrepresented states, mainly of core catastrophe (Bion) and unthinkable, unexperienced breakdown and madness (Winnicott).

Chapter 8—*"For You have returned my soul within me with compassion":* "Presencing," passion, and compassion in the depths of perversion, breakdown, despair, and deadness[3]—focuses on *compassion*, which is the analyst's specific way of "withnessing" or interconnectedness with the patient's agonizing states of deep distress, annihilation, and hopelessness. The clinical material here is taken from the analysis of the severely fetishistic-masochistic patient described in chapter 7 up to the cessation of his perverse practices in the third year. This led to an extreme collapse into profound devastation, emptiness, psychic death, and violent suicidal despair. Working within this collapse in analysis enabled the deep reason for the patient's breakdown in early life to unfold. And, most importantly, it engendered the crucial possibility that had never been experienced before, of reliving the patient's unbearable breakdown and deadness—this time patient-with-analyst t(w)ogether—and experientially coming through it differently. Yet it still remains without an ending of love.

Chapter 9—The "voice" of breakdown: On facing the unbearable traumatic experience in psychoanalytic work—weaves together three major contributions to the theory of trauma and repetition compulsion: Freud's (1920) reformulation in "Beyond the Pleasure Principle" of his metapsychological theory regarding the notion of trauma and the compulsion to repeat traumatic experiences and traumatic dreams; Cathy Caruth's (1996) elaboration in *Unclaimed Experience*, based on a dramatic story in Freud's article, of "the voice that cries out, a voice that is released through the double wound"; and Winnicott's unique ideas in "Fear of breakdown" (1974) and "The psychology of madness" (1965a) about the early unthinkable breakdown that has not yet been experienced and has to be experienced in analysis. I explore the clinical implications of the intricate relation between knowing and not-knowing in facing trauma. In particular, I relate to the profound difficulty of hearing the "voice" of breakdown that cries out from the belated "double wounding," the critical importance of experiencing the unexperienced *with* the analyst; and the immensity of the terror and hope that is at the heart of the reaching to the original unbearable traumatization in psychoanalytic work. I present three detailed clinical illustrations from various psychoanalytic writings and excerpts from an autobiographical essay by Virginia Woolf.

Chapter 10—From extension to revolutionary change in clinical psychoanalysis: The radical influence of Bion and Winnicott—addresses the profound departure of late Bion's and Winnicott's theoretical-clinical ideas and practices from traditional psychoanalytic work, that introduce revolutionary change in clinical psychoanalysis—a transition from "extension" to "scientific revolution" and "paradigm shift or paradigm change" in psychoanalysis (Kuhn, 1962). I underscore in both late Bion's and Winnicott's innovations, the radical ontological experience of patient-and-analyst being-in-oneness at a primordial point of origin, in order to reach and transform the patient's unknown and unknowable, unrepresented states, mainly of core catastrophe (Bion) and unthinkable breakdown and madness (Winnicott). I therefore suggest that the revolutionary approach that their clinical thinking introduced be termed "*quantum psychoanalysis*," and it may co-exist with classical psychoanalysis in the same way that classical physics co-exists with quantum physics.

Notes

1 For simplicity's sake, throughout this book, I will use the term "analyst" to refer to both analyst and therapist, unless I am describing a particular patient-therapist situation.
2 Ontology—the study of the nature of being.
3 "For You have returned my soul within me with compassion" is from the morning prayer that religious Jews recite daily.

Part I

Within the depths of being

Experiences in a new dimension

> No matter how deep our analytical experience, this is just the tip of the iceberg of that mystery. It is a mystery, and we are just starting to learn the mystery behind it.
>
> (Bion in Buenos Aires, 2018/1968)

> There is something about going into the depths, and even further, beyond what we think the depths can be.
>
> (Merle Molofsky, 2012)

Chapter 1

The heart

Or, what's *heart* got to do with it?

What does it mean to approach the heart of psychoanalytic work? In this chapter, I will delve, clinically and theoretically, into the essential meanings and experiences that this question carries for me.

A "hearing heart"

The peculiar biblical combination of a "hearing heart"—"לב שומע"—has captured my imagination and thinking and carved out a space in my clinical understanding over many years. As a child in primary school, I studied the biblical story of King Solomon asking God to give him a "hearing heart" to be able to judge the people (I Kings 3:9), and I was perplexed by this peculiar combination—how can a heart hear? The marvel of a "hearing heart" followed me into my first analytic paper on storytelling and listening in the analytic situation (1996). Later on, in my paper on containing (2002a [Hebrew], 2004a [English]), I emphasize the importance, even the necessity, of the analyst's "hearing heart"—hearing, listening, and understanding with one's heart—in the process of containing. And, more recently (2012a, 2015a, 2016a—chapter 9 in this book), once more, it forms a fundamental aspect of my thinking when facing the "voice" of trauma or breakdown.

When translating my 2002 paper on containing from Hebrew to English, I was surprised to discover that the standard translations of the Bible into English diminish the peculiarity of this combination by changing the "hearing heart" to "an understanding heart,"[1] "a discerning heart,"[2] "an understanding mind,"[3] and "a thoughtful mind."[4] Only the *Oxford Study Bible* comes closer to the original Hebrew—"a heart with skill to listen."

These translations miss a subtle yet crucial further occurrence in the Hebrew biblical narrative. Although King Solomon asks God for a "hearing heart" ("לב שומע"), he is given "a wise and an understanding heart" ("לב חכם ונבון"), and also "both riches and honour":

> Behold, I have done according to thy words: lo, I have given thee a wise and an understanding heart, so that there was none like thee before thee, neither after thee shall any arise like unto thee. And I have also given thee that which thou hast not asked, both riches and honour.
>
> (I Kings 3:12–13)

Thus, "the wisdom of God was in him" (3:28), yet *not a "hearing heart."*

What does this mean? Hazan (2008), who, too, relates the "hearing heart" to analytic listening, offers an intriguing explanation:

> It seems to me that buried in this ancient text is a unique insight into the essence of analytic listening, and, even if it is not found there, a contemporary listening to the text allows us to derive this insight from it. What I am saying is that it is referring to a wish that will always remain only partially fulfilled, and, at best, we must be satisfied with a wise and understanding heart, which is no small feat. But even if we do not receive a *hearing heart*, it exists there as a poetic ideal which constitutes part of who we are, and serves as a landmark which determines the azimuth according to which we listen.
>
> (p. 7, italics in original)

I understand this differently. I think that in the biblical text a "hearing heart" thus becomes a great human longing that cannot be obtained from without, not even through Divine giving; nor does it pertain to the realm of wisdom, even Divine wisdom. All of these may confer "a wise and an understanding heart."[5] The "hearing heart," however, can be attained only through *a willingness to dare to open one's heart and soul to another human being*. It is thus at the core of the analyst's difficult, sometimes exceedingly difficult, struggle to give himself/herself over—with all one's heart, soul, might (Eigen, 1981, based on Deuteronomy 6:5)—to being there within the troubled emotional experience of the patient's world—staying open and attuned, sensing, hearing, and feeling the "voice" of the patient's trauma or breakdown that cries out (Caruth, 1996; Eshel, 2015a, 2016a—chapter 9).

Tustin's "heart-break"—or, "Who needs a heart when a heart can be broken?"[6]

Then, into my "heart" thinking entered Frances Tustin's "heart-break." In the early 1990s, I became acquainted with Tustin's writings, and although I did not work with autistic children, they influenced the way I thought of and practiced psychoanalytic treatment, especially with severely disturbed patients. I was affected not only by her ideas, but also by the distinctive way in which she expressed them—in imagery that she carried over throughout all of her books: "the black hole of traumatic bodily separateness"[7] (1972, 1981/1992, 1986, 1990), "the protective shell against an original agony" (1990), "at root, there is such a terror of worse than death" (1972). And, in particular, I was enthralled by her words regarding "the heart-break which is at the centre of human existence" (1972). She wrote about it powerfully in her first book, ending on a somewhat enigmatic note:

> Distribution of largesse may seem like sympathy and kindness. Manipulation of materials, often of an extremely capable and skilful kind, may seem like creative activity. But these are not the works of creative imagination or caring. *For this to occur, the heart-break which is at the centre of human existence has to be experienced again and again in ever-widening contexts of developing maturity. The care of psychotic children demands people who have experienced this.*
>
> (Tustin, 1972, p. 83, my italics)

"*Who needs a heart when a heart can be broken?*" The words of Tina Turner's song resounded while I was reading Tustin's words. And, in Tustin's last book (1990), a very experienced medical director of a psychiatric clinic admonished a young psychiatrist regarding his patient, "You should never have taken such a patient. These patients break therapists' hearts." But Tustin, who over the years (1991, 1994) undauntedly discarded some of her early key ideas, retained the idea of "broken-heartedness"—from her first book in1972 to her last, 18 years later, in 1990. She recounts in the latter, that the young psychiatrist mentioned above, who was admonished by his director, had come to consult her about his patient, and as the result of what she had learned from autistic children, she

> . . . was able to help this psychiatrist to see that these patients threaten to break therapists' hearts because they themselves are 'heartbroken.' The 'heartbreak' goes beyond what we usually mean by the term. The feeling of brokenness goes into the very fabric of their being . . .. Their sense of 'being' was felt to be threatened. Annihilation stared them in the face, and very desperate steps had to be taken to combat it. To combat it and to cover their brokenness, they developed the plaster cast of autism. This concretized experience of encapsulation spells death to the psyche . . .. Understanding their sense of agony helps us.
>
> (1990, pp. 155–157)[8]

Tustin's years-long profound understanding of the "broken-heart" converges with my years-long journey regarding the significance of the "hearing heart" in psychoanalysis, becoming now *a meeting of hearts*.

Freud writes that the analyst "must turn his own unconscious like a receptive organ toward the transmitting unconscious of the patient. He must adjust himself to the patient as a telephone receiver is adjusted to the transmitting microphone" (1912, pp. 115–116). And Bion says, "If the analyst is prepared to listen, have his eye open, his ears open, his senses open, his intuition open, it has an effect upon the patient who seems to grow" (cited by F. Bion, 1995, p. 106). I see the "hearing heart" as an essential part of the analyst's increased receptive capacity, and emphasize the crucial necessity of the analyst's *openness of heart*. And adding Tustin's idea of "broken-heartedness," it is the analyst/therapist's heart that hears and "experiences again and again the heart-break which is at the centre of human existence," especially when the patient's transmission is unthinkably broken. In the Hebrew verse "With all one's heart, with all one's soul, and with all one's might" (Deuteronomy, 6:5), the word "heart" is spelled with a double letter *beit* ב—לבב *levav*—rather than the usual לב *lev* (that again, does not find *expression* in the English translation). It is this double "heartedness" that I put forward here. This very vital quality of the *analyst's hearing and experiencing "broken-heartedness"* engenders a different possibility for reaching and meeting the painful immensity of the brokenness of a human[e] psyche.

"I have called upon poets and writers to help me in this task . . . we need to be encircled by their integrating aesthetic embrace," writes Tustin (1986, p 12). I would now like to address the clinical meaning of hearing, experiencing, and staying with the heart-break through the tragic, horrifying story of Count Ugolino, told to Dante and Virgil in the depths of the *Inferno* (*The Divine Comedy*, 1320), and through my own case illustration. Let me begin with Dante.

Dante and Ugolino in the *Inferno*—the unmet weeping of the broken-heart

Dante's *Divine Comedy*, written 700 years ago and still widely considered one of the greatest classics of Western literature,[9] describes in the first-person Dante's journey through the three realms of the dead: *Inferno* (Hell), *Purgatorio* (Purgatory), and *Paradiso* (Paradise or Heaven). Dante is guided through Hell and Purgatory by Virgil, the great Roman poet he reveres, who protects him mentally and physically from the horrors of the journey, while his guide through Paradise is Beatrice, his ideal woman and the love of his youth.[10] But Dante does not want to write allegoric poetry; rather, he writes "a detailed and exact diary of a journey . . . [in which] the most prominent theme is the naturalist precision of the description" (Stav, 2007, p. 59), with tangible physical descriptions and a richness of visual imagery.

Dante and Virgil's journey through *Inferno* is narrated in onerous and excruciating detail, in over 34 cantos. They descend, circle by circle, through the nine circles of Hell, which are teeming with wickedness, horrifying tortures, and unending lamentation, and each of the nine circles represents increasing levels of evil, horrors, and agony. The last, bottommost circle of Hell, "the lowest point of all evil," is the circle of treachery—betrayal is the ultimate sin in the eyes of Dante—divided into four sections according to the type of betrayal: of blood relatives, of homeland or party, of one's guests, and of masters and benefactors. Depending on the form of their treachery, traitors are forever entrapped in varying degrees in the vast ever-frozen Lake Cocytus (from the Greek Κωκυτός, "lamentation"), filled with heartbroken voices. Here, in Canto 33—the penultimate canto of the journey through Hell—Count Ugolino tells Dante his gruesome story, the longest and most tragic story told by any of the characters in *Inferno*.

It is an appalling story that begins with a horrifying scene, in which Dante and Virgil (at the end of Canto 32) see in the frozen lake a man who is gnawing another man's head and neck from behind "as in hunger people will gnaw bread." Dante inquires what has warranted such cruelty, "O you who show by such a bestial mark/The hate you have for him whom you are eating,/Tell me why" (Canto 32, p. 185). The man raises his mouth from the bleeding skull and wipes his lips on his victim's hair. Identifying himself as Count Ugolino from Pisa and the other man as the Archbishop Ruggieri, who informed on him, he begins to tell of his "desperate grief, which presses on my heart." But although Ugolino is condemned to eternal damnation at the lowest circle of Hell for political treachery, he makes no attempt to exonerate himself of the crime; his story, instead, is about the terrible days during which he and his innocent children were cruelly killed, starving to death.

When imprisoned for treachery in a tall tower together with his four sons, he dreamed one night that a man, a lord and master, with hunting dogs, was chasing after a wolf and his cubs, the dogs catching them and tearing them to pieces. He woke up from this nightmare, feeling an imminent catastrophe, and hearing his famished sons crying out in their sleep. But when the morning came, they heard that instead of bringing them food, the gate to the tower prison had been locked and they were left to starve to death. Ugolino looked silently at his sons, his heart turning to stone as his sons cried, until his youngest son, Anselmo asked in fear: "Why do you stare so, father, what is the matter?" But Ugolino neither cried nor could reply that entire day and night. The next day, when he saw "on their faces the look that was in my own," he bit his hands in deep grief, and they thought that it was from hunger. They thus offered him to eat their bodies, the bodies he had given to them. Ugolino was silent in view of such suffering, and all of them remained silent for the next two days. On the fourth day of their torment, his son Gaddo threw himself at his father's feet, cried out for help, "My father, why do you not help us?" and died; the remaining three brothers died one after the other over the following two days. Ugolino who had turned "blind and crazy," groped over his dead children and for two days later called out their names; "And then, hunger had more force than grief." (Canto 33, pp. 186–188)

Ugolino's last statement that hunger proved stronger than grief has been interpreted in two ways: either that Ugolino devoured his children's corpses after being driven mad with hunger, or that starvation killed him after he had failed to die of grief. Whatever the case, Ugolino ends his story and resumes gnawing on Ruggieri's skull. "[W]ith his eyes bulging,/ He again seized the skull with his teeth,/Which, on the bone, were as strong as the dog's" (Canto 33, p. 188).

At this point, the text presents harsh but impersonal lines, cursing Pisa, wishing for its downfall, "For if Count Ugolino is supposed/to have betrayed you so that you lost your castles,/You had no right to put his sons to torture./ Their tender age made them innocent,/You modern Thebes!" (Canto 33, p. 188). And Dante and Virgil move on, passing to the third ring of traitors.

What has happened here? Why, after telling his dreadful story, does Ugolino immediately revert to the same cannibalistic behavior as before? In recent years, the notion of "*witness*" has increasingly gained currency in clinical psychoanalytic thinking, particularly in cases of trauma (Caruth, 1995; Grand, 2000; Reis, 2009a; Stern, 2012; Amir, 2012). The witness is an attentive presence that enables the traumatized person to face the traumatic. For the trauma leaves the survivor cut off, disconnected, lonely, and lost, with nobody to turn to—"The trauma survivor remains solitary in the moment of her [or his] own extinction . . . possessed in its impenetrable solitude" (Grand, 2000, p. 4). Reis (2009a) compellingly broadens the notion of witnessing and suggest that "it is the analytic encounter that allows traumatic repetition to take on the quality of a communication, an address to another, rather than remain meaningless reproduction" (p. 1359).

In Dante's classical text, the most essential features of witnessing are present: Dante's question to Ugolino is asked from a real wish to know—there is a concentrated listening. And at the end there is an angry outcry regarding the injustice of the dreadful punishment of Ugolino's innocent children. So, what is missing here? Why after all this does Ugolino immediately return to the relentless cannibalism of before?

Perhaps the answer lies in Ugolino's two moments of emotional relating to Dante: First, after being asked by Dante what has warranted his cruel cannibalistic behavior, Ugolino begins by saying:

> You are asking me to renew
> A desperate grief, which presses *on my heart*,
> Even to think of, and before I speak.
> But if my words are to be a seed

> Which may grow . . .
> You shall *see me speak and weep at the same time*.
> (Canto 33, p. 186, my italics)

But after telling Dante about his waking up terrified from the nightmare about the wolf and his cubs devoured by the hunting dogs, fearing an imminent catastrophe, and hearing his famished sons crying out in their sleep, he says to Dante:

> You must be cruel, if it does not *hurt you*
> To think of the apprehension *in my heart*;
> And *if you do not weep, what do you weep for?*
> (Canto 33, p. 187, my italics)

Thus, in the beginning, Ugolino's need is for Dante's listening as he spoke and wept while recounting the desperate grief of his heart. But, soon, this is transformed into Ugolino's yearning for a hearing, feeling, and experiencing human being who is willing and able to connect with a heart in pain, terror, and desperation, and also weep when he hears the voice of the broken-heart crying out (Caruth, 1996; Eshel, 2012a, 2015a, 2016a—chapter 9).

I suggest calling this deeper quality of relating "*withnessing*," rather than "witnessing" (Eshel, 2013a, 2016a—chapter 9)—to *be-with*, within the unbearable painful experience of the severely traumatized person through the deep and very fundamental quality of interconnectedness, psyche-to-psyche, heart-to-heart. It is the "*withnessing*" *presence*, not exoneration, that was needed here. But this is difficult—to allow the unbearable cry to touch us. And Dante, with Virgil protecting him mentally and physically in order to survive the horrifying journey through Hell, wanted to move on and end their passage through the dark depths of the Inferno because Dante's goal was to redeem his soul and be able to reach his eternal love and Heaven. It seems to me that the last weeping of Ugolino's broken-heart—the last cry just before hope was abandoned—remained unmet.

Case illustration: the gate of tears

I would now like to further address what it means to hear, experience, and stay with-in "the heart-break which is at the centre of human existence" by using my own case illustration.

Ben, a very tall, athletic, and strikingly handsome young man of twenty-eight came to me for psychoanalytic psychotherapy because of a prolonged depressive crisis over the preceding two years, centering on a girlfriend who had betrayed and left him. He had already been through two failed psychotherapies, which had terminated with a recommendation for medication.

In response to my questions, he vacantly described what had happened with the girl. There were always girls who had been interested in him, who had "come on to him," but after a night or two they would leave. Only this girl, Julie, had stayed, insisting on continuing the relationship, saying that she loved him. After three months together, she decided to go abroad. He did not object, and even felt relieved. She left, and about a month later the tonc of her letters changed—they became more sporadic, until they finally stopped. On her return three months later, she told him that while abroad she had had a relationship with someone else, and, although it had ended, she categorically refused to go back to Ben, despite his repeated entreaties that she come back and try again. From her point of view, Ben was a closed issue, she said. He began calling her day and night, sometimes speaking, pleading with her to come back, feeling humiliated but unable to stop, and other times not speaking at all. Each night he hung around her house for hours, drunk, drugged, in a daze, tracking her movements: Was she at home? What time did she switch off the light? What time did she go to bed? Did she have someone else?

Despite enrolling in a university, he barely attended lectures and throughout those two years repeatedly failed all his examinations. He sometimes did random, simple work, mainly at night, to partially cover his expenses. It was a major, all-encompassing emotional and functional crisis.

Having told me this, and after asking him a few more informational questions and receiving informational answers at the first sessions, there appeared to be nothing else to say, to talk about or relate to. Any effort of mine to go on asking and encouraging him to talk always ended up in the same meaningless, empty, futile place. "Does zilch for me," he would repeatedly respond to anything, his words addressed to no one. There was no area that interested him. His studies? "Zilch"—he had no interest in what he was studying, and no interest in any other field either. The long trip around the world he had taken after his military service and the places he had visited? "Zilch." Going out with friends? "Zilch." Work? "Zilch." The treatment? "Zilch," and anyway they'd told him everything in his previous treatments, which "also did zilch for me." When I gave up on my attempts to ask questions and encourage him to talk, a silence reigned that was no less hollow and dreary. It was not his non-speaking, but this "Zilch" that crept into speech and silence, into every corner, everywhere, limitless, with no way out. It was as if there was an irreparable fault in the aliveness of his psychic apparatus. "Zilch." A desolate emotional wasteland. There was only the nocturnal, disconnected, ceaseless, and despairing hanging around Julie's house, perhaps because she, by leaving him, was the only one who had broken through this nothingness.

After about two-and-a-half months of this, I thought that perhaps if he were in treatment with a younger female therapist, one closer to him in age and his world, something more libidinal, more alive, might evolve. And perhaps I had also become weary. Thus, I offered him this alternative. But he immediately replied that he had no intention of going to any other therapist, neither younger nor older, that this was the last treatment he was ever going to try, and, besides, he didn't know why he was still trying at all.

And so we continued treatment for another month. Gradually there was a significant diminishing of his nocturnal wanderings. And then, after being in treatment for almost four months, he told me that he saw no point in continuing. Nothing had changed, it was end-of-year-exam time, and it would be better to spend his time studying. After one further session, I accepted his decision, asking him only to call me if matters deteriorated. He called about three weeks later. He told me that he had failed all of his exams, that he hadn't even sat for some of them, and that he had resumed his nocturnal wanderings around Julie's house.

We resumed treatment.

During this next period in treatment, Ben tried something different. He brought the letters Julie had written him from abroad and read them to me, trying to seek and discover with me what had happened and when: when had she stopped loving him, what had gone wrong, and why. He brought photographs of the two of them that had been taken before she went abroad. They showed a handsome couple, with Julie looking at him very affectionately.

During these months, his "wanderings" around Julie in the treatment hours replaced his nocturnal wanderings around her house. He struck up a relationship with a new girl, but she, too, terminated it after two weeks. Once again, a relationship that was terminated abruptly. Once again there was this terrible gap between his remarkably attractive appearance, and the incomprehensible and unavoidable collapse of any relationship.

After about three months into this stage of treatment, he came to a session looking very tired. He said he had hardly slept that night because he had been with a woman several years older than he, whom he had met at a pub, but he didn't want to continue the relationship with her. He didn't want to hurt her because she wanted something serious. She was as desperate as he was when he wanted someone. Perhaps he would go out with her a few more times when he was lonely and drunk. He added that he was not attending lectures, he didn't feel like it, didn't want anything. He asked if he could lie down on the couch in my room. He lay down and asked, "Can't see you?" Then he lay silent and motionless until the hour was up, looking very long and stiff. I thought (although I did not know for sure) that he had closed his eyes. He awoke himself just before the session was over and left.

At the following session, he did not utter a single word. I felt that he had been frightened by his letting go at the previous session. The day before the next session he called to say he would not be coming. He didn't want to continue treatment. I asked him to come so that we could talk about it.

He came and stated at the outset that he didn't want to be in treatment any longer. It ran counter to the macho image he had been raised to assume—it annoyed him. Then he fell silent. Later he said that he had called Julie that week and she had told him that she didn't want to speak to him, that he was no longer part of her life, and then she had hung up on him. He didn't want to be in treatment. I said that he couldn't leave treatment like this, without something improving for him, in some area—in his studies, at work, in love. "It doesn't matter, I'll go somewhere or other," he said. But I felt that he could not go in this state. And in stark contrast to the previous time he had wanted to leave treatment, now I was fighting for this failed treatment with a stubbornness incomprehensible to me, telling him that I couldn't let him go like that, to nowhere, despairing, and destructive, that this ran counter to my professional and human responsibility. And as I spoke, I felt tears coming into my eyes.

He looked at me, seeing my distress, and said, almost feelingly (I thought), "You're the only one who cares about me, of all the psychologists. I know it's not a matter of ego with you. But you just don't understand—I'm lost. I'm lost. There's no chance. No chance at all."

"Give me, give the treatment, a year," I said. "You came to treatment at the beginning of April. So stay in treatment until next April, and if it doesn't help you, I won't say another word if you want to go."

"I came at the beginning of April?" he asked. "That's when I was born." We checked my appointment book, and indeed found that he had come for the first time one day after his birthday.

Something in this new, surprising, and tangible feeling of time, which had thus entered the treatment, drew my attention to the fact that every three or four months a crisis would arise in treatment. Julie, too, had gone abroad after three months with him, and had betrayed him after four. As he had come to treatment at the time of his birth, had something happened during his first year of life, after four months? Had something been stopped and cut off at that time? But what?

I suggested something that I do not usually do—that he ask his mother what had happened when he was about four months old. At first he refused, saying "What would be the use of my asking? And anyhow, what's the use of my telling you things?" I told him that now I know him differently, now that I have come to know his suffering and distress, after seeing the letters and getting to know the recurrent and incomprehensible collapse of every relationship.

He said that he "had scenes in his head" that he couldn't relate. But when I ask him what's on his mind, he can't stand it; I shouldn't ask him, I should say what I think and he'll correct me. We agreed to this. Was he telling me about the inability to think/mind the unthinkable, I asked myself later when I read these words.

He came to the next sessions without having asked his mother. I waited. "How can I ask questions like that, it's weird, what would I say to her?" he finally said. I suggested that he tell her "The therapist asked me to ask." When he did ask her, he came back and said that his mother had been astonished by his question, and told him that, at that time, terrible things had happened that she had never spoken about. She wanted to tell him now, but he did not want to hear, and then she asked his and my permission to tell me directly. He gave his permission, and I gave mine. I subsequently received a long, poignant letter from her in which she recounted that when Ben was three months old, he had contracted spastic bronchitis. She spent the nights walking around holding him in her arms, frightened for his life, while he struggled to breathe, wheezing, almost suffocating. A month later, when he was four months old, his brother, who was a year older, contracted meningitis. His condition was critical, and she sat at his bedside in the hospital for three weeks without going home and without seeing Ben during that entire period. When she finally came back home, Ben neither cried nor was happy. He was not ill, but completely quiet, and she thought that everything had passed satisfactorily. And, she added, she herself had been too tired to think about anything. During the subsequent months she herself had undergone a period of terrible fatigue and depression. She had been unable to bear anything more.

I read the letter and realized that it was here that he had given up forever, had emotionally died out, had become this "Does zilch for me." But when I related-read to Ben what she had written, he sat there with a blank, immobile face. "I see that this moves you," he said at the end, "but it makes no difference to me. It was a long time ago. It's nothing. It does zilch for me."

During the period in treatment that followed, however, things flowed a little more freely. He spoke more, bringing up "the idea of self-destruction—to hurt yourself in order to hurt the person who had hurt you, that you're angry at them, that they should feel bad, that they should feel that it's their responsibility." But at the end of March, toward the end of the four-month extension that had been granted, he gradually withdrew and shut down. His words dried up. And at the beginning of April, he told me that a year had gone by, there had been no change, and he was stopping treatment.

This time I did not argue. "You kept to the agreement and I am thankful for that," I said, and added softly, "I'm very sorry that despite the great effort we both made, I didn't manage to help you."

The treatment was terminated.

About five months later, Ben called to tell me that he was taking summer semester at the university. At first, I did not grasp the significance of this, but then he added that he was taking the summer semester because he wanted to complete his studies by March of the following year, as this time he had passed all of his end-of-year exams. I realized that a change was taking place.

He called again three months later. He told me that he had successfully completed summer semester, and that he would finish his studies in March. He called again in March, after passing all his final examinations. He had begun a relationship with a new girl, and again she terminated it a week later. He thought he should resume treatment. We arranged to begin again in April, this time on the day before his (thirtieth) birthday.

At the first session back in treatment, he quietly recited-sang a song by Israeli singer Ehud Ba'nai that I hadn't heard before, "The boy is thirty, he's got a high fever, he's out of work and love." And when he reached the chorus, there were tears in his eyes:

> Please hurry, put a bandage on my heart
> Before you lay me down to sleep
> And tell me of the child I once was,
> How joyful I was at the first rain.

The treatment has continued ever since for years (after another year it turned into analysis, at his request)—heavy, difficult, draining, but surviving.

Concluding thoughts: heartbreak and breakthrough

It is difficult to convey in words this quality of feeling-with or experiencing-with another human being "the heart-break which is at the centre of human existence," and later not to undermine it by offering explanations. But I believe that it is this very specific quality of the analyst/therapist's presence that is vital to create a profound change.

Like Ben in my case illustration, "heartbroken" patients bear the inscription of an early breakdown (Tustin, 1990; Winnicott, 1974, 1965a, 1967a; Ogden, 2014), in which massive defense organization has shut down and decimated the experience of unthinkable agony and terror. It thus lurks within the psyche as an unexperienced, unlived, and dead part, deeply woven into the psychological fabric of their being. Hence, the critical importance in the treatment of the analyst's being there with-in, experiencing the unexperienced brokenness. This feeling-with or "withnessing" presence creates the fundamental possibility of patient-with-analyst to undergo the unbearable heart-breaking that made it impossible for the patient to be there and experience it alone. Using Mitrani's concept of "taking the transference" (2001, 2015), I would say that the analyst/therapist "takes" the heart-break. Perhaps our capacity to take the transference is never so important as it is with these patients.

In my patient Ben's infancy, his mother's inability to suffer the agony of her abandoned baby and the tormenting life situation at that time led to an inner brokenness and emotional desolation within him that went into the very fabric of his being and relating. The emphasis thus lies in allowing the unthinkable agony to be gradually experienced and suffered in the treatment situation—where the analyst bears and experiences with the patient and for the patient the feelings of pain, dread, loss, brokenheartedness, and despair that already happened but could not be experienced and suffered. Ben found his vanished last cry in my cry for him. He had slowly become able to face the naked terrible heart-break buried under his all-encompassing, incessant "Zilch" through my heart-hearing and experiencing of it.

"The intuited suffering of a broken heart is something that needs . . . well, to be suffered," writes Hinshelwood (2018, p. xviii). So in closing, let me add to the biblical "hearing heart" and to Frances Tustin's "heart-break" the concluding sentences of Eigen's (1993) book, *The Electrified Tightrope*, written in his own unique way:

> I wonder if all therapists feel the sacred element of this work. I suspect many do, in one way or another. In this business we deal with broken lives and heartbreak, and we do so with our own broken hearts. Yet we discover, within our patients and ourselves, *heart within heart within heart* . . . what a breathtaking experience to discover such richness at the null point, always more than we can take.
>
> (pp. 277–278, my italics)

Hear—heart—here.

Worlds of meaning and clinical experience converge here at the heart's center of psychoanalytic work. They will continue to reverberate throughout this book concerning the crucial being-with, hearing, and experiencing in treatment "the heart-break at the center of human existence [that] has to be experienced again and again in ever-widening contexts of developing maturity"—this time patient-with-analyst bearing the experience t(w)ogether, and coming through it differently.

Notes

1 *King James Bible; American King James Version; The Jewish Publication Society; New American Standard Bible; Darby Bible Translation; Webster's Bible Translation.*

2 *The New International Version Study Bible.*

3 *New Living.*
4 James Moffat Translation.
5 This brings to mind Alvarez's most interesting three-level conception of "the thinking heart" (2012).
6 From "What's love got to do with it" (Tina Turner, 1984).
7 I write about this later (Eshel, 1998, 2016b, now chapter 3 in this book).
8 Tustin's words about the agony of the "heartbroken" patients who developed the plaster cast of autism to cover their brokenness relate closely to Winnicott's ideas on early breakdown or madness (1974, 1965a, 1967a). Tustin, herself, refers to the "Fear of breakdown" thinking of Winnicott (1990, pp. 154, 156.)
9 The adjective "Divine" was added later by Boccaccio, author of *The Decameron.*
10 In the last stage of Paradise, Dante is guided by St. Bernard of Clairvaux.

Chapter 2

Two-in-oneness

Transformations in "O"

Ever since I began working as a young clinical psychologist at a psychiatric hospital, and especially over the last 30 years since I qualified as an analyst, I have come to realize the essential significance of the analyst's presence. The process of doing analysis has slowly given birth to the analyst who I have become, and am still becoming, to "being an analyst." Over these years, new experiences and understandings have come my way, and they have shaped, deepened, and altered how I view analytic treatment. The most profound and continuous impact has come from the lived experience with my patients. Along with this, psychoanalytic theoretical and clinical influences have provided me with important ways of delving into the nature and meaning of these analytic experiences. Yet, even from the very beginning of my early therapeutic work with patients—without the later elaboration of theory—I felt, deep inside, that the fundamental core from which everything originates and grows, and to which it returns, is the essential role of the analyst's presence, a presence that is critical and indispensable. It was a profound and basic felt sense, emerging already in those early days, that there is no possibility for true emotional living, nor a true possibility for treatment, without the presence of another psyche. The human psyche cannot exist and thrive, nor can the repair of the psyche occur in an alive and true manner, within a state of privation, isolation, and loneliness. The analyst's ability and willingness to "be there" within—this deep availability and "absorption" (Phillips, 1997) into the patient's experience so that patient and analyst live the experience t(w)ogether (Winnicott, 1945)—has become for me a fundamental means of treatment.

With time and experience, I realized that psychoanalytic work that is grounded in the analytic presence, and the ensuing patient–analyst interconnectedness or "withnessing," opens up yet another dimension of analytic functioning—a fundamental dimension involving a more encompassing model of analytic work. And it engenders new possibilities for extending the reach of the psychoanalytic treatment, particularly with more disturbed patients.

What kind of analytic presence and "withnessing" would that be?

"Presencing" or being-within

I will now introduce and elaborate the key terms of this new dimension of analytic functioning. The starting point is the analyst's "being there" or "presencing" within (and with-in) the patient's experiential world and within the grip of the analytic process. I first developed this approach with regard to massive acting out, acting in, and enactment, based on my experience that the fate of these acting situations in the therapeutic work is determined largely by the analyst's willingness and ability to give him/herself over to "being there," staying within the intense impact of the acting situation, and communing with it (1998a, 1998b). Later, I expanded these ideas to the treatment of difficult-to-reach schizoid, narcissistic, and severely perverse patients, as well as various difficult treatment situations (2005, 2007a, 2009, 2010, 2012b, 2013a, 2013b; now chapters 5, 7, 8 in this book).

Essentially, "presencing" is the analyst's deep acceptance of the necessity of becoming an embedded, elemental, and sustaining functioning presence within the treatment process—thereby experiencing, withstanding, processing, and gradually transforming, *from within*, the repetitive cycle of pathological self–other relations and defenses. While "presencing" may develop into its full potential in the treatment of difficult-to-treat patients and in difficult treatment situations and enactments, it is a part of every analytic situation. It is a primary quality of presence—a multiple-function presence or deep availability—that focuses on experience-near attunement, receptivity, holding, containing, emotional responsiveness, and protection, rather than proffering interpretations of the analytic relationships and especially of patient–analyst separateness. I believe that while "presencing" involves the above capacities and functions, the experience of "presencing" is a quality that is superordinate to these capacities and functions and must be considered as an aspect of the analytic experience in its own terms. It is primarily an *interconnected* relatedness rather than an interactive relationship, and it concentrates on the *ontological (being) quality* of the analytic experience that is lived through *with* the analyst rather than the epistemological and interpretive qualities. In this respect, it is similar to Ferro's description of "the analyst's way of being in the session . . . without any particular interpretive caesura" (2005, p. 44). The analyst gives himself over to becoming part of the patient's ongoing emotional reality and mental processes.[1] Patient and analyst "*live an experience together*" (Winnicott 1945, p. 152, italics in original; see also Ogden, 2001[2]).

Winnicott's and Green's unique words come to mind in this regard, adding compelling arguments for the analyst's presence or "*being*" at the core of the clinical situation. Winnicott (1971a), in a memorable interpretation to his patient after two hours into a long session, poetically and simply expresses this "presencing" quality:

> All sorts of things happen and they wither. This is the myriad deaths you have died. But if someone is there, someone who can give you back what has happened, then the details dealt with in this way become part of you, and do not die.
>
> (p. 71)

And in the footnote, he adds: "That is, the sense of self . . . is lost unless observed and mirrored back by someone who is trusted and who justifies the trust and meets the dependence" (p. 71).

Forty years later, Green (2010), in his last article, uses this passage to elaborate on the concept of *being* in Winnicott's work and, in particular, the vital aspect of how *being* develops in opposition to destruction, dying, or non-being. Green leads us to realize that this is much more than either holding or containing. Drawing on Winnicott's latest posthumous writings, Green emphasizes

> . . . a connection between dying and reflection as a form of resurrection, through the presence of the other, felt as an opportunity for survival—the other having integrated the dead fragments into a new,

> living unity . . . sending back the situation with what has been newly integrated by him or her . . .
>
> In this situation, the other tries to stay as close as possible to the subject, without being confused with him . . . . But in an earlier stage, there is no difference between subject and object.
>
> (2010, pp. 14–15)

These powerful words on the experience of *being*—and its standing in opposition to destruction, dying, and non-being—are especially relevant for patients who overwhelm their analysts and themselves with physical and/or psychic death and non-being.

In this regard, Bion, in his autobiography *All My Sins Remembered* (1985), and later Francesca Bion (1995), make special mention of Dr Wilfred Trotter, the distinguished brain surgeon whom Bion admired during his medical studies at University College Hospital in London. Bion was particularly impressed by his quality of presence with the patients. He writes that Trotter

> listened with unassumed interest as if the patient's contributions flowed from the fount of knowledge itself. It took me years of experience before I learned that this was in fact the case. . . . the doctor from whom help is being sought is being given the chance of seeing and hearing for himself the origin of the pain.
>
> (Bion, 1985, p. 38)

For me, the analyst being there, within the patient's experience, attending closely to the patient, hearing and seeing "the origin of the pain," is, indeed, "the fount of knowledge."

Patient–analyst interconnectedness or "withnessing"

Through the analyst's "presencing within" (and the often-evolving therapeutic regression, in Winnicott's [1954a, b] and Balint's [1968] sense), patient and analyst enter another realm of experience—of patient–analyst interconnectedness or "withnessing." The patient is able to transfer-project unbearable, split-off inner experiences into another psyche that is there to be used as an *area of experiencing, processing, and transformation*. Patient-with-analyst thereby forge a deep experiential-emotional interconnectedness and, thus, a living therapeutic entity that is fundamentally inseparable into its two participants. Viewed in this way, it is not a one- or two-person psychology, but a process whereby the analyst and the patient interconnect psychically and become an emergent new entity that goes beyond the confines of their separate subjectivities and the simple summation of the two—an entity (unit or being) of interconnectedness, "withnessing," or "t(w)ogetherness." *Two-in-oneness*—a oneness that transcends the duality of patient and analyst, transference and countertransference.

This puts the emphasis not so much on the "difficult-to-reach patient," but rather on the "difficult-to-reach *interconnectedness or withnessing* of patient-and-analyst." Such interconnection means changing the patient's (and analyst's) already existing psychic space. Their interconnected psychic being—arising from the analyst's readiness to be given over to this interconnection—creates an actual, *nonlinear* (synergic[3] and transcendent) *new possibility* of getting in touch with, withnessing, experiencing, containing, and affecting hitherto unknown, dissociated, split-off, unthinkable areas of being and relating—hence, its importance, even its necessity, in working with more disturbed patients and difficult treatment situations (Eshel, 1998a, 2001, 2004a, 2004b, 2005, 2006, 2009a, 2009b, 2010, 2012b, 2013a, 2013b; now chapters 1 through 8 of this book). The patient-with-analyst becomes able to experience, tolerate, and go through the anxieties that were unbearable and unthinkable in their original setting, as the analyst bears and experiences with the patient and for the patient the relived early traumatization.

Furthermore, "presencing" and interconnectedness go beyond the level of interactions and patient–analyst relationships (object or subject relationships)—even beyond intersubjectivity—offering the opportunity for getting in touch with basic (environmental) relatedness and formative experiences of being and becoming, for correcting early past experiences, and for enabling nascent emotional development. To use Winnicott's (1954a) words on therapeutic regression, it

> . . . reaches and provides a starting-place, what I would call a *place* from which to operate. The self is reached. The subject becomes in touch with the *basic self-processes* that constitute true development, and what happens from here is felt as real.
>
> (p. 290, author's and my italics, respectively)

Over the last decade, I have further developed this dimension of patient–analyst interconnected being and experiencing and expanded it beyond recent analytic notions of intersubjectivity and witnessing to more radical *patient–analyst deep-level interconnectedness or "withnessing" that grows into at-one-ment*. Supported by late Bion's and Winnicott's posthumous writings, I have emphasized the radical ontological experience of patient-and-analyst being-in-oneness at a primordial point of origin, in order to be able to reach and transform the patient's most extremely dissociated, unknown, unrepresented states—mainly of nameless dread and catastrophe (Bion) and unthinkable, unexperienced breakdown and madness (Winnicott). I came to learn from within my analytic experience that only this radical kind of analytic oneness makes it possible to reach the most traumatic dark depths in which the unthinkable, unexperienced breakdown and the vanished last scream can come into being (2015b, c, 2017a, b, c; also see Part II of this book).

I have also called this process of patient–analyst deep interconnectedness "quantum interconnectedness," drawn from physicist David Bohm's (1980) phrase "the quantum interconnectedness of distant systems," in order to convey the profound implications of this quantum-like psychoanalytic quality of experience. For patient–analyst deep interconnectedness evokes the revolutionary ideas[4] of quantum physics concepts of inseparability of observer and observed, the crucial formative effect of the process and the conditions of observation, and the unbroken wholeness that underlies our perceived world of separateness at the particle level (Bohm, 1980; Godwin, 1991; Sucharov, 1992; Field, 1996; Mayer, 1996a; Kulka, 1997; Botella and Botella, 2005; Eshel, 2002b, 2005, 2006, 2010, 2013a, 2013c, 2016b, 2017a—chapter 10 in this book; Gargiulo, 2016; Suchet, 2017). This unified counterpart in psychoanalysis may be described as the "implicate order" (Bohm, 1980) of psychoanalysis.

As in quantum reality, treatment thus *creates* psychic reality, and goes beyond the exposing or deciphering of the patient's already existing repressed or concealed emotional reality. This point of view focuses predominantly on a different kind of knowledge, experience, and way of being in the analytic process—not that of a patient-centered one-person mode or an interactive two-person mode, but on the knowledge, experience, and powerful effects that come into being when the analyst interconnects with the patient's psyche in living through (or being unable to live through) the process.

In just a few words, T. S. Eliot (1940) conveys the essence of this movement into deep interconnectedness:

> Into another intensity
> For a further union, a deeper communion
> Through the dark cold and the empty desolation . . .
>
> (*East Coker*, p. 204).

Clinical illustration: saying it for the first time

Each chapter in this book describes in some specific way my clinical experiences of being-within the grip of the process, and the eventual emergence of interconnectedness or "withnessing" that enabled a transformation within me-and–the-patient. Here, I would like to describe the first time I expressed to someone these nascent thoughts that were developing within me, and maybe even to myself. I hope it is true to that private, intense struggle.

Dan, a 40-year-old man, came to me for psychoanalytic treatment because he was suffering from prolonged depression. Over the years the periods of depression became longer and more frequent, primarily because for years, in spite of being regarded as gifted and brilliant in his field, he was unable to complete a single project at work, not even the simplest, least demanding, least creative ones. Each project, however willingly and enthusiastically begun, was put off or dropped by him, as though each time he was abandoning or being abandoned.

He had been married and divorced three times and had three children—one from each wife. His first marriage lasted five years, but three years into the marriage, after the birth of his first daughter, he formed a relationship with another woman and lived with her intermittently. This relationship broke up shortly after his divorce. His other two marriages lasted some two years each. When he came to me for treatment, it was just after yet another relationship had abruptly ended. Yet, he claimed that it was his depression and his inability to function at work, rather than his relationships with women, that had led him to seek help.

Before coming to me, he had undergone two previous treatments, each lasting about a year and a half and terminating without alleviating his depression. At the start of treatment, he informed me that in two-and-a-half years' time he was scheduled to spend a year abroad working on a project to which he was already committed, but would be able to resume treatment upon his return.

As it is beyond the scope of this description to give a detailed account of the treatment, I describe only its main points. In the course of the treatment, toward the beginning of the second year, it came out, first in passing, that around the time of Dan's birth, his father had been appointed to a diplomatic post abroad and left the country for several years. Then, when Dan was around two years of age, his mother joined his father, leaving Dan behind with her sister, whose children were close to him in age. When she returned, probably some seven months later, she was in an advanced stage of pregnancy with his younger brother. These details were not told as if they held any special significance, but came out when I questioned him further. He did not know how old he was when his mother left, how long she was away, and how old he was when she returned. He did not feel it held any emotional significance for him, he said. His aunt was a kind woman and took good care of him, he added, and anyhow he was only a child, so why should they say anything. In his previous therapies, this had not become an issue! And, indeed, it was difficult to turn it into an issue of any further inquiry, reflection, or meaning. When I tried to relate it to his relationships with women, to the projects abruptly dropped, to the treatment that was due to be interrupted after two-and-a-half years, or to issues in the treatment, he responded without any real interest, any relating, any affective resonance, or without it having any emotional significance for him. "Yes, that sounds reasonable," or even "That sounds interesting," he would say politely and wearily. "So what?" Nonetheless, he attended treatment regularly and conscientiously, and during the first two years of treatment he gradually came out of the deep depression that had been so manifest initially and suffered no further bouts of depression. He also began having new ideas and enthusiasm for new projects, and enjoyed telling me about them, although he did not put them into effect.

After two years, the issue of his approaching departure for a year came to the fore. He referred to it matter-of-factly, as a foregone conclusion. At the same time, with the laconic detachment that was typical of his way of relating, he said that it was perhaps a pity to leave now because he felt the treatment was helping him, "helping his depression." In addition, over the previous months he had formed a new relationship with a woman, after a year of no relationships, not even casual ones.

Consequently, he made a concerted effort to shorten his scheduled stay abroad, and managed to reduce it to six months, even though this meant that it would be far more intensive and strenuous and less rewarding financially. Yet, in spite of this being a serious undertaking, he talked about it laconically in the sessions, as if delivering a factual report, detached from any emotional context, almost surreptitiously, as if, to a certain extent, it had taken him by surprise—not understandable, unrelatable either to him or to me. "I don't feel it," he would say, closing the issue when I tried relating to it.

While he was speaking and reacting in his emotionless way, I, for my part, was *feeling*. In the three months prior to the planned interruption of the treatment, my mind was totally flooded with him. He seemed to seep into every pore of my thoughts—I can find no other way of describing it. Mostly, these were not thoughts with content, but rather images. Repeatedly, I saw him, his face, his expressions, his look, the things he had said at our last meeting. It was as if something in my thoughts and feelings was being drawn toward him, over and over again.

A month before his departure, at the height of this flooding, I attended a weekend conference in London (a short, also previously planned interruption of the treatment). While there, I went to a senior colleague, Mrs. Irma Brenman Pick, for a supervisory consultation and told her about it. She listened and told me that, without delay, I have to interpret to him that he was about to leave me in the same way that he had left all his previous women—once again he was leaving a woman with his child. I said spontaneously, "No," trying to collect my thoughts and feelings and put them into words, "I don't think that will reach him. These are familiar things he knows, things that have been said to him many times before, by women and by therapists. Perhaps, if I allow myself to feel these feelings, if I listen to them and think them, I would learn something from within myself, other than the familiar words, something from within, from the real, poignant feelings of being forsaken and abandoned, which he himself is unable to feel."

She listened and said, "You are a brave analyst!" and then we talked at length, differently, not about what should be quickly interpreted, but about inner wounds, painful feelings of abandonment, and fear of breaking down and disintegration—about a child who wanted his mother to be with him and not forsake him, to speak to him, to relate to his feelings, that at least somebody should relate to them. But he was abandoned, without being related to, and without being able to internalize a feeling, empathic adult who longed for him or related to his abandonment. And since then, not-feeling had become the only way of defending himself, of not being driven insane by abandonment, of not shattering and breaking down, of not being there again. Never again.

It was already evening when I left. A London rain was falling, and I walked along, engrossed in my thoughts. I was not sure that I was "brave," although it was nice to hear it. Had my own actual life been full of abandonments, perhaps I would not have been able to withstand such overwhelming feelings of being abandoned. But I felt that I had said something true, both to myself and to her, which had found such lucid expression within me for the first time—about a different kind of reaching and knowing, from within, of feelings that the patient perhaps could not feel, but that I, the analyst, could feel and listen to, words from and into the abandonment. And she listened.

There are things that one can know only through interconnecting with the other—both in treatment and in supervision.

I would say that my patient's painful, unbearable, expelled, and denied feelings of loss, longing, and vengefulness—that profound past inner rupture, so powerful and painfully tangible—were projected into me "to repose there long enough" for my psyche to experience and modify them, thus enabling the patient to take back and reintroject them (Bion, 1959). And I took them into myself, into my being, my longings, with all their intensity and flooding, as a real, fresh, high tide of feelings in me, becoming "reconciled to the feelings that we are on the verge of a breakdown, or some kind of mental disaster" (Bion, 1975, p. 206)—thus integrating within me, in the present, separation, abandonment, and longings, as a longing child, a longing mother.

I believe that my patient's psyche sensed-knew-absorbed this, without interpretations, without words. In the six months he spent abroad, he managed, for the first time in years, to complete a project, and for the first time he experienced longing. On resuming treatment, which lasted another five-and-a-half years, he slowly developed the capacity to carry out tasks and finish them and, subsequently, even do projects that he wanted and loved to do. With memory and passion. And, gradually, at first almost surreptitiously and without expressing emotion, he solidified the relationship with his woman friend, which had begun before his going abroad, and it became the first stable, close, and only relationship in his life, and has remained so ever since.

Further thoughts: transformations in "O"neness

I would now like to elaborate further my main contention that the analyst's willingness and capacity to be-with the patient and to risk moving out of a known, prescribed, internally separated stance, ushers patient-with-analyst into dimensions of experience that are deeply emotionally informative, even mysterious, and truly transformative.

Over the years, I have encountered various terms used by a number of psychoanalysts that emphasize profound forms of patient–analyst connectedness: Grinberg's "state of 'convergence'" (1991, 1997); Symington's "corporate personality" or "corporate entity" (1986); Little's "basic unity" (1986); Searles's "symbiotic relatedness," "symbiotic involvement," and "therapeutic symbiosis" (1965, 1979); Racker's "psychological symbiosis" and "unity[5] (1968); and Ogden's "the intersubjective analytic third" and "the subjugating analytic third" (1994).

More recent contributions include Ogden's (2009) formulation of Bion that "It takes two minds to think one's most disturbing, previously unthinkable thoughts" (pp. 97, 100); Botella and Botella's (2005) description of the analyst's "functioning or working as a double," which goes beyond "already known" countertransference meaning and thus gives access to the patient's unrepresentable areas that would otherwise remain traumatically unknown and unreachable (pp. 82–83); De M'Uzan's (2006) conception of "psychological chimera"—a new "monstrous" entity that emerges from the intertwining of unconscious minds of the analysand and the analyst" (p. 19); and, the conceptualizations of the Barangers' *Work of Confluence* (translated into English in 2009) and Ferro's "*bi-personal field*" (1999, 2009, 2010; Ferro and Basile, 2009), which emphasize the formation of a new identity—the analytic field—that unconsciously is created between patient and analyst within the unit that they form in the session. Ferro (2010) says, "Such a description illustrates the fundamental point that the field must get ill with the patient's own illness in order to be then cured of it" (p. 418).

Here, I would like to point out how the dimension of analytic oneness that I suggest converges with and differs from intersubjectivity and analytic field theories. While I agree with Ferro's fundamental point cited above, the analytic experience of "presencing" and of "withnessing" or interconnectedness is not located *between* the patient and analyst but is as much as possible *within* the patient's world. In a similar vein, with regard to Ogden's "intersubjective analytic third," I share his thinking when he says, "I do not view transference and countertransference as separate entities that arise in response to one another; rather, I understand these terms to refer to aspects of a single intersubjective totality" (1995, p. 696f). However, I differ from Ogden in the emphasis that he places on the analyst's own subjective past experiences and memories, which are evoked in the analyst's mind in the session. I reach out toward the analyst's embeddedness in the patient's subjective reality, especially as a necessary functioning presence, by suspending his/her own subjective reality and letting the patient's subjective reality impose itself on him/her. The analyst thus becomes part of the patient's state of being and experiencing, to the extent of becoming psychically akin to a transplant or to chimeric antibodies (Eshel, 2012b; now chapter 5 in this book). Or, to put it differently, the analyst's being with-in the patient's subjective reality is akin to receding towards the "vanishing point" in a perspective drawing. It is this very specific ontological quality of the analyst's "presencing" and interconnectedness or "withnessing" that engenders a new possibility for being and experiencing, where that possibility had been absent or foreclosed.

To further support this thinking, I would add Vermote's (2013) integrative model of psychic functioning for dealing with the unknown or the unthought. Drawing on Matte Blanco's and Bion's writings, Vermote identifies three distinct *zones or modes* of psychic functioning to describe the scope of psychoanalytic work and the range of possible psychic changes, each characterized by varying degrees of differentiation, different major psychoanalytic models, and different clinical implications for the analyst:

> Mode 1—Reason (reason as a secondary process)—Oedipal, understanding Ucs system (Freud, Klein).
>
> Mode 2—Transformation in K (knowledge)—Container-contained, reverie, dream-work, alpha-function (Bion, Marty, de M'Uzan, Bollas, Botella and Botella, Ogden, Ferro).
>
> Mode 3—Transformation in O—when dealing with the most unthought, unknown, undifferentiated zone of psychic functioning (Winnicott, Milner, late Bion, late Lacan).

> Real, life-giving psychic change occurs at this level of radical experience, unrepresented and unknowable (called "O" by Bion, for "Origin"),[6] while the epistemological exploration of the unknown in Mode 2 of transformation in Knowledge or dream-thought, remains at the level of representations. Thus, Mode 2, "Transformation in Knowledge," is a thought for something that was not thought yet, and Mode 3, "Transformation in O" is a *new experience* that happens, that can only "be 'become', but it cannot be 'known'" (Bion, 1970, p. 26).[7]

I believe that working within the dimension of analytic presence, and the ensuing patient–analyst deep interconnectedness or "withnessing" that grows into at-one-ment, reaches down *from transformations in K to transformations in O* the third, most undifferentiated and fundamental mode of analytic functioning. For me, this radical mode of analytic at-one-ment with the patient's most unknown emotional reality-O has become connected mainly with unthinkable early breakdown (Winnicott) and mental catastrophe (Bion) (see chapter 10 in this book). The unthinkable cannot be thought, but only relived and gone through with the analyst. I call this *transformations in Oneness*.

The shift in contemporary psychoanalysis over the last decades has been from classical one-person psychology (Mode 1) to the intersubjective domain and the theories of the analytic field generated between the subjectivities of patient and analyst (Mode 2). But my way of thinking goes further, beyond intersubjectivity and analytic field theories, to a more radical *patient–analyst being-in-oneness*. While the shift from an intrapsychic to an intersubjective model has required a leap out of the assumptions of a one-person psychology, I am suggesting that we leap again, this time out of the assumptions of a model in which the field is limited to what is generated dyadically (Tennes, 2007; Eshel, 2014, 2016b, 2017a) to a mode of at-one-ment and be(com)ing-in-oneness that is fundamentally inseparable into its two participants (Grotstein, 2010)—an analytic oneness at a primordial point of origin. This is a shift from getting to know the emotional reality of the patient's experience (K) to becoming at-one-with the emotional reality of the patient's experience (O) as the crucial point. Different worlds of experience open with these different modes of approach, and they keep opening the more we open to them.

I will conclude with three intriguing viewpoints, which, although very different in style, are profoundly relevant to patient–analyst deep interconnectedness and its qualities of experience. First, Nacht and Viderman's (1960) inclusive conception of "the analytic situation as a whole" and "the pre-object universe in the transference situation" encompasses the movement towards a more primal form of analytic experience:

> Sometimes, in the course of analysis we reach a deeper, more secret and unchanging level of the psychic structure, characterized by an intense need for absolute *union* . . . let us accept that the same aspiration . . . remains buried and unknown in recesses of each individual psychic structure. . . . We agree that the dynamic of transference, in the strict sense of the word, is drawn from man's perpetual search for object relationships. . . . But the analytic situation as a whole goes beyond the elementary dynamic of transference perhaps to include the original primitive experience of Being and to express its essence. From this point of view, it is legitimate to describe the analytic situation as an *ontological experience*.
>
> (pp. 385–386, authors' and my italics, respectively)

At that time, Fromm (2000), in his New York lectures in 1959, emphasizes "a *central relatedness*" between analyst and patient:

> I can explain the other person as another ego, as another thing, and then look at him as I look at my car, my house, my neurosis, whatever it may be. Or I can relate to this other person in the sense of being him, in the sense of experiencing, feeling this other person. Then I do not think about myself, then my ego does not stand in my way. But something entirely different happens. There is what I call a *central relatedness* between me and him . . .
>
> When I use the concept "central relatedness" I mean the relatedness from center to center instead of the relatedness from periphery to periphery . . . . What happens is that I have a sense of union, of sharing, of oneness.
>
> (pp. 174, 177, 178)

And nearly 50 years later, Adam Philips, in acknowledging the dimension of deep connectedness, says in his very particular style:

> But just consider it—the Oedipal taboo was nothing. Compared to the taboo invoked by this quality of connectedness—now, *there's* a taboo.

> It suggests a capacity for connection that's far more fearful in implication than Oedipal love. It's far deeper, far more radical. Where are the boundaries? Where's Freud's concept of ego? It's overwhelming. Fascinating and full of promise but overwhelming.
>
> (Cited in Mayer, 2007, p. 270)

A closing note of fiction

In attempting to further convey the essence of the "becoming" of deep interconnectedness and at-one-ment, I turn once again to the imaginative concise words of the Bible and Dante's *Inferno* that come to mind in connection with these ideas.

In Exodus, in the description of God's relating to the crying out of the children of Israel from their slavery in Egypt, we can see a kind of undifferentiated "becoming":

> . . . and the children of Israel sighed from the labor, and they cried out, and their cry ascended to God from the labor. And God heard their cry, and God remembered His covenant with Abraham, with Isaac, and with Jacob. And God saw the children of Israel, and God knew.
>
> (Exodus 2: 23–25)

These verses contain a sequence of verbs, moving from "God *heard* their cry," "God r*emembered* His covenant," "God *saw* the children of Israel," to the last one, "God *knew*"—"וידע אלוהים"—which, unlike the other verbs, has no object following it (my italics). I understand this to mean that when a deep knowing of a traumatic state is reached, there is no longer a differentiation or divisibility between subject (God) and object (the children of Israel).

And, ultimately, Dante (1320) in the *Inferno*, most vividly captures the essence of the presence and "withnessing" that I have been describing in this chapter. Dante is guided and protected throughout the *Inferno* by the Roman poet Virgil in their descent, circle by circle, through the nine dreadful circles of Hell. It is a most critical moment of Dante-with-Virgil interconnection, when Virgil and Dante, "more afraid of death than ever," had to be lowered by the giant Antaeus into the last, bottom circle of hell—"the lowest point of all evil." Virgil, already in the grasp of the giant's hand, called out to a horrified Dante, "'Come close, so that I can take you'; Then made one bundle of himself and me [Dante]"

(Canto 31, pp. 134-135, 181). And the giant thus placed them in the bottom pit. Similarly, I would suggest that the analyst and the patient *become one bundle* in order to go through the "collapse into being with the deepest states" (Eigen, 2006, p. 138) of the patient's emotional reality, mostly unknown, unthinkable, and unexperienced—a terror too terrifying to be experienced alone.

Notes

1 In this context, I would like to add Bollas's (1987) distinction between two fundamental genres of transference: One involves the patient and his objects; the other derives from a receptive capacity (in both analyst and patient). It is a state of being in which the analyst functions as a part of the patient's mental process, and that facilitates the creation of new internal objects and self experiences. "The psychoanalyst's countertransference task within this transference is to allow himself to be assumed by the patient and not to interpret unless the patient needs it" (p. 256). I find that working with this kind of countertransference is closely related to my idea of "presencing."

2 Ogden (2001a) beautifully amplifies this aspect of Winnicott's thinking: "*Live an experience together"* [Winnicott 1945, p. 152]—what makes the phrase remarkable is the unexpected word "live." They do not "take part in," "share," "participate in," or "enter into" an experience together: they live an experience together. In this single phrase, Winnicott is suggesting (though I think he is not fully aware of this as he writes this paper) that he is in the process of transforming psychoanalysis, both as a theory and as a therapeutic relationship" (pp. 226–227, italics in original).

3 Synergia/synergism/synergy (from the Greek: *syn* -together + *ergon* -work)—coordinated or correlated action of two or more structures, agents, or physiological processes so that the combined action is greater than that of each acting separately (*Stedman's Medical Dictionary*, p. 1540).

4 Elsewhere (Eshel, 2002b), I have elaborated on the specific significance of this "quantum process." Whereas classical physics (and classical psychoanalysis) are based on the assumptions of linear causation, determinism, continuity, and sharp separation of observer and the object under observation, quantum physics is based on essential inseparability and indeterminacy at the most fundamental levels of particles. Thus, the fundamental claim of quantum physics finds its counterpart in this dimension of the analytic process in which patient and analyst form an interconnected unit that is, in principle, inseparable (also see chapter 10 here).

5 "A kind of unity the analyst must achieve in the countertransference, especially with what the patient rejects or splits off from himself, enabling the patient to establish a unity within his psychic structure" (Racker, 1968, p. 174).

6 Bion, 1965, p. 15. According to Neville Symington (2016), it is called O by Bion, for "Ontology" (private seminar, Tel Aviv). Winnicott (probably in 1968) joins these two words by writing about "ontological origin" (p. 213).

7 Let me add here Matte Blanco's (1975) words: "If the attention of the observer remains focused on the first level, that of consciousness, then he will only be aware of the concrete individual; and *if he lets himself be permeated by the underlying levels*, this infinity will unfold itself before him, though in an unconscious manner. Embracing this infinite series (sequence) there is one unity: the class or the set. This, in its turn, is lived as one unity" (1975, p. 175, my italics).

Chapter 3

Into the depths of a "black hole" and deadness

> And when you look long into an abyss, the abyss also looks into you.
> (Nietzsche, *Beyond Good and Evil*, 1886, p. 279)

This chapter explores the vicissitudes of a difficult analytic encounter with massive, devouring deadness in the self-m/other relatedness, which I have named and characterized metaphorically as the astrophysical *"black hole" of interpersonal psychic space*. I will present the analysis of a patient who opened up unfathomable depths of deadness and emptiness, and describe my search and struggle to meet this "black hole" experience and to find a deep understanding and analytical survival *within* these overwhelming depths of deadness and emptiness. The emphasis here is on the patient–analyst's survival of the deadening, destructive processes in the analysis, and the analyst's capacity (and struggle) to be there and remain alive, while experiencing and going through annihilation and death along with the patient—a years-long struggle that could not be completed without reaching a moment of "at-one-ment" with the patient's desperate and painful innermost experience.

A theoretical-clinical context

"Black holes"

The term "black hole" has acquired meaning in the fields of psychoanalysis (Akhtar, 2009) and astrophysics (Hawking, 1988, 1993; Gribbin, 1992). The origin of the term can be traced back many years earlier to a dungeon in Calcutta, India, where on June 20, 1756, 146 captured soldiers were imprisoned and 125 died overnight. This horrific prison, a point of no return, was designated as a black hole.

I will first relate to the black hole as used in psychoanalysis, and then elaborate on the astrophysical black hole and particularly its metaphorical use in this chapter.

Black holes in psychoanalysis

The term black hole as used by Tustin and Grotstein refers to the nature of early infantile traumatizations and the collapse into nothingness and meaninglessness, which result in primitive mental disturbances. "Black hole" was first applied clinically by Bion (1970) in reference to the "infantile catastrophe" of the psychotic. Tustin, and later Grotstein, both analysands of Bion, developed and broadened the use of this term: Tustin to autistic children and Grotstein to psychotics and borderlines.

Tustin (1972, 1986, 1990, 1992) regards the "black hole" experience as a very significant element in psychogenic autism. She describes having learned about the black hole from her four-year-old autistic patient, John,[1] to whom she refers to in all of her books. Tustin views autism as a reaction to a very early trauma of premature bodily separateness from the primal mother, experienced by the infant as an unbearable rupture, leaving a black hole of depression, despair, rage, terror, helplessness and hopelessness. Autistic encapsulation and entanglement arise as protective reactions against the black hole type of depression, which these children plug with autistic objects or shapes or with confusional objects.

Grotstein (1986, 1989, 1990a, 1990b, 1990c, 1993), following Tustin's ideas, further developed the black hole experience and applied it to adult patients with primitive mental disorders, adding concepts from astrophysics ("singularity" and "event horizon") which emphasize the "awesome force" of the black hole. He regards the black hole phenomenon as the fundamental experience of the psychotic internal mental space of these patients—an endless, bottomless void of primary meaninglessness, nothingness, disorganization, chaos, and nameless dread where the mother used to be and was prematurely ripped away. Whereas the psychotic patient seems to have already fallen (metaphorically) into the black hole and become devastated by this cataclysmic experience, the borderline patient appears to exist on its borders, continuously experiencing the threat and the pull of falling over its edge into its horrific interior.

Later, I (Eshel, 1998a) expanded the metaphorical analytic application of the astrophysical black hole and the "event horizon" to an interpersonal phenomenon with regard to less disturbed individuals, whose *interpersonal/intersubjective psychic space* is dominated by a *central object that is experienced essentially as a black hole*. In this regard, the astrophysical black hole and the event horizon (Hawking, 1988, 1993; Gribbin, 1992) became for me a most apt metaphor, as I will now describe.

Black holes in astrophysics

The astrophysical term black hole, describing an idea about dark, invisible stars that was first speculated upon as early as 1783, was introduced by the American physicist John Wheeler in 1968, stimulating astrophysical research and theory as well as science fiction. "This was a stroke of genius: the name ensured that black holes entered the mythology of science fiction. It also stimulated scientific research by providing a definite name for something that previously had not had a satisfactory title" (Hawking, 1993, p. 105).

A black hole is the set of events caused by the massive collapse of a dying star. Eventually, when the star shrinks to a certain critical radius of infinitesimal size and almost infinite density ("singularity"), its gravitational field becomes so strong that light can no longer escape—hence its blackness. According to the theory of relativity, nothing travels faster than light; therefore, if light cannot escape, neither can anything else. Everything is dragged back by the gravitational field, "producing a region of space-time where infinitely strong gravitational forces literally squeeze matter and photons out of existence" (Penrose, 1973, cited in Gribbin, 1992, p. 142).

The boundary of the black hole—the "event horizon"—is formed by the paths in space-time of light rays that just fail to escape from the black hole, hovering forever on its edge.

> Another way of seeing this is that the event horizon, the boundary of the black hole, is like the edge of a shadow – the shadow of impending doom . . . The event horizon acts rather like a one-way membrane around the black hole: objects, such as unwary astronauts, can fall through the event horizon into the black hole, but nothing can ever get out of the black hole through the event horizon. One could say of the event horizon what the poet Dante said of the entrance to Hell:

> 'All hope abandon ye who enter here.' Anything or anyone who falls through the event horizon will soon reach the region of infinite density and the end of time.
>
> (Hawking, 1988, pp. 98–99, 110)

Falling into a black hole has therefore become one of the horrors of science fiction.

I find that the metaphorical use of the astrophysical black hole and the event horizon captures the fundamental experience of individuals whose *interpersonal/intersubjective psychic space* is dominated by a *central object that is experienced essentially as a black hole*. They are either gripped by its enormous, compelling pull, or are petrified in their interpersonal psychic space, out of fear of being pulled over its edge. My usage of this term differs from Tustin's and Grotstein's formulations of the black hole. They describe the nature of internal mental space in primitive mental disorders resulting from an infantile catastrophe of very early separateness from the primal mother. Unlike them, I apply the astrophysical black hole metaphorically to an interpersonal phenomenon. I use it to illustrate the nature of the black hole experience as "the shadow of impending doom" in the area of emotional closeness, love, and intimate relationships of individuals, who otherwise generally function in their social and professional life. This shadow evokes here "the shadow of the object" (Freud, 1917, adopted by Bollas, 1987), "the shadow [of the basic fault] which has been cast over one's whole life" (Balint, 1968, p. 183), and especially "the shadow of the mother's [psychic] absence" (Green, 1986, p. 154).

The "dead" mother as a black hole

In my clinical work, as powerfully illustrated in the analysis I will shortly present, I came to realize that the black hole experience in the interpersonal psychic space is caused mainly by the shadow or the impact of a psychically "dead" parent, particularly "the dead mother" (Green, 1986). The essential element in the case of the psychically "dead" mother is not a traumatic, precocious interruption of the mother's presence by her real, sudden death or separation, but that the child grows up in the *presence* of a mother absorbed in an inner world of blank bereavement, depression, and deadness. The mother's blank mourning brings about in the child a massive decathexis of the maternal object, resulting in a "psychical hole in the texture of object-relations with the mother" (p. 151) and unconscious identification with her, while secondary hatred and erotic excitation teem on the edge of an abyss of emptiness. This carries in its wake, besides loss of love, the loss of meaning because of the totally unexplainable gap between what the child has done and the maternal reaction. Thus, the child "might imagine this fault to be linked with his manner of being rather than with some forbidden wish; in fact, it becomes forbidden for him to be" (p. 152).

This experience takes on full impact in light of the enormous importance of the mother and the mother–child relationship in the development of the child's emotional and interpersonal world and their self- and object-representations, which find numerous expressions in various theories (Stern, 1985; Benjamin, 1988). In the case of the "dead" mother, these fundamental needs are not met by a mother who is emotionally able to listen and relate, to take in and process the infant's fear of dying (Bion, 1959) and respond with attuned, reliable holding and containing; by a mother who can provide feelings, love, life and responsiveness. On the contrary, the child's interpersonal/intersubjective emotional space is centered upon and dominated by the "dead" mother. Under the impact of the mother's emotional and psychic deadness and overwhelming feelings of blankness and emptiness, the child forms a desperate, intense need to revive the mother and himself. He strives to cure her, to bring her back to life. The yearning to repair this central, fundamental relationship, and through it himself and his self, is enormous. He is "under the empire of the dead mother . . . prisoner to her economy of survival," in Green's words (ibid., p. 156).

It is this powerful impact of the "dead" mother that led me to describe it by using the metaphor of the astrophysical black hole—the black hole formed by the massive collapse of a dying star, from which it is impossible to escape because its enormous gravitational pull sucks into it and annihilates everything that gets close to it. I use the metaphor of the black hole in interpersonal psychic space, rather than Green's psychical hole of blankness or Quinodoz's non-existent "hole object" (1996), to capture this gripping, pulling, annihilating hole experience rather than a static hole caused by a lifeless mother. Individuals under the impact of their "dead" mother are either held and trapped in her devouring, deadening inner world, or if they succeed in detaching themselves from her grip, are petrified and paralyzed in their interpersonal space, because of the imminent threat of being drawn back again into the mother's deadness. Consequently, they are unable to form relationships of closeness, love, and intimacy. In Green's view (1986), this is "because [their] love is still mortgaged to the dead mother . . . the place is occupied, in its center, by the dead mother" (p. 154). I would add that every close contact evokes the overwhelming experiences which she imprinted in them psychically and somatically.

According to the astrophysical metaphor, those individuals who are in the grip of the "dead" mother can be regarded as trapped inside the black hole, unable to escape its destructive processes; whereas those who succeed in detaching themselves, remain "hovering forever" on its edge, in the area of the event horizon, paralyzed by the threat of being pulled back over the edge into the black hole which is so central to their interpersonal world. However, an observer who remains at a distance would not in any way be affected by the black hole, since neither light nor any other signal from it will reach him.

The metaphorical use of the astrophysical black hole embodies and emphasizes the questions which I feel are crucial to the analysis of these patients. Can analysis provide the enormous counter-forces needed for freeing and extricating these patients from the powerful, gripping, destructive forces of the black hole, of the "dead" mother? And can the analyst (when not a remote observer) survive and influence in this devouring, annihilating world of deadness?

I will now describe an analysis in which I found myself grappling with these questions, and offer a more complete discussion of these questions after illustrating what I was and was not able to be and to do in this analytic encounter with the intense grip of devouring deadness, nothingness, and death.

The analysis

Introductory comment

In Israel, as a result of the Holocaust and numerous wars, many analyses and psychotherapies involve people who grew up with psychically dead extinguished parents. There are many "dead" mothers who for a while, around the time of birth, felt that there was a breakthrough and a victory over death, but soon afterwards sank again into an abyss of depression, blankness, and deadness. Often there was also enormous aggression, because of the absence of other mechanisms for handling emotions; and their children grew up in a world of devastation, deadness, and a struggle for survival, in which they were the ones who had to provide the love, aliveness, commiseration, and compensation for the catastrophes and cruelties of life. The following is an analysis of a person who grew up with a "dead" mother, with all its massive implications regarding his ability to love and develop emotional closeness and intimacy.

****

Adam, a 33-year-old oncologist, came to analysis because of his profound inability to form an ongoing relationship with a woman. After reaching the age of 30, he began to feel vaguely disturbed by this, although he was uncertain whether it was due to society's expectations or his own. As he was good looking and very intelligent, he had no difficulty finding women with whom to spend the night, but these relationships would last no more than a night or two, after which he would end them, and if occasionally they were renewed, they were again quickly ended.

He described himself as professional and efficient in his work, though emotionally detached. However, he saw this as characteristic of his profession.

Adam was an only child. His mother had gone through the Holocaust in Europe, but he knew almost nothing of what had occurred to her during those years. It was only in the seventh year of analysis that he dared ask her some details about her family. On that occasion, he discovered that she had had a brother who had been drafted and disappeared, and that her mother, who he always thought had been killed during the Holocaust, had in fact remained in Europe after the war. Contact with her was lost, until news arrived of her death from cancer when he was six years old.

His mother did not breastfeed him. When he was born, she became afflicted with severe eczema on her hands, and therefore hardly touched him, except to clean him. She was always sick, suffering from an ulcer, hyperthyroidism, high blood pressure, chronic constipation, and nightmares. What he remembered most about his childhood was his mother screaming at night from nightmares for many years. He would then steal into the kitchen to eat cookies that she kept hidden. This made her very angry and she would call him bad and heartless. For many years, beginning in childhood, he had a recurring dream about *a clock ticking like a metronome, with his mother's screams reverberating in the background.*

His mother was compulsive about cleanliness. Upon entering the house, he had to change his clothes, remove his shoes, and wash his hands over and over again. She would often quarrel with the neighbors, with his father's relatives (she had no family of her own), and with his father who she felt sided with them. He recalled how he would try to stop her screams and fits of weeping, to distract her and calm her down, out of fear and shame that she might be heard outside.

Adam's father was absorbed in his work, working long hours and coming home very late. For several years he worked far from home, and came home only at weekends. Thus, Adam was frequently at home alone with his mother, subjected to her moods, illnesses, outbursts, pain, and loneliness, afraid of bringing friends home and also afraid of going to their homes and leaving her at home alone.

When he began his army service he left home; after the army he went to study in another city, and never came back to live in his parents' house again.

****

The analysis (of four times a week) lasted seven years. Here, I will focus on the facet of the sick, dying, "black hole" mother, which was central to the analysis.

About a year into analysis, Adam became less emotionally detached. This began to express itself slowly in his relationship with women, and most dramatically in his attitude towards his hospital patients. It became particularly striking in his involvement with one patient—a young woman, terminally ill with cancer. He tried to tie her to life, to the will to live. He complimented her on her beautiful eyes, so prominent in her emaciated face and bald head. He made contact with her family, and became distressed when her small son asked about her illness and he couldn't tell him how serious her condition was because the family insisted that he not tell the boy. When she died, he attended the funeral and had a severe depressive reaction, which was new to him.

Then a dam seemed to burst within him. After several months he developed a strong attachment to two other female patients—first to a young woman, and then to an older woman—both suffering from cancer and undergoing intensive chemotherapy. He accompanied them to all their treatments and examinations, even in other hospitals. He supported them, tried to bolster their physical and mental strength, and came whenever they called, at any time of day or night.

Towards the end of the third year of analysis, a lonely older woman, a physician, came to the hospital for surgery and chemotherapy, and she became the supreme object of Adam's total dedication. He devoted himself completely to her care, spent hours at her bedside when she was in the hospital or when she went to another hospital for a new treatment, and read every bit of available information about her illness. When she was in remission, he accompanied her on a farewell trip to the land of her birth, together visiting people and vistas from her past. Later, when her condition worsened, he was with her constantly in the hospital, even when she received treatment in other departments. He spent every spare moment with her, drawn into her illness, her death throes, her dying.

All his time, concern, feelings, passion, and commitment were devoted only to her—to the sick, dying woman, to the fight for her life. As she became weaker, sinking into apathy and deadness, her eyes closed, he was unable to bear the feeling that she was drifting away from him, that she was going to die, that she was "allowing herself to die." He pleaded with her to open her eyes, to look at him, not to die, not to leave him. The life and death struggle was absolute.

The battle for her life, and Adam's total absorption in it, continued for over a year. During that entire time, the analysis seemed to have become devoid of meaning, even though he attended each session. It seemed that I could only be swept along by the course of events, to just be there, within the host of details related to the cancer treatments. I felt that there was nothing I could say that would be really meaningful. Was I carrying the desperate effort and the paralyzed inability of a child struggling to be taken in by a mother whose mind and body were filled with sickness and death? My interpretations sounded more and more inconsequential, worthless, hollow—words that failed to reach or touch, that fell into a void without emotional resonance. It seemed that there could be no relating, no way of communicating, no place for understanding and reflecting in this analysis. Nothing could compete with or break into this closed world of the struggle with death. And I eventually became silenced, wordless.

With time, however, I felt and knew with growing clarity that it was the holding, the protection, and the containing provided by analysis that was enabling Adam to totally plunge himself into this world of dying and death as he had never before dared to do; that made possible the massive re-enactment of the traumatic past locked inside him, where the shadow of the other who was ill and dying overwhelmed, engulfed, and stifled the very existence and right to live of anyone connected to it; that made possible the actualization of the deep-seated fantasy of saving and restoring the dying woman to life.

In actuality, this was told to me only once, after a particularly difficult session. This session took place after Adam had returned to the hospital from two weeks of reserve duty to find, in addition to his three patients whose condition had worsened, a childhood female friend, his classmate throughout elementary and high school, who was also diagnosed with cancer. He spent the entire day running from one sickbed to the other, and when he came to analysis said feverishly, "All the women I know have cancer." I felt his world, consisting entirely of women with cancer fighting for their lives, sweep down upon me with enormous intensity, perhaps even more so because I had been away from it for two weeks. I found myself drawing back, pressing hard against the back of my chair as if trying to distance myself from him and this world of sickness and death, trying to move away and remove myself from the impact of this horror on my body and psyche. I said, "The room today is full of cancer."

When Adam arrived the next day, he appeared ill and pale. He said, "Yesterday I sensed your alarm when you said, 'The room is full of cancer.' I felt sick all night, I couldn't sleep, I was burning with fever. I was afraid that you would disappear, leave me, that you would want to walk away from this treatment. You are with me, close to my soul . . . I need you in order to get through this."

Adam needed me here as an *availing and sustaining, existing presence*, with no needs or demands of my own for him to be concerned about; to absorb, bear, and work through for him, within myself, alone, his unbearable projections and his (and my) world of death. And that is what I became.

The battle for Adam's patient's life was all-consuming, and he was totally immersed in it, tirelessly, unremittingly, to the end . . . And when she finally died, he remained empty, defeated, cheated, but no longer guilty. He felt that he had done everything that was within his power to do. The deep archaic guilt was gone.

For months after his patient's death there was nothingness, as if nothing remained of his enormous effort—only a sense of futility and loss of direction. And then the relationship with a young female doctor who had helped him throughout the past year began to develop. The two of them spent much time together; they talked about themselves and about their relationship, even harshly at times, but with the feeling that they were able to talk to one another. They began living together, got married; then she became pregnant. Each of these steps involved difficulties and doubts for him, but he felt that there was much love, concern, and strength in this woman and in her relationship to him, and that they had a good relationship.

During the pregnancy they decided to stop working in oncology because they felt that raising children and oncology do not go together. They decided to go abroad a year later to specialize in another field. Life appeared to be gently but inexorably seeping into Adam's world, and the pull of death was lessening.

Although none of this diminished Adam's profound commitment to his patients, he was now dedicated to them in a different way, without the same all-consuming time and emotion. And the younger of the two cancer patients who had been with him longest, sensed this and reacted to it. Before he left for a week's vacation at the time of his marriage, she looked at him as he sat at her bedside, and even though she knew nothing of the events in his life, she remarked poignantly, "You went to live." He attempted to blunt her penetrating words somewhat, saying, "Isn't that what we all try to do—to live?" She insisted however, "But you have learned to live."

Another year remained before the analysis ended, and during that year a second encounter with the black hole of the "dead" mother took place—a further chapter, also massive yet different. While the first encounter was with her dying, this time it was with the enormous, unfathomable emptiness that her motherhood had left in him, and the hunger and longing for a different kind of motherhood. This encounter focused entirely on his relationship with me. Whereas previously, in Grotstein's terms (1993), there had been "background transference," there was now "foreground transference," in which the analyst is clearly and obviously in front as a satisfying and/or rejecting, frustrating object.

Throughout this year, Adam concentrated entirely and endlessly on demanding that I tell him what I was feeling, at least towards him. Now that he was no longer operating under the overwhelming passion to save the sick woman from death, and the task of building a joint life had eased, he was confronted by a sense of emptiness and nothingness inside him. He had no strong emotion, no passion. His "love is brittle" and he "lost all passion," and he felt that analysis had not resolved this matter of missing passion and feelings, as I had not told him my feelings. He said, "I have to hear you speak feelings so that I can feel, so that I can experience having feelings and being moved by them. How can I feel, how can I identify with feelings, if you don't feel? You've given me so much—your attention, your caring, your stability, so why won't you give me this as well? For six-and-a-half years you were able to give, and now not?!"

Working under this enormous strain, which continued incessantly throughout the first half of the seventh year of analysis, my response to Adam's demands for my feelings took several main channels of interpretation: first, that his insistence that I tell him my feelings stemmed from the reliving of his need as a child whose mother never told him herself, a mother whose past and whose feelings were blocked, and whose touch was missing. Therefore, he had to know that I was alive, feeling, and responding to him. Adam reacted to this by attempting to talk to his mother about her past, and did actually gather new information about her brother and mother (as described earlier), but this was quickly stopped by his father who feared that returning to the past would upset the mother. In any event, even when he spoke to his mother, Adam felt that the great longing inside him to hear *me* speak *my* feelings was not reduced. The need for the absent touch was not quelled. He needed "contact with [my] feelings," and a massive emotional response; he needed "feeling that would be the repair of all feelings," and if I wouldn't speak my feelings he would remain with the deadness and the nothingness that was inside him.

A second channel of interpretation that I offered was that he was placing me in a situation similar to the one he was in as a child, of having incessant demands made upon him that he do something to fill the emptiness existing in the other. Now he was making me face, as he had, an empty, sucking, demanding figure.

A third channel was that due to the impending ending of analysis and the approaching separation from me, he was afraid that my presence would diminish and fade, that once again the demanding, ravaged Holocaust mother would dominate him internally. He therefore had to take something from me that would stay with him in a most concrete way.

Another interpretive approach which I attempted was that he was afraid of his feelings, of the emotional awakening inside him, of pain, dependence, of wanting someone, and he therefore wanted me to be the one who felt and revealed feelings.

Adam listened to these interpretations and to many similar ones, sometimes confirming them, at times even adding to them. But nothing changed in his unrelenting, demanding clinging to me, to my feelings, and in his total, suffocating insistence to hear my feelings, which I experienced as intrusive, symbiotic, and at times, overwhelming and intolerable. This would occur particularly when I made a connection between the difficulty he had with my "not speaking of feelings" and the lack of speech and the emotional vacuum that had been in his life. "That's exactly it," he said, "I cannot bear another abyss here. Emotion is to the soul like blood to the body. I need your feeling for me to have feeling . . . I need the touch of feeling to feeling . . . Perhaps if I were to go mad, fall apart, smash into smithereens, you would respond differently, you would become emotional. Perhaps it's because of the psychoanalytical training, the things you learned—that you mustn't tell your feelings to a patient."

I will now describe the session which I believe was the turning point in this endless, all-encompassing, suffocating neediness and demandingness towards me. It was in the second half of the session, and Adam was speaking excitedly. "You don't tell me your feelings. I once said, and you agreed, that a change in the patient brings about a change in the analyst. Where is the change in you? From the beginning you were understanding and empathic, but you never gave me your feelings. Put your analytic defenses aside. A flower must have water, light, in order to develop. I must have your feelings in order to continue to develop. I read in a book that the mother gives emotion and gives it a name, and the baby links up to her emotions. My mother couldn't do that. I'm empty. *It has to be here*! I must have your feelings! I'm on the verge of tears and I don't even know if you're aware of it if I don't tell you." He sounded highly emotional.

When he spoke these emotionally laden words, I felt my own inner response changing. This time, more than ever before, his words reached me in a different, unfamiliar, moving way—not as unchanging, unending, stifling demandingness, but convincing me more and more of their rightness, justification, essentialness, of the poignant, desperate, deep longing for a feeling, alive mother—and they *touched my heart*. In the silence which then descended upon the room, I searched for a way to formulate these feelings within me, for myself as well, and then said, "I feel that you are absolutely right. *It's just that I can't*." I said this with sorrow, feeling deeply the pain, the deprivation, the loss, that I wished I could undo, but could not.

There was silence until the session ended, and when Adam got up to leave, he stumbled and almost fell as he reached the door.

He was very emotional when he came to the next session, and immediately asked me why I couldn't. "I'm not asking you for love, I'm only asking you to speak feelings."

He told me that the previous evening he had been terribly excited and suspicious. "Excited, because if you understood my feelings, it's possible to go on, it's possible to give myself." He also, for the first time, felt love for his as yet unborn baby. But he felt suspicious, ". . . because perhaps you now want to appease me since we're at the end, and I'm very afraid of being led astray. I couldn't bear that! This is much too important to me. You saw how I reacted."

From this point onwards, Adam spoke very differently. His enormous demandingness and pressure were tempered; intense neediness no longer met a void. Things that I had said before now began to resonate in him, perhaps just as what he said had reached, touched, and affected me. Although he kept talking about his need for my feelings, there was a sad acceptance in his words. There was pain, loss, and real mourning for what he never had with his mother, and for the feelings that he needed, in the way that he needed, which I too could not give him, because this was an analytic relationship. He said, "I feel calmer now about these things, but it's difficult. If I wanted my mother's touch, her milk, her responding to me—it was impossible. It was just a disaster for me. So then I didn't want anything. I just gave everyone my touch, my niceness, but inside I was blocked. Here, with you, I once again opened up the child who needs, who desperately wants a hug and love, and it hurts me that here too it can't happen . . . It's like a blockage to the heart that has to be bypassed. There are alternative ways, but it's difficult and insufficient."

Analysis was now a place of lack and mourning for the things that were not and would not be, but there was no longer nothingness and total death. The nothingness had been transformed into "no-thingness," an absence where feelings and thoughts may enter, to be felt and thought about (Bion, 1970; Grotstein, 1990a). In the sessions, I was keenly aware that there were no longer the fundamental feelings of emptiness and hollowness associated with both his and my own attempts to experience something that felt significant and real.

Feelings of separation were now able to come to the fore. "You have disarmed me. I have no more complaints, nothing more to cry about. But now the other cries are beginning to be heard—the fear of being alone. I'm afraid of what it will be like without this kind of being with you that you are such a magician at. Here I'm not laid bare, I'm not shocked by everything. You're the buffer and I'm protected."

And towards the end, "I'll miss hearing your quiet breathing behind me. Your smiling, even laughing, at things I say . . . I breathe and live the things that this fantasy with you has done for me, has built in me, revived in me, saved me."

At the end of the year analysis ended; during the last month before he went abroad, the two cancer patients that had been with Adam longest—the younger and the older—died. Their death demonstrated in the most final and concrete way how difficult is the release from the "dead" mother and how entwined it is with anguished feelings of guilt, abandonment, pain, anxiety, and grief. And yet, perhaps because life and the right to live had already taken such a firm hold inside him, he could move on.

The night before his departure, Adam wrote me a farewell letter in which he quoted a poem by Dylan Thomas, "And Death Shall Have No Dominion," which held particular significance for me regarding him, the analysis, and myself:

> And death shall have no dominion . . .
> Split all ends up they shan't crack;
> And death shall have no dominion.
> (1933, p. 55)

Discussion

Within the depths of a black hole and deadness

I. Survival and living-through t(w)ogether

"Having begun an analysis I expect to continue with it, to survive it and to end it," wrote Winnicott (1962, p. 166). I have recounted an analysis that I began, continued with, survived, and ended, or rather—one that we, the patient and I, began, continued with, survived, and ended, "*livi[ing] an experience 't[w]ogether*" (Winnicott, 1945, p. 152, italics in original).

I will first elaborate on the idea of both patient and analyst analytically surviving and living-through the patient's internal world of deadness and destructiveness, and primarily the analyst's experiencing and surviving the deadness and the destructiveness of the analysis. The analyst's close contact with the patient's internal world has been an important theme of different psychoanalytic schools over the years, beginning with Freud's (1910) statement that psychoanalysis should take place in "the neighbourhood" of the patient's feelings and repressed material. In this regard, crucial questions arise: how can the analyst be in "the neighborhood" (Freud, 1910) or "experience-near" (Kohut, 1984; Ornstein and Ornstein, 1985); how can the analyst be affected (Brenman Pick, 1988), invaded by, take in, experience (Bion, 1959), feel, think and share as if they were a part of his/her own self (Grinberg, 1991) the patient's pain, terror, unbearable inner objects, and psychic illness, when facing a black hole experience—the experience of being gripped, devoured, distorted, and annihilated by enormous forces of deadness and death?

The analyst's inner struggle over being influenced by the patient's world is an intense one in the case of those patients who engulf the analyst with the "black hole" and "dead" mother experience. Being near or within this world means becoming trapped and devoured in the world of deadness. Remaining at a distance means that there is no emotional contact with the patient's deadening world and deep, annihilating core experience; it means remaining outside, distant, unaffected, and, in my opinion, no change can then take place.

Green (1986) addresses primarily technical issues with regard to these overwhelming, deadening situations. He suggests modifying "even the analytic technique" regarding patients with "dead" mothers, because the analyst's silence "only perpetuates the transference of the blank mourning for the mother," and interpretations of destructiveness and hatred are secondary and "never approach the primary core of this constellation—the central decathexis of the maternal primary object" that resulted in the "psychical hole" (p. 146). He prefers "Winnicott's (1971a) position, as it is expressed in his article "The Use of an Object." Only in a single paragraph does Green relate emotionally and exceptionally sharply to the analyst's feelings:

> The dead mother refuses to die a second death. Very often, the analyst says to himself: "This time it's done, the old woman is really dead, he (or she) will finally be able to live, and I shall be able to breathe a little." Then a small traumatism appears in the transference or in life which gives the maternal image renewed vitality, if I may put it this way. It is because she is a thousand-headed hydra whom one believes

> one has beheaded with each blow; whereas in fact only one of its heads has been struck off. Where then is the beast's neck?
>
> (Green, 1986, p. 158)

Returning to the clinical illustration of Adam, I have no doubt that in this analysis the enormous power of the "dead" mother—described by Green as the thousand-headed hydra, for whom any small traumatization in the transference or in life gives her renewed vitality—was curbed and perhaps even overcome. This was so both in terms of her intense grip and compelling pull on the patient and in terms of the patient's ability to actually free himself in order to build a life for himself; and it withstood the traumatizations which he experienced with me in the analysis, and in reality.

However, the use of the experience of deadness in the analyst's countertransference, to generate verbally symbolized meanings that are eventually offered to the patient in the form of interpretation (Ogden, 1995), did not occur here—particularly not during that most difficult period of more than a year when the patient was completely immersed in the struggle for the life of his dying cancer patient. I was caught, silenced, and paralyzed by that black hole of deadness, dying, and struggle to rescue, which completely dominated the analysis. It seems that "[S]omething more than an interpretation was required to be the agent of psychic change in this patient" (Stewart, 1992, p. 138).

And so, what actually worked here? I will attempt to put into words feelings and thoughts which I had during the analysis and afterwards—thoughts of the essential dynamic role of the *experience of surviving and remaining alive analytically*.

The patient in this analysis was a child who grew up with a "dead" mother—an emotionally and physically ill mother, and was subjected from infancy to the influence of her inner world of illness and deadness, like a black hole which pulls, distorts, devours, and annihilates. To protect himself from the intense grip of the "dead" mother, he froze his self-experience and his longing and neediness for her love, feelings, and responsiveness:

> Along with this goes an unconscious assumption (which can become a conscious hope) that opportunity will occur at a later date for a renewed experience, in which the failure situation will be able to be unfrozen and re-experienced, with the individual in a regressed state, in an environment that is making adequate adaptation.
>
> (Winnicott, 1954a, p. 281)

And indeed, within the holding environment provided by analysis, Adam came out of his detached, frozen self-state, and reopened the deepest, fiercest, and most terrifying passion of his inner life—the long-buried yearning to repair his primary relationship, to rescue the mother from death in the most concrete, absolute way, and thus, rescue his self. I became involved and eventually totally engulfed in the world of dying and deadness that was at the very heart of his experience. He compelled me to know and feel what it is like to be in the presence of a sick, dying woman; to feel my paralyzed inability when faced with a person who could not be reached through understanding, through contact, through interpretation, but only by facing actual dying and acting; to feel overwhelmed by the deadness, by somatic and psychic fears which dominated me and the analysis, and by the helplessness that comes from realizing that nothing could stop what was happening. This was a very real knowing and experiencing of the grip of deadness and dying, of being caught and trapped in a black hole experience. There was nothing left but the raw, fateful interplay between death and survival.

I now realize that this was a very deep experiential converging with the patient's self and object world and history. This interconnected presence is crucial to the analytic process because the analyst who is there, receptive to the patient's devastating experiences without closing up or avoiding them, who struggles to tolerate and to work through distressing countertransferential feelings and deadness and survives, eventually changes the patient's basic experience of being and relating. The devouring deadness of the black hole becomes something that is felt, stayed with, and slowly, with time and effort, contained, lived through, and recovered from, within the interconnected experience of self-with-other (Eshel, 2013a, 2016a; now chapters 8 and 9).

But will the patient feel that he is not alone, that the analyst is there with him, when all possibilities for verbal and emotional expression are petrified and deadened during this battle between death and survival? Is being there with the patient, surviving his annihilating world in a way that is not bound or justified by interpretations, sufficient?

I believe it is. To my thinking, such experiences do not only represent, they *present* something fundamental. I met, *experienced*, and was deeply affected by the patient's destructiveness—first by the massive, deadening destructiveness of his object world, and then by his needy emptiness—without retaliating and without escaping or denying it (Winnicott, 1971a). I was not a distant observer, standing outside the black hole experience.

I was there, "with-in," affected, touched. *It was this intersecting of my being deeply affected and remaining alive that made contact, survival and living—both his and mine—an existing fact and emotional reality in the analytic experience of self-with-other.*

In this way, the cumulative analytic experience gradually provided and actualized an alternative lived interconnectedness, in which the patient was not incessantly driven by anxiety and deadness, by the dread of being destroyed or destructive, and by guilt for the object. It thus influenced and transformed the black hole paradigm that derived from his history of self–other relations, and that has lived on as the central scene of his being and relating—what Stern (1995) calls "Schemas-of-being-with-other" and "Schemas-of-being-with-self" which are formed from subjectively lived experiences of being-with the other.

I find these thoughts captured powerfully in Margaret Little's (1981) words:

> In a state in which everything relates to survival or non-survival . . . only a series of experiences which have for the patient the psychic reality of annihilation, and yet in which he discovers the actual survival both of himself and the object he is related to (in analysis—the analyst), can alter this state in any degree whatever" (p. 139). To analyze these areas means to go back to a not-yet-personalized state and *to allow time for the psychic work to be done, which means experientially going through annihilation and death and coming forward again, but differently.*
>
> (p. 152, my italics)

"Experientially going through annihilation and death and coming forward again, but differently"—these words summarize for me the central experience of this analysis: the transformative experience which evolves by dint of the analyst's holding and containing presence, while experiencing and going through annihilation and death along with the patient. Astrophysicists and science fiction writers would use the term "wormhole" here—an interior tunnel leading through the annihilating forces of the black hole that makes it possible to pass through the black hole and come out alive in another place in space. This seems to me an intriguing analogy between the inner journey through annihilation and deadness in analysis, held and contained by the sustaining analytic functioning, and the wormhole which, according to those astrophysicists, will require intense effort and perseverance to construct or to keep open, stable, and traversable.

I have come to believe that being-with-in and surviving analytically through space and time—this "waiting without" of the analyst's, which holds the faith, the hope and the love (Eliot, "East Coker," 1949, p. 200)—are what charge the treatment and the patient with the force of life, in the face of annihilating deadness and dying.

II. The possibility of rescue and a moment of "at-one-ment"

Yet, something was still missing after this years-long struggle to hold, contain, and survive the massive, overwhelming world of deadness and dying that flooded both life and treatment during the first five years of the treatment. Throughout the first half of the seventh year of analysis, we struggled with the enormous, unfathomable emptiness and nothingness that Adam felt his mother's deadness had left in him, and his great hunger and longing for a different kind of motherhood. It seemed that we still had not reached "the primary core of this constellation" (Green, 1986, p. 146). Or, in Tustin's (1972, 1990) words, the *heart-break* which is at the center of his being had yet to be experienced.

Bion (2005a), in his second Rome seminar (July 9, 1977), describes movingly the awakening of "the possibility of rescue," and the patient's terror lest this possibility be missed:

> So the analyst, in the midst of the noises of distress, the failure of analysis, the uselessness of that kind of conversation, still needs to be able to hear the sound of *this terror which indicates the position of a person beginning to hope that he might be rescued* . . . . Previously the terror had been sunk, so to speak, in the overwhelming depths of depression and despair."
>
> (p. 21, my italics)

Adam demanded unrelentingly that I repair his emptiness by telling him my feelings, and, in spite of the many interpretations I offered, nothing changed in this suffocating needy insistence. Was "all that said," as Bion contends, "in a vague hope that somebody or something will turn up who will be able to understand what he is communicating and will be able to supply the correct mental nourishment" (p. 20)?

This unrelenting, suffocating insistence only changed when I became totally with him within his desperate cry for emotional survival and said, "I feel that you are absolutely right. *It's just that I can't.*" Was this a moment that *met his hope* that there is somebody who really understands and *that he might be rescued?*

I have received many thoughtful and interesting responses and interpretations regarding this session. These included viewing it as a "moment of meeting" (Stern et al., 1998); as a moment of emotional experience in which I felt and said the longed-for and long-lacking words his mother could not (Marcus, 1999, personal communication); or that I became, in the treatment relationship, the overwhelmed child, struggling with his mother's world of sickness and dying and demandingness, and now I was carrying out an "act of freedom" that Adam himself was unable to do (Ofarim, 1998, personal communication). For me, however, it is first and foremost *a moment of "at-one-ment,"* a profound interconnectedness that grew into being *at-one with Adam's innermost emotional core reality* of emptiness and desperate plea for a feeling mother. When I said to him, "I feel that you are absolutely right. *It's just that I can't,*" in essence I was saying that I wish I could, I am sorry that I can't, because I felt—my heart felt—the depths of his loss, pain, lack, broken-heartedness, and despair, and that what he said he needed was truly most right, most needed, most essential. It is "a way of experiencing which is undertaken with one's whole being, 'with all one's heart, with all one's soul, and with all one's might'" (Eigen, 1981, p. 413)—a work of Faith as the only state of being that meets catastrophic impacts, faith in O (Eigen, 2012).

Grotstein (2010), in writing on infantile trauma and chronic resistance, maintains that unlike the treatment of the healthier personality, the course of treatment of the split-off, "castaway patients . . . involves the indivisibility of the transference-countertransference in the analyst's reverie, his or her capacity to '*become*' the patient's anguish and agony . . . Bion terms this phenomenon 'transformations in O within the analyst'" (p. 25, italics in original).

Indeed, the analyst's profound interconnectedness with the patient and "becoming" at-one with the patient's innermost emotional reality-O may develop into its full transformational potential with more disturbed patients and very difficult treatment situations, thus offering new possibilities for extending the reach of psychoanalytic treatment. For only the great intensity of be(com)ing at-one-with the patient's unsolvable agony can reach these innermost *annihilated-annihilating states, and create a new experience* within the depths of black hole and deadness. Yet, I wonder, do not all analytic treatments have to reach *a moment of at-one-ment with the patient's experience*, a moment of patient–analyst profound interconnectedness, which provides a mode of transformation that relationships and transformation in Knowledge cannot offer at deep levels of primary core experience?

Note

1 According to Tustin and her followers (Spensley, 1995), John, the little autistic boy, used this term some years before physicist John Wheeler introduced the term in 1968.

Chapter 4

Whose sleep is it, anyway?

Or, *Night Moves*[1]

> But in each event—in the living act, the undoubted deed—there, some unknown but still reasoning thing puts forth the mouldings of its features from behind the unreasoning mask. If man will strike through the mask! How can the prisoner reach outside except by thrusting through the wall?
>
> (Herman Melville, *Moby Dick*, 1851)

Over the years, I have come to think of extreme experiences in the clinical situation as a challenge to one's technique and complacent knowing. They evoke search and struggle, ingenuity and creative moves, at times leading us to extend, and even go beyond, the boundaries of our understanding and knowledge. They are an internal Rubicon that we have to cross.

Yet, writing about my own extreme experience of sleeping during treatment made me face, more so than with any other subject that I have written about, the conflict and deliberation over self-exposure and concealment; the wish, on the one hand, to communicate, share and rethink a therapeutic experience that intrigued and puzzled me, and on the other hand the misgivings, the feeling that it is safer to remain silent, to hold back the more personal, private truth. Therefore, I shall begin by quoting McLaughlin's encouraging sentences at the end of his paper "The sleepy analyst":

> I think we stand to learn much more about the way we work and the vicissitudes of the analyzing instrument if we can become freer to talk about and study the full range of our reactions. The continuum of vigilance-to-sleep experienced by the analyst during his working day hold rich content for this dialogue.
>
> (1975, p. 381)

However, at the same time, other voices come to mind; much more ambivalent, hesitant, cautious are Eigen's (1996) expressive words:

> Will our professional milieu survive us and we it if we make our fullest and truest offerings? To what extent do professional interchanges . . . contribute to the real growth of personality and culture? We need each other to bounce off, fight with, communicate and non-communicate with, interact with, gain real confirmation/disconfirmation. But how much exposure can we bear? How much do we dare or have the right to dare?
>
> (p. 84)

And Bion (2005a) in his sixth Rome seminar (on 16 July 1977—Morning), at age 80, says:

> It seems to me that the analyst who actually participates in the experience has a chance of decicing whether to try to communicate—as he is doing here—and whether we would be capable of hearing and understanding the communication. If he is to communicate the experience, which language is he to talk? Will articulate speech do? . . . In any case it require courage if he is going to dare to make public, to communicate to somebody not himself, his experience. It may take a long time . . .
>
> (p. 64)

This chapter grew out of the tension between these differing voices. It was written in a hopeful attempt to foster dialog between analysts, based on their own authentic, troubling reactions and experiences in extreme analytic situations (see also Searles, 1959, p. 285; Marcus, 1997, p. 240; Coen, 2000, p. 449). But more essentially, it was written out of my profound interest, even awe and fascination, with the gripping intensity of the analytic process, which is (re)created and found, again and again, in each psychoanalytic endeavor and patient–analyst relation—in a way that is particular and unique, often unexpected and unknown, and sometimes even mysterious—sweeping its two participants into it, involving and affecting them.

"In the grip of the process"

These words, taken from Searles, capture and powerfully articulate for me the essential element in the experience of analytic "presencing," that is central to my thinking about the treatment process.

Searles (1965) writes:

> . . .[S]till more essentially, to see the extent to which both patient and therapist become immersed in and swept forward by the current, the process, of treatment . . . not only the patient, but he [the therapist] also is in the grip of the process, the therapeutic process . . . which . . . is far too powerful for either the patient or himself to be able at all easily to deflect it . . . away from the confluent channel which it is tending . . . to form for itself.
>
> (pp. 36–37)

The complex, difficult, and intriguing nature of being "in the grip of the process;" the ensuing patient–analyst deep interconnectedness as an intrinsic feature of the analytic process, and, particularly, the profound impact of the patient's inner world upon the analyst, comprise the broader and basic context underlying my thinking about the analyst's sleepiness during treatment (when it is not just the analyst's personal fatigue).

From this broader and basic introductory context, I will proceed to the subject of this chapter—the analyst's "sleep." I will first let the clinical material speak, describing a clinical sequence in which my sleeping during the sessions became an open issue, and closely follow my experience of being in the grip of this process as the treatment unfolded. I will then return to that sleepiness in the discussion, in an attempt to understand it more fully.

Clinical material

Background

Clari came to me unwillingly for treatment, after undergoing two years of twice-weekly face-to-face therapy with a female psychotherapist to whom she had become considerably attached. Clari, then in her early 30s, was born in South America, and was the second of three daughters born at three-year intervals. Her younger sister had been very ill from the age of six months. She was kept alive for nine years, a vegetable, until her death when Clari was 12 years old, two years after the family immigrated to Israel, leaving the child behind in an institution. Clari married at 20, but her relationship with her husband was difficult and sexually frightening.

She left him and, for nine years, lived with a woman in a stable but stagnant relationship dominated by her partner's obsessive-compulsive preoccupations. She originally sought therapy because of severe anxiety attacks during the Gulf War. The therapy was warm and supportive, in the best sense of the word, and led to a turnabout in her life: she decided she wanted to have children, but thought that children should grow up with a mother and a father. She therefore decided to leave the woman with whom she had been living and establish a relationship with a man.

It was at this point that Clari's psychotherapist was informed that, unexpectedly, she would be leaving Israel within a few months for family reasons. Therefore, she asked me to accept Clari for treatment, as she was concerned about abandoning her at such a stage of critical decision-making. I was unable to accept Clari then, since I had no vacancy, and suggested referring her to another therapist, but Clari's psychotherapist pressed me to take her because she felt I was strong enough to treat Clari during this angry, stormy time. I finally agreed, on the condition that the treatment begin in six months' time.

Before committing ourselves to treatment, Clari and I met once, at her suggestion. During that session, she expressed a reluctant and rejecting attitude toward me, glancing suspiciously at the couch—even though she would be coming for twice-weekly face-to-face therapy, as in the therapy she had been undergoing—saying that she would never have gone to a psychoanalyst for treatment, and the only reason that she came was because her therapist had recommended me so warmly. I said only that I understood it was hard to change treatment in this way. At the end of the session, after Clari checked that I had no long-term plans to leave the country over the next few years, we set a date for starting treatment, and I asked her to phone me a month beforehand. However, when she did call me five months later, as arranged, I was still unable to begin the treatment on the date we had set and could only begin two months later.

When Clari came in to start treatment, she appeared lost and depressed, unlike how she appeared at our first meeting. Over the previous few months, she had been very lonely, both because her therapy had ended and because her relationship with her woman friend had ended, and her friend had already formed a new relationship with another woman. She calmed down soon after treatment began, and it became apparent that the fact that treatment was taking place made her feel more held.

During the first two years of treatment that followed, she was very lonely, cut off from her former circle of women (lesbian) friends, yet resolute in her decision to establish a serious relationship with a man. Little by little, she told me that she had been repeatedly dreaming what she called "dreams of force"—horrific dreams she had had before but which were now recurring with increasing frequency. In these dreams she was always in the familiar surroundings of her home and bedroom, when suddenly, everything would go dark, with an overpowering, sinister feeling of terror. She would usually try to do something—get up, switch on the light—without success, becoming slower, paralyzed. Then she would be gripped and overcome by a tremendous force exerting a terrible, crushing pressure on her chest and especially on her head, and she would be unable to move. She knew that there was no point in struggling; all she could do was submit and lie still until it passed, so that it would spare her and not kill her, and try to just continue breathing—to just survive.[2]

Despite sleeping very lightly, she could not avoid the dreams, which occurred even when she slept during the day. But gradually, over the first two years of treatment with me, the frequency of the dreams decreased, and her numerous physical pains also diminished. Clari settled into a new job and studies, and in the third year of treatment, after unsuccessfully dating several men, her relationship with her estranged husband, who over the years would phone her once a year on her birthday, was slowly and cautiously renewed. They experienced many difficulties at first; each time they quarreled she would become frightened and threaten to end the relationship. They again encountered sexual problems, but her husband, who over the years had undergone psychotherapy, was given great, direct encouragement by his therapist to persevere in the relationship, and he showed a determination and patience that he had not had in previous years. The relationship stabilized, and they moved in together, hoping to start a family.

Twilight zone

In moving from the description of the *events* in Clari's treatment to the treatment itself and the quality and texture of the therapeutic relationship, I enter another realm, opaque and shadowy—a twilight zone.

From our first session in treatment, Clari spoke in a manner that was spare, restrained, vague, unclear—it is difficult for me even to find the word that might precisely describe the way she spoke. Often, I could not hear or understand what she was saying. Initially, I thought and interpreted that she found it difficult to talk to me because she had come to me for treatment against her will (and, in fact, against mine, too); but as treatment continued, there was no change. Later on, I thought that perhaps she was afraid of evolving erotic transference, or that I was afraid of it, but I quickly realized that these were rather simplistic, external interpretations. Something was strangling her capacity to communicate, but what was it?

She seemed just to need my presence there. She attended treatment regularly, never missing a session or arriving late. At the beginning of the session she would examine me closely, and then begin talking in her vague, stiff, disconnected way, her face immobile. After ten or fifteen minutes, my laborious attentiveness would gradually diminish, and I would become detached. It was not that my thoughts wandered or that I was bored. Nothing. Blank. Absent. I ceased to exist as a person who listened, thought, and responded. I would sometimes become numb and sleepy. Then, in the last ten minutes of the session, I would come out of it and become myself again, listening, relating, responding.

This pattern bore little relation to my feelings of fatigue. While at the beginning fatigue would hasten the process, later on it made no real difference.

By the beginning of the fourth year of treatment, after the decisions and changes described earlier in Clari's life had been discussed in the treatment and actually made, and were thus less central to the therapeutic discourse, this situation became particularly acute, so that after the first ten to fifteen minutes of listening and responding, I would fall into a deep sleep, totally devoid of feeling. Then, in the last ten minutes, I would wake up. This was all while sitting facing her, thus I was unable to conceal it and, in fact, I did not try to.

When I first began falling asleep, Clari was very surprised that I dared close my eyes and be with her in a situation in which I was "so very unprotected and exposed." She repeatedly said that even with her woman friend, during their long relationship, over all the years of knowing each other and living together, neither ever closed her eyes in the presence of the other, not even during their intimate games and sex, because they were afraid of each other. She said that her woman friend would say that she was afraid of a streak of cold cruelty in Clari. Clari herself never dared fall soundly sleep. "As far back as I can remember, I would never sleep at night," she said.

She then began to fear that I would decide to terminate the treatment because of what was happening. Thereupon I told her that, *indeed, something very strange was happening to me, and I could only suggest that we let things be until we could better understand what was going on.* (This was what I truly thought and felt.) Clari was silent for a moment, and then said, "All right," in a voice I could barely hear, and she appeared very pensive and far less tense; her entire body seemed to relax. Much later she would tell me that, throughout this entire period, up until I said this, she had been terrified that "the situation would become so unbearable that you would be unable to endure it, that you would stop breathing or stop the treatment, or that I would go mad." She was convinced that I was about to tell her that after trying years of treatment with her, it was clear that there was no point in continuing, and that she should see another therapist. She would not be able to argue with this, as it was completely logical, but for her, it would be fatal. In her own words, "Then all is lost. We won't be saved. Death." (This, however, was only said to me much later—after shifting from psychotherapy to analysis.)

But, at this stage, things continued in the same way for several months, and my direct efforts to understand my recurring sleeping, to discuss and consult, were to no avail. I examined various ideas, but felt unable to really understand or change it. I did not seem to have an inner clue for comprehending what was happening to me.[3] My only feeling was that of a massive sinking into sleep, without emotions, without understanding, without thoughts (at the time, I didn't even ask myself or Clari what was happening to her while I was asleep). It was like something dissociative, or like being under anesthesia after receiving a sleep-inducing injection. I therefore felt that I could only rely on the truth and the necessity of the treatment process, on its hidden meaning and order, and on its own reality. So I let things be and waited to see what would evolve.

This continued until one session, while still in this deep sleep, I saw a kind of schematic drawing of a bright tunnel with a small black dot moving up and down in its center. That was the first time that I saw or felt something while in this state, and I awoke with an unfamiliar sense of relief.

When Clari came to the following session, she was extremely troubled, sitting pale and silent. I waited and then remarked that she seemed troubled. She said, "No," probably because she thought I was referring to her reaction to my recurring sleeping, "Your tiredness is sometimes hard for me, but *after last time*, I thought that we are both stubborn, and when one of us weakens, the other keeps holding, and vice versa." "Yes," I said, and she gave a faint smile of relief. She fell silent again, very much within herself, and then said that she had dreamt a dream or, perhaps, hadn't dreamt at all. Perhaps it had been a kind of fantasy or a memory-scene.

> *It was dark, she got up to pee, and then she saw this scene. She heard someone shouting, "No, no, no, no," a terrible cry, and she suddenly understood that it was her. Then she saw a baby, swollen from beatings, being put in a crib, a baby dressed in threadbare clothing, looking like a corpse. She saw the shadow of the person who was laying the baby down, perhaps the shadow of a woman, and she, as a little girl, was climbing up the crib's rail to see.*

This profoundly frightened her. *Who was it? Was it memory or fantasy?* It had seemed so very real—"no feeling of a dream." Was the baby her sister, who at the age of six months had become a vegetable, who would lie in bed, hooked up to feeding tubes because she didn't eat? Had something happened to her? But her mother had said that even earlier she felt there was something wrong with the baby, and had taken her to all kinds of doctors. Since her sister was three years younger than she was, it seemed to fit the dream . . . was she herself the baby? There were the threadbare clothes, white trousers, a flannel shirt. She used to wear shabby clothes . . . there was an orphanage near their home, so perhaps it was something she saw there (Clari's speech was very fragmented). But, if it were her, how was she able to see it all? It was like a split within her. This frightened her greatly. She was unable to go back to sleep. She thought that this memory—the horribly battered baby—explained all the pain and the terrible somatic things she had experienced in the past: the pains in her arms and hands, the illnesses at the beginning of her marriage, the other terrible pains. Her whole body had been sick and in pain for years.

The next time she dreamt, it was again a dream of darkness, as though darkness had had erupted and taken over her entire world:

> *I am outside, in the neighborhood, in a park, and suddenly it turns dark. A feeling of a power failure, and then a light failure. I can't see a thing, there's this total darkness, with no stars, no light at all. I tell myself I must go home, but it's impossible even to know which way to go, because everything is so terribly dark. There is a feeling that*

something dangerous is about to happen, something evil . . . and I woke up terrified, my heart pounding wildly. Darkness like the darkness before I saw the scene of the baby, like in the dream of force.

It's obvious that the darkness is an omen of bad things to come. I have to remind myself that there is life, because in some strange way, if I don't remember, if I don't hold on to reality, I'll become smaller and smaller and disappear into something like that, something dark, and empty, and suffocating. I think that the baby in the dream is me. That explains a lot of things, all the terrible somatic things. When I tell myself this, it's with a horrific feeling, of death, because it was dying, and then to live, you have to hold on to having to breathe, otherwise you'll stop. Living. Just to go on breathing. A sensation that gives me the feeling it could be reality. Not even panic, not to move, just being aware of having to breathe.

Dreams and dream-thoughts

In the period that followed, her dreams, their images, the experiences they expressed and their sequence enabled us to get into and explore the ongoing brutal seesawing between holding and falling, hope and destruction; to recognize Clari's longing and struggle to work her way towards feeling that trust was a valid response to catastrophe. For the first time, she began dreaming different dreams, dreams of hope, of being helped and of a helping figure. And then, in the nights that immediately followed, again, unbearable dreams, with scenes of horror and disaster. In the first different, new dream,

She goes to sleep, and in their bedroom, there is a little girl of about three, curled up and dressed only in panties. She [Clari] gets up, because she understands that if she doesn't take care of the child, no one will. She takes the child's hand and leads her into a room of her own—all is very dark, a wind is blowing and the curtains flying—and she dresses her in a nightgown. The child is happy, gets into bed, and before she falls asleep says, "I thought the whole house was going to collapse, but it's only Grandma who died."

Clari was deeply moved and fought back tears—which appeared for the first time during the treatment—when we talked about the dream.

"My feeling is always kind of hazy. I have a lot of stumps," she said. "All of life is built on something that isn't there. It's like in movie cartoons—you keep going on nothing, you look down and then you see that the ground isn't there, that you've been running on air."

Yet, each hopeful dream was immediately followed by dreams of catastrophe in which hope, change, prospects, and her sleep were attacked and shattered—although in these dreams, too, amid the shattering, now there were the beginnings of struggles for help, either in the dream, or in the waking up that followed it. The night after telling me the preceding hopeful dream, Clari was thrown back into a harrowing "dream of force," in which she was in bed, and a sensation of paralysis and pressure began, particularly in her head, which was big, swollen, and heavy. She got up to turn on the light, and there was no electricity. Horrified, she tried over and over to turn on other lights, with no success, her entire body gradually becoming incapable of movement. She woke up confused and disorientated. The sensation continued for a long time; she didn't know who she was. She said to me,

> *I remembered you before I remembered me. And then I said to you, to me, 'Just a second, I'm Clari, I'm 35 years old. There's Ron [her husband].' And then I told myself where I am in my life, where I work, and where I live. I almost called to tell you that something evil was about to happen, and then I realized that it wasn't real. But the sensation and the swelling in my head continued. I felt a need to eat, and I sat down and ate.*

In another disastrous dream, the little girl from the previous hopeful dream was drowning, as though the good dream could not be supported for long:

> *Clari is with her husband and the little girl near a water reservoir, and the girl falls into the water. And when she falls in, she stops breathing, doesn't do a thing, curls up, and begins to sink . . . the water is very deep. Clari yells to her husband to jump in and save her because the girl isn't breathing, isn't breathing. Ron begins undressing to jump into the water but has problems with his laces, and then she jumps into the water with her clothes on and begins to dive deeper underwater, but she cannot reach the little girl because the reservoir is very deep. She comes*

> *up for air and tries to dive down again, but it is clear to her that she cannot save the child. She thinks: Why doesn't Ron jump in, maybe he can reach her? It's not clear whether he jumped in or not.*

Again, the agonizing inability to be saved and to save, although there was a desperate attempt by Clari at saving.

Were the dreams heading towards a null point, a breakdown, the collapse of a new beginning?

On the threshold of analysis: between the darkness and the dread to know

Two months after the scene of the mortally battered baby, Clari asked to switch to analysis. She said she felt that she "needed to be in more treatment at this time." I agreed, but would only be able to begin analysis six months later.

Then, in the following session, a very significant one, there was a recurrence of my massive falling asleep. Clari began the session by saying, "Now that we like each other more,"—I was surprised because she had never previously used any words expressing such feelings—"I want to tell you something else." She told me that when she was a little girl, she felt she was a boy, a hyperactive boy; she would go to the bathroom and pee through a tube. She never told this to anyone, but there was something very confused in her, causing her learning difficulties and memory problems in school in spite of her great efforts at studying. I heard her up to this point, and then I fell into a deep sleep, awaking for the last ten minutes of the session. Clari said that she was observing me "from outside," as though she were seeing the little girl sinking in the dream, as though she were seeing herself as a boy. This boy had been there since she was three years old, since nursery school. When they hit her, he was strong, so they couldn't trample her.

There was something so palpable in her words that I found myself asking, "And what was his name?"

"Johnny," she said.

I said, "You needed trust to tell me this." Apparently, I had said too much.

Clari shrank back and responded cuttingly, "Trust is needed to be here for such a long time while you sleep." She was silent; then she said, "Yes, I really never, ever told anyone about him, ever."

From this point on, she began to sleep more soundly at night, and I, during the sessions, was becoming less and less sleepy; maybe it began before, but now it was clear. The mixture of good and terrifying dreams continued, but these were dreams with a frightening content and no longer "dreams of force" in which "there is only sensation; no content." She said, "There's no getting out of a dream of force. I'm in it; it's a horror that I can't even think. But now, when the anxiety overwhelms me, I think and come out of it."

In addition, she would now scream in her sleep, out of the terror of the frightening dreams, screaming for help. Even when her mouth was paralyzed and only sounds emanated, her husband would hear, wake up, and wake her. Now there was a scream and there was someone who heard.

Then there was another change. While on the border between sleep and wakefulness, she felt herself entering her own body, and it surrounded her like a thick, flexible, safe, protective tire, whereas previously she had observed her body and kept it protected from without

She joined her mother on a family visit to the country of her birth, and there she went to the house where she had been born, but did not dare go inside. She also did not dare to sleep during the entire journey, until her return to Israel, and treatment.

On her return, strange, unknown details of her early childhood were suddenly revealed, following a question that she asked her parents about her childhood. Her father related that when Clari was six months old, her mother suddenly developed a strange illness that tests were unable to identify, "as though life seeped out of her." He took her to the maternal grandmother's house, and he returned home and to his work. The mother was put in the cellar, in the dark, while Clari was moved to the top floor. He said that her mother would constantly ask, "Where's Clari? Where's Clari?"

What went on there? Who looked after Clari? Where was the older sister? This all remained unfathomable, unresolved, and unanswered, flooded with fantasies. The conversation caused her mother and sister great anxiety, and it was impossible to ask any further questions.

At the end of these months, prior to the shift to analysis, Clari dreamt two dreams that strongly recapitulated the motifs of falling asleep, darkness, and terror. I will conclude the clinical illustration by describing them in Clari's own words.

The first dream took place before I left for a month-long vacation, some two months before the shift to analysis; in it there was a close connection between her being able to fall asleep, despite the dark, in face-to-face togetherness with me, and her capacity for separating afterwards.

> *It is terribly dark in here. I am lying on the couch, covered with a blanket from home, and you are sitting on a chair next to me, and then at some point you think I've fallen asleep, and you slowly get onto the couch and cover yourself. We are both lying on our sides, face-to-face, and then, in that position, I really do fall asleep, until at some point you wake me, and you're in a hurry, you have to leave, and there are all kinds of things that I dropped that you give me—car keys, my earrings, and some other things. We leave and you turn right, assuming that I'm going with you. There's a big parking lot there, but I say, "No, no, I parked on the left," and then we part.*

The second dream was just before the transition to analysis, after the session in which we finalized the two additional hours of analysis:

> *I am in my grandmother's house. The maid takes me into a room, the one that used to be mine, and when she switches on the light, the bulb burns out. It's a room that hasn't been used for a long time. She goes to get a bulb and leaves me in the dark, and I'm frightened. I ask her to take me first to the living room where everyone else is, but she already left. In the dark, I try to walk along the length of the wall, but I can't find the wall, as though there is a void all around; and yet I continue walking, with my arms out in front of me, searching for a wall, and the more I walk, the more frightening it becomes. I walk more and more slowly—these things from the dream of force, where everything begins to slow down. Eventually I can't move, I'm becoming paralyzed, with a feeling of approaching danger. By then I'm crawling and I open a door that I find. Apparently, it's the front door of the house. And then I'm even more terrified, because it's dark and I'm alone, and who knows who might come in, and I try to close the door and I can't, because I'm paralyzed. And I start to scream and scream from fear. And then someone comes in through the door, in a short skirt. She bends down and hugs me, and I see that it's my mother, and she's terribly upset, as though something very bad has*

> *happened, she's suffering a lot, and then she begins telling me that she wanted to tell the servants before she left that . . . and I wake myself up because I'm so terrified, so I don't have to hear. I know that there have been times in a dream when I woke myself up, so that I wouldn't hear something.*

I thought of her desperate struggle to break through the horrific, dark void and of the moment of the encounter she described in her dream. She had forged her way out from the terror of the darkness and the void-with-no-objects in which she was left alone, and from the grip of the paralysis, and finally reached her mother. But the mother, who could have contained and mitigated the horror, was herself very upset and overwhelmed (and overwhelming) by her own distress, and Clari fears knowing her. At the threshold of the door that she now opened, on the threshold of analysis, amid the desperate helplessness, neediness, and the yearning to be helped, she fears that something unbearable has come in and will seize her through the contact with the motherly other.

Loneliness and longing, hope and dread (and the immense tension between them)—now, between the darkness and the dread to know, on the threshold of analysis . . .

Discussion

Whose sleep is it, anyway?

I will begin this discussion by reviewing the psychoanalytic literature on the analyst sleeping during sessions, and then focus on exploring the clinical illustration of my own sleeping.

There is little mention of the analyst's "sleep" in the psychoanalytic literature. More is written about the analyst's drowsiness or sleepiness, but even then, it is usually not the main subject of the article. However, it seems these experiences actually occur more often than they are described in the literature (Dickes, 1965; McLaughlin, 1975; Brown, 1977; Alexander, 1981; Rittenberg, 1987). Scott (1975) comments that this is because the analyst who becomes bored and sleepy may feel so guilty that curiosity about these experiences is forgotten. Alexander adds that besides feelings of guilt, the experience is acutely unpleasant, distressful, and puzzling for the analyst, and therefore is also "prone to be forgotten" (1981, p. 46). He also mentions McLaughlin's (1975) reference to "superego/ego-ideal pressures" in these situations.

The following review is based on four papers that were written specifically on this subject (Dean, 1957; McLaughlin, 1975; Brown, 1977; Alexander, 1981) and on various mentions, both brief and lengthy, in the psychoanalytic literature over the years.

McLaughlin's comprehensive paper (1975) views the states of consciousness of the analyst at work as a continuum, ranging between extremes of vigilance and deep sleep, and attributes the analyst's sleepiness to the dynamics of the analytic atmosphere, the analyst, and the patient. However, his clinical examples, taken from Boyer (1979) and, more recently, from Renik (1991), describe the analyst's falling asleep in a *specific session* and not *recurring* sleep, as was my own sleep in the clinical illustration with Clari.

The analyst's *recurring* drowsiness or sleepiness is illustrated by Dean (1957), Brown (1977), and Alexander (1981) as the main subject under discussion, and also addressed by Grinberg (1962), Pacheco (1980), Rittenberg (1987), Kelman (1987), Brenner (1994), Wolfenstein (1985), and Little (1985).

At first, the emphasis was on the patient's resistance and the patient's and analyst's withdrawal: Ferenczi (1919) commented on the analyst's dozing as an unconscious withdrawal reaction "to the emptiness and the worthlessness of the associations" and his awakening "at the first idea of the patient's that in any way concerns the treatment" (p. 180). Much later, Racker (1968) extended it to the patient's and analyst's "mutual withdrawal" and the analyst's "talionic response" to the withdrawal of the patient (p. 139). In a pioneering, short, and straightforward paper, Dean (1957) described struggling with his drowsiness with two analytic patients and attributed it to his passive analytic attitude and failure to actively analyze the tenacious resistance of obsessive-compulsive patients. Alexander (1981) also described the analyst's "sleep" with certain withdrawn patients as a way "to further avoid the frustrating nature of the situation" (p. 49).

Brown's paper offers a further understanding of recurring countertransference drowsiness "*as a response to the patient not being present in some important sense*" (1977, p. 490, my italics). Although this can be a transference resistance, he feels that

> most fundamentally, it represents a primitive splitting in which *a whole part of the self is dissociated.* By a process of projective identification, *the analyst feels depleted or half-alive*, and thus disorientated and out of touch with the basis of what is most alive, or would be most alive at that time if the patient were truly there.
>
> (p. 490, my italics)

This view comes close to my own thoughts, as I will discuss later.

The patient's excessive, violent projective identification (related to infantile experiences) is emphasized by Grinberg (1962) and by Pacheco (1980) as the cause of intense drowsiness in the analyst. Rittenberg (1987), Kelman (1987), and Brenner (1994) suggest additional conceptual contexts for the analyst's sleepiness: Rittenberg attributes it to the "charm" of certain patients, which casts a spell over the analyst. Kelman relates his drowsy withdrawal to "resonant cognition (by induction)" of the emotional impact of the patient's sleepy, unavailable mother. Brenner refers to it as patients with "dissociative character"—dissociation is described as a defensive altered state of consciousness due to autohypnosis, augmenting repression, or splitting—and describes a case in which the patient slept for months in analysis, and her analyst "found himself becoming sleepy and fantasizing about research grants to study the effects of analysis on narcolepsy!" (1994, p. 826). This brings to mind Isakower's notion of "near-identical" regressed states of mind of analysand and analyst that constitute "the analyzing instrument," and may induce sleep in the analyst (Balter et al., 1980). However, in my clinical illustration, the patient did not fall asleep; I did.

In this respect, Wolfenstein's (1985) intriguing paper does describe an experience of falling asleep that is very similar to mine in Clari's treatment, particularly in the sudden, invasive, and overwhelming nature of the onset of the sleep "as if I had been injected with a sleep-making drug." But his subsequent struggle with his sleepiness—"find[ing himself] trapped between antithetical imperatives: I must go to sleep! I must stay awake!" (1985, p. 83) and, later on, "Within the half-sleep induced by the analytic interaction, I would find myself in the company of various visual images, fragments of poetry, snatches of songs, myths, and stories" (p. 88)—are very different from the massive sleep, completely devoid of feelings and content, into which I sank without a struggle. Thinking about this now, was my own sleep the state of mind that Bion (1970) advocated and Wolfenstein quotes in his paper, in which "the nearer the analyst comes to achieving the suppression of desire, memory and understanding, the more likely he is to fall into a sleep akin to stupor" (p. 47)?

In addition, neither Wolfenstein nor any of the articles above regarding the analyst's recurring sleep mention that either the analyst or the patient related to the analyst's sleeping within the analytic interaction; they probably didn't. This is very different from the direct way in which my sleep was approached in Clari's treatment.

Only Margaret Little (1985), as the patient, brings recurring sleep into the province of the analytic dialog, when she relates to Winnicott's sleepiness during her analysis, while holding her:

> Literally, through many long hours he held my two hands clasped between his, almost like an umbilical cord, while I lay, often hidden beneath the blanket, silent, inert, withdrawn, in panic, rage or tears, asleep and sometimes dreaming. Sometimes he would become drowsy, fall asleep and wake with a jerk, to which I would react with anger, terrified and feeling as if I had been hit . . . He must have suffered much boredom and exhaustion in these hours, and sometimes even pain in his hands. We could speak of it later.
>
> (p. 21)

But Little does not write what they spoke of later . . .

Having reviewed the literature, let me reflect further. I felt that the various descriptions and explanations in the literature on the analyst's sleepiness during sessions do not yield the satisfactory, decisive understanding that I was seeking for my puzzling sleeping during Clari's treatment (although, as already mentioned, I found some of them particularly meaningful).

I then gave closer consideration to my own experiences of withdrawal, disconnectedness, fatigue, and even sleepiness in the course of my clinical work over the years. This provided me with a broader view of my personal susceptibility to these kinds of reactions and to the specific situations that evoke them, particularly situations laden with deadness and depleting "terminal objects" (in Bollas's sense, 1995, p. 76). But I still felt that I had not really come to understand my recurring sleeping in Clari's treatment and its peculiar, intense nature. I therefore tried to focus more on the experience, and find within myself an understanding of what it was that made me sleep during this particular treatment, taking into account all of the above. I felt that this attempt at understanding was both intriguing and also part of my professional task following such an extreme experience.

The explanation that I have arrived at is open to further probing and discussion, which is partly why the title of this chapter and the discussion—"Whose sleep is it, anyway?"—is framed as a question. However, the effort of formulating the explanation became very meaningful to me, as it touched upon and expressed my deep, basic assumptions regarding the psychoanalytic process.

In discussing it further, I will proceed along two interrelated axes: the profound presence of the uncanny in Clari's world, and patient and analyst converging into a state of deep interconnectedness.

I. In the grip of the uncanny

The "uncanny"—"*Das Unheimliche*" (Freud, 1919b)—"is that class of the frightening which leads back to what is known of old and long familiar"—a lived experience ("*Erlebnis*"). The German word *unheimlich* contains the word *heimlich*, which is primarily its opposite. *Heimlich* usually means "homey, belonging to the house or family, familiar, intimate, friendly, comfortable" (as does *heimisch*); but it might also mean "concealed, kept from sight . . . withheld from others." This last, different shade of *heimlich's* meaning comes close to *unheimlich*, which means "ought to have remained secret and hidden," but in addition "eerie, weird, arousing gruesome fear" (Freud, 1919b, pp. 222–225). For Freud, the uncanny is the return of something that has already been experienced and repressed. It is as if the experience of the uncanny is a sort of dialectic between remembering and forgetting.

With this in mind, I will return to Clari and to the overpowering presence of the uncanny in her world. Clari's dreams of horror always began in her familiar environment: the repeated, dreadful, overwhelming "dreams of force" occurred in the real and familiar situation of her home and bedroom; the dream/memory-scene of the mortally battered baby is seen when she "got up to pee" there; and the dream of total darkness and disorientation which immediately follows it occurs in her familiar neighborhood. All of these gripping horror situations occur when deep darkness descends upon her familiar world—*heimlich* that becomes *unheimlich*,[4] when the texture of her real, familiar, homey environment violently and abruptly collapses into something awful, unthinkable, without meaning and without mercy—something that cannot be stopped or resisted; into a complete loss of safety, confidence, protectiveness, and orientation; into near-death.

Is this striking shift from the familiar environment to darkness, void and repetitive horror devoid of content, an expression of an awful, extremely traumatic rupture of *unthinkable anxiety*, of *nameless dread*? Or is it also a defensive reorganization of the traumatic, horrific contents hidden in her familiar world?[5]

As mentioned earlier, Clari told me later in the treatment that from a very young age, probably from the age of three, she regarded herself as a boy, a hyperactive, powerful boy, and this made her feel both strong and very confused. This takes me to Freud's description of the "double" in the "uncanny," which can be

> marked by the fact that the subject identifies himself with someone else, so that he is in doubt as to which is his self, or he substitutes the extraneous self for his own . . . for the "double" was originally an insurance against the destruction of the ego, an "energetic denial of the power of death."
>
> (Freud, 1919b, pp. 234–235)

This immense presence of the uncanny in Clari's world coincides with Bleger's notion (as presented in Gampel, 1996) that "the uncanny is . . . a state of disorganization or reorganization which the ego suffers . . . . Bleger speaks of a break, a split between the "me" and the "not-me," and not just a simple return of the repressed" (pp. 86–87).

In this respect, the uncanny corresponds to Winnicott's "fear of breakdown" (1986), the fear of the unthinkable original agony that caused the patient's massive defense organization. As Winnicott puts it,

> The breakdown has already happened. . . . The patient needs to "remember" this but it is not possible to remember something that has not yet happened, and this thing of the past has not happened yet because the patient was not there for it to happen to.
>
> (p. 105)

Similarly, Lichtenberg et al. (1992) emphasize

> *the gap in continuity of experience* . . . . In instances of abuse, especially acute traumatic abuse . . . cognitive-affective paralysis occurs and with it a gap of information processing . . . the person is apt to be left with a vulnerability to dissociative self-states.
>
> (pp. 167–168, my italics)

Having drawn the trajectory of "the uncanny"—"fear of breakdown"—"gap in continuity of experience"—"dissociative self-states," I will conclude with Mollon's (1997) extensive description of dissociation:

> Dissociation is primarily the defensive response of distancing or detachment from an overwhelming trauma, usually of exogenous origin. The detachment of observing and experiencing ego may then proceed further into multiple dissociations and dissociative identity states . . . involves the use of the imagination or pretense, along with capacities for spontaneous self-hypnosis, in an effort to cope with overwhelming mental or physical pain, terror or severe emotional injury or extreme isolation . . . Dissociative patients usually appeared to have minds that have been *violated*. They are extremely vulnerable. Their distrust is fundamental and profound.
>
> (pp. 3–4, italics in original)

I think about the relevance of all of the above to Clari, particularly "the detachment of observing and experiencing ego" and her observing from without, which recurs again and again, in the dream/memory-scene of the mortally battered baby, in the dream of the drowning little girl, in observing herself as a boy, in watching and protecting her body from without, and while looking at me sleeping during the sessions.

II. Interconnectedness

The very last point leads me to the second axis in the understanding of my sleeping during Clari's treatment—the converging of patient and analyst in the process into a therapeutic entity or being of deep interconnectedness or "withnessing" that goes beyond the confines of their separate subjectivities and the simple summation of the two.

As I wrote earlier, this way of thinking goes far beyond the mere participation of the analyst/therapist in the patient's inner experience. It involves changing the patient's inner space (as well as the analyst's) by providing and creating the opportunity, *via experiential deep patient–analyst interconnectedness*, to get in touch with, experience, know, contain, and influence the unknown, dissociated, unthinkable aspects of being and relating.

Thus, Searles (1965) regards "symbiotic relatedness between patient and therapist [as] a necessary phase in . . . successful therapy with either psychotic or neurotic patients, although it is particularly prominent in the former group" (p. 524). He believes that "the patient can never become deeply a whole person unless he has his chance . . . to identify with the therapist who survives the fullest intensity of this kind of attack to which the patient was exposed in childhood" (p. 536).

Searles himself, in looking back on his own analysis, came to understand that "all several years of craving [in his analysis] had actually represented my determined effort to make *him* [his analyst] feel *my* feelings—the feelings repressed in me which I myself had been afraid to experience" (1965, p. 20, italics in original).

On the basis of these ideas, I would like to return to the question of what made me sleep during Clari's treatment. But first, was this a "sleep"? I would like to draw upon a passage in Winnicott's letter to Clifford Scott about "regression to sleep" in Scott's presentation to the British Psycho-Analytical Society (January 27, 1954). Winnicott wonders whether sleep is the "right word" to be used for this sort of sleep: "The sort of sleep that you are referring to seems to me to be more in the nature of a depersonalization or an extreme dissociation or something awfully near to the unconsciousness belonging to a fit" (Rodman 1987, p. 56).

In a similar vein, Dickes and Papernik (1977) argue that sleeplike states of patient or analyst during treatment are hypnoid or hypnotic states and not ordinary sleep. They are often a repetition of childhood hypnoid states that occurred as a defense or refuge from intolerable feelings resulting from traumatic overstimulation and abuse (Dickes, 1965).

I, too, regard my "sleep" during Clari's treatment in these terms of "extreme dissociation" (Winnicott), "hypnoid state" (Dickes and Papernik), or "cognitive-affective paralysis with a gap in continuity of experience" (Lichtenberg et al.). *My self-experience became dissociated.*

In Clari's inner world, the traumatic, terrifying early experiences were massively dissociated, their contents warded off. She was caught within a persistent nightmarish scene of raw horror, with repeated, uncanny scenarios of utter darkness, loneliness, and desperation, while being in the grip of an overwhelming, inescapable anti-life force. She was crushed and stifled nearly to death, emotionally and somatically, depending for existence itself on a whim—a scene of total helplessness, of dissociated, unspeakable abuse and longing, and mere physical survival. There was also the retraumatization with which Clari came to me for treatment because of her former therapist's departure.

As the treatment evolved, Clari increasingly projected these basic, central elements of her inner world into me—the coercive extreme dissociation of self-experience; the cognitive-affective paralysis with the gap in continuity of experience; the absence. Now, the experience of being inside a dissociative, blank process was occurring in *me—a vicarious self-state dissociation*, thus detaching and distancing it from her while she observed from without. But when I let it affect me, allowing it to be and become me,[6] without understanding it but also without dread, carrying in me the knowledge from experience of having been repeatedly dissociated and absent—yet staying there, in the treatment, surviving, trying to think and contain the experience—it gradually became a therapeutic experience. The dissociation very slowly became a new kind of dissociation—*an attenuated, deferred dissociation*, because the dissociation in me—or, more precisely, in the interconnected therapeutic entity of her and me—was no longer the extremely lonely, unmediated, life-defending dissociative self-experience of her, but a dissociative experience that was held differently within me, and within a human process—a massive yet sustained and tolerable one.

This externalization and mitigation of the dissociation with and through me, and being within an interconnected, expanded, more contained therapeutic space, enabled Clari to dare approach, observe, and experience the dread of her inner self-other experiences. She could begin to think, dream, and imagine, to risk exploring the traumatic contents of her massive uncanniness, which, until now, had been unknowable, unthinkable, extremely dissociated, and unapproachable, threatening her with desperation, collapse, madness, and dying. Fact-finding became self-finding. In this way, we went through and beyond the dissociation.

Bion's (1970) words come to mind here:

> If the analyst can take certain steps that enable him to "see" what the patient sees, it is reasonable to suppose that the patient has likewise "taken steps," though not necessarily the same ones, to enable him to "see" what he sees.
>
> (p. 40)

In my own personal associations and images, the reflection of Clari's petrifying dissociation in me resembled the reflection of the mythological Gorgon Medusa in Perseus's mirror-shield, given to him by Athena, which enabled him to approach the Medusa without looking her directly in her petrifying face, and overcome her, while all who looked directly at her turned to stone.

It can also be said, following Freud's thinking in "The uncanny" (1919b), that I became the "double"—a human, alive, real, and present "double" in Clari's uncanniness " by mental processes leaping from one . . . to another—by what we should call telepathy—so that the one possesses knowledge, feelings and experience in common with the other . . . there is a doubling, dividing and interchanging of the self" (p. 234). Botella and Botella (2005) expand on the idea of the analyst's "functioning or working as a double," which goes beyond "already known" countertransference meaning and thus gives access to the patient's unrepresentable areas that would otherwise remain traumatically unknown and unreachable (pp. 82–83).

Perhaps in order to enter and become implanted inside Clari's impervious, inaccessible, yet needy inner world, I had to be in an unprotected, vulnerable, paralyzed state, to match the quality of her own core vulnerability.

Finally, still along this line of deep therapeutic interconnectedness, but looking at my "sleep" from a very different perspective—my sleep during Clari's treatment could be regarded as regression in the countertransference to a "good sleep" (suggested by Bollas, 1997, personal communication). When I actualized the capacity to fall asleep for Clari, she, too, was able to let herself fall soundly asleep (as in the dream of her falling asleep, in spite of the dark, in face-to-face togetherness with me). She could hold the hand of the terrified, lost little girl within herself and put her to bed, as in the first good dream that she dreamt, and begin to actualize "dream-space" (Khan, 1972) and inner space for remembering, which she was robbed of by her traumatic childhood. This is a "good sleep" that is created with and through another person. This point resonates with Ferenzci's (1932) earlier words: "A sleeping person is defenseless: When one is asleep, one relies on the safety of the house and the environment, otherwise one could not fall asleep" (p. 45).

Perhaps, therefore, at the end of all the explanations and beyond all explanations, I would dare to say that in this treatment, without knowing it at the time, amid the depths of not understanding and not knowing, there came into being an "*act of faith*" (Bion, 1970) and "area of faith" (Eigen, 1981)—out of my fundamental, profound belief and trust in the psychoanalytic process, in the deep connection between patient and analyst, in holding and being held, in containing and reverie; in myself as an analyst.

Also, given the state of deep patient–analyst interconnectedness and interpenetrating influence, the "act of faith" came into being within the interconnected therapeutic entity of me-and-Clari, Clari-and-me.

Concluding thoughts

Night Moves

I gave this chapter a subtitle, *Night Moves*, because "moves" in the darkness of night and in the darkness of unknowing were very significant in this treatment; and because of Berman's (1998) paper: "Arthur Penn's *Night Moves*: a film that interprets us," which touches upon thoughts that I had about Clari's treatment, particularly at the time of the transition from psychotherapy to analysis.

The film *Night Moves* (1975) describes detective Harry Mosby's attempts to decipher the disappearance and later the violent death of an adolescent girl, Delly G. He initially succeeds in finding the girl and bringing her home, but when he later learns of her violent death-murder, he embarks on a second search in order to discover the truth. Berman regards the detective's search as a metaphor for the psychoanalyst's quest, and speaks of "The two analyses of Delly G:" The "first analysis" is seemingly successful, but then proves insufficient and fatal; a "second analysis" is needed, in search of a fuller truth, external and internal. Now the detective-psychoanalyst has to grapple with questions that he had previously evaded about himself, his personal and professional identity. At the end of this second, perilous, more daring and more penetrating search, he arrives at the truth, but he is shot and seriously wounded, and it is not clear at the end of the film whether or not he survives.

I pondered Clari's two therapies and the upcoming analysis: the first therapy, with her former therapist—a straightforward and more ordinary therapy—and the second therapy with me—opaque and shadowy, moving in the dark, entering into uncanny states, dissociation, and my peculiar sleep. What would have happened in Clari's treatment had she not been forced to change therapists? How far should we go—and dare we go—in search of a fuller and deeper truth, into unknown recesses of the uncanny, into deep and regressive levels of transference-countertransference. And at what price?

I thought about Clari's persistence in treatment and her great determination to intensify it, despite the dread that was strongly expressed in her dream just prior to the transition to analysis, as she opened the door to the unknown and to something dreadful in the contact with the motherly other—so terrifying that she woke herself up to avoid knowing it. Then, on the threshold of the deeper analytic endeavor, at the threshold of the opened door and the entering of uncanny trepidation and the dread to know—faced with the opened Pandora's box—I reminded-reassured myself that in the mythological story of Pandora, all kinds of misery and evil burst out of the opened box, but in its depth—and for the first time—there was also Hope.

Afterword

In this account, I have restricted myself to what I experienced, came to know, and did not know about my "sleeping"—during the course of Clari's psychotherapy and shortly afterwards, at the beginning of the analysis. I chose not to use material from later in the analysis because I wanted to convey the quality of the experience for me at the time—its grip, its experiential vicissitudes, its unknowns and unfoldings. Yet, I would like to add that during the analysis, I no longer experienced "sleeping." It seems that this was a phase in the treatment that Clari and I had already lived through. *T(w)ogether*.

Notes

1 *Night Moves* (1975), directed by Arthur Penn, will be referenced here later.
2 While writing this chapter, I encountered an article in *The New York Times* that described phenomena such as a sensed presence, terror, strong immobility, a

crushing pressure, and struggle for breath as the mysterious "sleep paralysis" (Kristof, 1999).

3 It was after writing this that I read Bion's (1992) words, which resonated with my experience at that time: "It means that I am forced to have an emotional experience and that I have to have it in such a way that I am unable to learn from it . . . I am not allowed to comprehend it. Then I cannot learn by the emotional experience, and I cannot remember it" (p. 220). Years later, I also read Francesca Bion's description that Bion "often talked to her about his feelings of being totally in the dark . . . He would say, . . .'It's beyond me,' or, 'I can't make head or tail of it.'" (1995, p. 96).

4 When I asked a native German speaker to explain the word *unheimlich*, she said, "It is a child in darkness, a lurking danger."

5 Grotstein has argued that the "dead child within" is universally ensconced in abused and traumatized patients and is transformed into the "undead child," the one who relentlessly haunts them for their having made a Faustian bargain with an internal dark force in order to survive (2000, p. 229).

6 I am using the words "*be*" and "*become*" because I also associate them with Bion's late writing on the primacy of the analyst's "being" and "becoming" the patient's innermost emotional reality-O that is unknown and unknowable, which enable the deepest form of psychoanalytic reaching, rooted as it is in experience: "He [the analyst] must *be it* [O] . . . In so far as the analyst becomes O, he is able to know the events that are the *evolutions* of O. Restating this in terms of psycho-analytic experience, the psycho-analyst can know what the patient says, does, and appears to be, but cannot know the O of which the patient is an evolution: he can only 'be' it" (Bion, 1970, p. 27, italics in original).

Chapter 5

A beam of "chimeric" darkness

Presence, interconnectedness, and transformation in the psychoanalytic treatment of a patient convicted of sex offenses

In my endeavor to grasp, explore, and embrace the true nature of the analyst's "presencing" and interconnectedness or withnessing, I will focus in this chapter on the "chimeric" element or quality of patient–analyst interconnectedness. I have chosen the term "chimeric" for its wealth of mythological, genetic, biological, biomedicinal (chimeric proteins), and psychoanalytical associations, which serve to highlight the complex quality involved in patient–analyst deep interconnectedness, especially in difficult, psychotic, psychically foreclosed, profoundly dissociated, and perverse states.

The "chimeric" element in interconnectedness

The term *chimera* or *chimerism* has its origin in Greek mythology, the chimera being a monstrous creature with a lion's head, a goat's body, and a dragon's or serpent's tail. Occasionally, it has been depicted as three-headed—the head of a lion, a goat, and a dragon, one or more spewing fire.

In modern sciences such as biology, genetics, and botany, the term "chimera" or "chimerism" denotes an organism that is made up of genetically different cell populations with two distinct DNA systems. This condition may develop when two zygotes (fertilized ova) fuse, or as a result of organ transplants, especially bone marrow transplants. In modern medicine, effective chimeric protein drugs (for example, in cancer treatment) are based on chimeric antibodies that bind to the antigen to fight the pathogen, but without triggering the immune reaction in the body generally triggered by regular antibodies toward what they perceive as "foreign" elements. These characteristics are closely related to the nature of the interconnection that is described in this chapter.

In contemporary psychoanalytic literature, de M'Uzan (2006) coined the term "psychological chimera" for the "emergence, almost the birth . . . of a new 'monstrous' entity . . . comparable to an *immaterial being*, . . . [that] emanates from the imbricated or enmeshed activities of the unconscious minds of the analysand and the analyst" (p. 19). This emerges during a process of depersonalization in the analyst. De M'Uzan emphasizes that "the psychoanalytic process has the fundamental task of pushing back the limits well beyond the margins imposed by *reality-testing* (italics in original)," and therefore he attaches "crucial importance" to the power of this "fabulous," "nocturnal existence" that induces "one of the strangest powers of which the analytic situation disposes" (p. 19).

Bach's (2010) "chimeras" draw an analogy between the functioning of the immune system and the functioning of the narcissistic system, both in keeping the other or non-self at bay or in allowing for its eventual, gradual, and non-threatening assimilation and metabolization in the course of any analysis. Ithier (2016) brings together de M'Uzan's conception of the chimera and Ogden's "intersubjective analytic third," and proposes the chimera as a particular intersubjective third, engendered by unknown affinities (not differences) between traumatic zones in patient and analyst.

I would like to use the term "chimerism" to highlight and describe the complex quality of the analyst's "presencing" and interconnecting with the patient's psyche, especially in difficult and threatening, severely dissociated, perverse, or psychotic states—"to try to approach what is radically other, what the other feels as being foreign, but from which they cannot escape" in Pontalis's words (2003, p. 11). It is in these daunting, expelled, or deadening states that the full extent, meaning and potential of the chimerism entailed in the patient–analyst interconnectedness, comes into being. Perhaps only this difficult, strange, monstrously enmeshed patient–analyst chimeric entity can offer the sense of one corporate psyche working to enable new experiencing, processing, and transformation there. This is an intricate interconnectedness; its essence, significance and compatibility should be such that the analyst's functioning presence—like a transplant or chimeric antibodies—is not identified as a foreign body by the psyche's defense system and is therefore not attacked and rejected by it, but is able to become an interconnected entity, *a new, chimeric possibility*.

I will present the first years of a long treatment, which started more than three decades ago (Eshel, 1987, 2009b), because the crux of the work was being done—and had to be done—within the extreme chimerism that this difficult treatment entailed. This detailed clinical account from my early therapeutic work conveys the crucial significance of the analyst/therapist's "presencing" and interconnecting with the patient in a most extreme way. These ideas have continued to develop and crystallize in me over the years, but they originated there, within that very early, intuitive, and powerfully effective treatment. The focus here is on the nature, the extent, and the emotional meaning of the complex chimeric element involved in patient–analyst interconnectedness, particularly in difficult, psychotic, psychically foreclosed, extremely dissociated, and perverse states.

Case illustration

> If thou wilt go with me, then I will go; but if thou wilt not go with me, I will not go.
>
> (Judges 4:8)

The patient I describe was in treatment with me for over ten years, separated by two intervals, so that taken together spanned a period of more than 15 years. The following account focuses on the first two years, and mainly the second year, of the first treatment period (a four-year period).

Referral for treatment

Reuben was referred to me for compulsory intensive psychotherapy in the state psychiatric hospital where I was working. He was hospitalized there in order to undergo intensive psychotherapy, based on a court verdict and by order of the Commissioner of Prisons, in lieu of being sent to prison. Reuben was 30 years old, good-looking, beginning a doctoral degree. He was sentenced to five years' imprisonment for sex offenses involving four girls aged twelve to thirteen over a period of three months, beginning when his second wife left him. According to the evidence, in each incident he would invite the girl into his car with the excuse that he was searching for an address, take her to the same place, force her to engage in oral and anal intercourse, masturbate in front of her and take her back home. Thus, when he brought the fourth girl back home in his car, the police were waiting, and apprehended him.

Before the trial, he was interned in the psychiatric hospital for approximately five months for observation and preparation of a psychiatric expert opinion for the court. During this period, his smiling, cooperative manner was regarded by the hospital staff as superficial. He expressed no feelings of remorse or guilt about his behavior towards the girls in spite of great pressure to do so. He claimed that he did not remember what he had done, was unable to remember the girls' faces, could not explain his behavior, and asserted that it had not been premeditated. But he also insisted that he had only committed indecent acts and not actual rape. By contrast, he repeatedly expressed concern about his future, lest the hospitalization and his emotional state cause his intellectual ability to deteriorate.

The summary of the psychiatric expert opinion submitted to the court stated:

A The accused is capable of following the court proceedings and participating in his defense.
B At the time of the alleged incident, the accused was not mentally ill, but mentally disturbed and, as such, knew right from wrong. He acted under a strong, unconscious urge that, given his mental condition (compulsive states in a state of depersonalization), was hard to resist. However, at the time of the incident, he was not suffering from a mental illness.
C Although he is capable of serving any sentence, it seems to us that in this specific case there are strong grounds for allowing the accused to serve all or part of his sentence incarcerated in a psychiatric hospital, so as to permit intensive psychotherapy.

The psychological evaluation included in the expert opinion emphasized Reuben's rigid defense system with massive use of intellectualization, rationalization, and dissociation for dealing with feelings of abandonment and rejection in interpersonal relationships, and its collapse into vengeful perverse destructiveness. The evaluation also stressed the need for intensive psychotherapy to help him better understand his emotional world and the motives underlying his deeds.

During this period there were two unsuccessful attempts at psychotherapy, the first with a private psychologist (brought in by the family), who after several sessions felt she could not continue treatment because the patient was emotionally "flat" and "full of resistance." The second attempt was by the hospital's ward psychologist, who also felt that it was impossible to form a real therapeutic relationship. After the court sentence, and after the patient, under court order, had been sent back to the hospital for psychotherapy, I was asked to take the case. There was great concern that since Reuben had already been sentenced, even his superficial willingness to undergo psychotherapy would disappear.

Background

Although Reuben had apparently grown up in harsh emotional circumstances, when he spoke about his life at the start of treatment, everything was always "fine," and he "got along well with everyone."

Reuben was the second of two children. His sister was two years older. An older brother had died when he was two months old. Reuben's parents were born in Germany. They left Germany before World War II, moving to one country and then to another (when Reuben was about three years old). Their financial state was sound, but family relationships were very bad (which Reuben claimed he knew nothing about until his mother revealed this in the hospital). His father had frequently been away from home on business, and had relationships with other women. His mother made extended visits to her family in Israel when Reuben was four, six, and eight years old. When Reuben was four and eight years old she took the children with her (but at age eight, when they stayed for half a year, she placed him in a religious kibbutz, despite his secular upbringing); when Reuben was six, the children remained with the father. When they returned from their last long visit, the father complained of feeling unwell and was soon diagnosed with cancer. He was hospitalized and died half a year later. He was 42 years old when he died, and the mother was 36, "beautiful and imposing" (in Reuben's words). The mother sold their house and belongings, discovered that there were many debts, and immigrated to Israel with the children that same year. Reuben was ten years old at the time, and from then on he no longer lived at home. The mother lived with her older brother—a businessman with whom she was particularly close—and she placed Reuben and his sister in a residential institution for underprivileged children. Two years later she moved into a flat of her own, bringing the sister, who was an outstanding pupil, back home, claiming that she was too gifted to be left in an institution. Reuben, on the other hand, remained there and was a most unmanageable pupil. During those years, he visited his mother only during vacations, and she and her brother (the businessman uncle) visited him only sporadically.

At age 18 Reuben enlisted in the paratroopers, an elite army unit. After finishing his army service, he worked in construction for a while, lived with his mother, and took his matriculation exams. He then went to a university in a different city, fought actively in the Six Day War, and married a girl who had been a casual girlfriend from his earlier army days. The marriage was unsuccessful; his wife left him after a year and a half, and later they divorced.

After the divorce Reuben completed his bachelors and masters degrees. He met a girl who was a student at a university in another city, and became immediately and rapidly involved. In spite of a crisis during their second year together, they decided to marry. She switched universities, continuing her doctoral studies in the city in which Reuben was studying; they married, and he, too, started doctoral studies. After the marriage, great tension developed between the couple. Reuben's wife claimed that he was irritable and detached, and although he attended to practical household matters, she felt he was far away. He also interfered with her studies. After less than three months, she suddenly announced that she wanted to leave and move into the student dormitories, packed her bags, and left home. An attempt at marriage counseling was unsuccessful, and the counselor recommended a temporary separation. During this period Reuben became very restless, was unable to concentrate on his work and studies, and frequently went to his wife at her dormitory and work, pleading with her to come back to him. It was on the way back from these visits that the incidents with the girls began, until he was caught with the fourth girl. After he was transferred from prison to the psychiatric hospital for observation, his wife demanded a divorce.

The above information was provided mainly by his mother, uncle, sister, and wife. Reuben's speech was emotionally flat and fragmented. He remembered almost nothing of his childhood before age ten—until his father's death and the family's immigration to Israel. In fact, his clearer memories were only from the time they immigrated to Israel, when he was placed in the youth institution (a youth village). He stated repeatedly that his time there had been a good time of mischief and driving tractors, never mentioning the abandonment and neglect, and the fact that his sister had been returned home while he had not. He stressed that he had never been envious of his sister, but admired her for her academic achievements, and he also was not envious of his cousins, the children of his businessman uncle, who lived at home in luxury. All told, he was never envious. He stressed his successful army service. As for the action he saw in the war, he remarked that even though there had been many casualties on both sides, he had felt nothing, that "they ate breakfast alongside the dead bodies."

He stated that his first marriage had been unimportant and he saw no need to think about it any further. He regarded his second marriage as very important, but was unable to explain what had happened between him and his wife that led to the break and her wish to leave. He had tried to ignore the tension that had developed between them after their marriage and go on as if nothing was amiss.

As mentioned, he remembered almost nothing about the "incidents with the girls," and he was unable to understand what had happened to him.

Given the compulsory circumstances of the treatment, his level of personality organization, and way of providing information, Reuben's willingness and capacity to undergo dynamic psychotherapy and to relate reflectively and affectively to his inner world and relationships appeared to be minimal.

The treatment

The first two years of treatment—four-times-a-week (face-to-face) intensive psychotherapy—were marked by frequent disruptions in verbal communication, ranging from Reuben's general difficulty in speaking to lapses into complete silence. During the first year of treatment, these silences would last an entire session or several consecutive sessions. In the second year, the silence was long and massive, and lasted for over four months.

I will now describe these ruptures in communication, especially the long silence in the second year, and the breakthrough after two years of treatment.

The first session was laden with anxiety. Reuben shifted restlessly in his chair until he almost fell off, gazed at pictures on the wall, asked "Have to undress already?" and spoke in a vague, fragmented way about his relationships with his two wives and his mother, and about the "incidents with the girls." Beginning with the second session, he became withdrawn and barely communicated.

The sessions dragged on heavily; he would not speak spontaneously, and when he did speak, it was mostly to answer my questions in a stultified, dull way. Often he would not answer at all. Over and over he would say, "Again your annoying questions," immediately followed by "Are you angry?" Or he would say that he had not heard my question, and that his ears were ringing. He claimed that when he was in the army, a bazooka had been fired right next to his ear, causing it partial deafness. It was evident, however, that his hearing problems increased when the questions were more difficult for him to deal with. Later on, he began suffering from pain in his abdomen, hugging his stomach, his body contorted; he worried that he had an ulcer, until medical tests were conducted, which turned out negative.

After two months, Reuben gradually began to talk in a more detailed, emotional way. And then the silences burst forth. Any openness or emotional relating on his part was immediately followed by great tension, by angry outbursts at me that lately what I say "annoys" him and that I "distort things," by having difficulty remaining until the sessions ended, and by silences. He would sit tensely, his hands tightly gripping the arms of the chair, his face contorted, half crying, half shouting: "I don't know what's happening, I can't talk to you." When I said that the difficulty was perhaps rendered by our talking and connection, he smiled sadly and remained silent until the end of the session. The next session he spoke, but in the sessions that followed, the difficulty in speaking continued and worsened. He would speak little during the sessions, sit silently, his fingers fidgeting nervously with his lips and the tip of his nose, or he would draw squares on the sheets of paper that were on the table, applying great pressure on the pencil, filling in the squares with crisscross lines resembling prison bars. Sometimes he would begin by writing his name in a florid hand, then completely cover it with the crisscrosses. Or he would surround himself with objects, as if erecting a wall around himself—a pack of cigarettes, an ashtray, a matchbox and a pencil—covering his mouth with his hand, while his eyes watched alertly. He would sleep a lot before the sessions, and go to sleep immediately afterwards; during the sessions he would say that he was tired, that he had only just gotten up, that he could not concentrate, and that he could not think on his own between sessions. Questions about his thoughts or feelings only intensified his silences. My interventions and suggestions concerning these reactions evoked great tension and anger. Nonetheless, at the end of the sessions he would leave slowly, saying, "It's hard to come and hard to go."

It was at this time that the issue of recollecting the "incidents with the girls" resurfaced, after not being referred to since the beginning of treatment. Reuben began inquiring into the possibility of taking hospital leave one afternoon a week to study, and he was told that it would not be granted until he gained a better recollection and understanding of what had occurred with the girls, in order to increase his self-control. In the session with me he reiterated that he could not recall what he had done, and repeated what he had already said in the same vague, partial (only the ride in the car to and from the place), affectless manner. He again stressed that he was certain there had been no rape, repeating that he could recall nothing else, and fell silent. But at the end of the session, when I told him that the session was over, he burst out saying I should stay with him until evening so that he would remember—that I end the sessions whenever I feel like ending them, that he always has to come and remember and talk when I want him to and not when he wants and is able to, that I dominate him, and he left very angrily.

The next time he arrived quieter, saying that he understood and accepted that hospital leave was conditional upon his remembering and understanding the incidents with the girls, and since he wanted to be granted the leave, and was also interested in relieving himself of the matter but could do nothing more, he requested an injection of Pentothal. He was insistent about receiving the injection the next morning. I told him that it was not just a matter of providing information, but of his ability to recollect it on his own and with another person, of struggling with inner obstacles to knowing. Therefore, it was important that he remembers on his own, rather than a passive, forced remembering induced by Pentothal. Then suddenly, for the first time, he told me a dream he had dreamt in the youth institution when he was 11 to 12 years old. *He was pursued by wolves, and running, fell softly into an abyss ahead of him—an abyss with beautiful, shining stars alongside it.* He came to the following session feeling relieved that the idea of using Pentothal had been dropped. But there was no progress in his recollection of the incidents with the girls. He said that there are things which psychologists might want people to know, but people will *break down, go crazy*.

At the end of the first year of treatment I took a four-week vacation. Soon after I returned, a lengthy silence began that lasted over four months. This silence was directly related to Reuben's relationship with me. When I returned from vacation, he was awaiting me excitedly at the gate of the hospital. During the sessions he spoke about strong feelings of "loneliness and distress," of his fear of becoming dependent on me, of needing me, and that without me he felt great emptiness; he poignantly recalled a tree at the youth institution, under which he would sit alone and cry, and then spoke again of having no control over his relationship with me. Then, his tension and anger mounted; he asked himself over and over again, after the sessions, why he had told me all these very personal things, and had no answers. He left a session before it ended, saying in the next session that it had been because of a dream he had dreamt several days earlier, which he remembered in the previous session. In the dream,

> *he causes my husband's death, comes to my house, and I, totally unaware, greet him joyfully, looking softer than usual in a skirt and blouse. It is a one-story house with antique furniture and a door of pale wood, and many people are there.*

Reuben said the dream was terrifying because in it he causes death in order to get closer to me, and also because he has harmed me and I don't even know it. He said that he recounted the dream in this session and not the previous one because that session had been towards evening, and now it was early afternoon. Then he said anxiously that a dam had suddenly burst and his fantasies were beginning to run wild. I talked about the difference between fantasy and reality, thought and action. I said that if all the people killed in fantasy were to be dead, the world would be full of dead people. He appeared somewhat calmer. (Parenthetically, I would add that unlike other interventions in this treatment, today I would not have offered this interpretation because it was too experience-far from his acute sense of impending danger and dread of his destructiveness.)

In the following session, he said that he remembered something connected to one of the girls, which he had not remembered earlier. When he took her home, the girl asked him, "Nothing happened to me, right?" and he answered, "Nothing," and feeling extremely uncomfortable, brusquely opened the car door for her to get out, without looking at her.

At the next session, he said that he had told me too many thoughts and fantasies, that he had reached his limit. And then, silence reigned for over four months.

During these many sessions of silence Reuben sat very tensely, pulling apart paper clips and breaking them, tearing up paper that was on the table, breaking pencils and a ruler—first taking apart its metal ends and then bending and breaking the ruler into small bits. Then, he spent hours burning matches. He would light a match, and when it was almost all burnt, would get hold of the other end until the entire match was burnt and black, then place it in the ashtray and light another. My attempts to speak to him, to relate to his fidgeting with objects and playing with fire, to offer interpretations or help him speak, were received with absolute silence or with sharp cries of "Don't nag," "Don't fuck my mind," "You're pretending." It was only when I said I felt he wanted me to disappear, because in his world I had become very frightening, that he said, "You finally understand," but then went silent again. He sat hidden, with his leg up on the chair, his hand over his mouth as if to hold back the words, with only his eyes peeking out tensely, saying it was boring. The next time that he said it was boring, he pointedly took out a newspaper to read, but his eyes did not follow the lines. Then he took a day's hospital leave in place of our session, leaving the hospital a few minutes before the session was to begin. At each session during this long silence, he would repeat just one sentence—standing at the door, before leaving, he would ask or point out the day and time of our next session: "You'll come on . . . at . . . o'clock."

What stood out during all of these sessions was that, despite his seemingly complete detachment and fidgeting, he was inexplicably very sensitive to my every movement, and if I shifted in my seat or looked elsewhere, he would suddenly shout, "You're fed up, I can see that you're fed up with me and this whole treatment."

As for my own reaction, I was surprised at my abiding patience for him during these continuous hours of silence. At times I was anxious about his emotional state; occasionally I became impatient with his detached, obdurate, provocative reactions; but mostly I sat there quietly, engrossed patiently and resolutely in him and in that massive, intensive something that was going on inside him. Waiting in silence.

Reuben came to the session following the one he had skipped for hospital leave looking pale, a rash covering his face. He began by saying he was tired, depressed, in a bad mood, and couldn't sleep, attributing it to our meetings. He said he wanted to stay at a distance from me because relating to me, especially his feelings and fantasies, was difficult, and he also wanted to try things on his own, so that he wouldn't have to tell everything. He said, "I'm afraid it'll get burnt," didn't explain, but suddenly appeared more relaxed. Then he said, "But you aren't leaving yet," and sank limply into his chair, appearing to be sleeping quietly until the end of the session. After that session he resumed talking—and spoke continuously for hours about the youth institution, his feelings of abandonment and rejection, terrible earaches at night, the physical abuse there, and his aggressiveness. He said fearfully that he was "destroying the only home he had ever had, the idyllic picture," but still continued talking. After another hospital leave, he spoke emotionally about his feelings when he visited his rich uncle and family, that they were all very disturbed, hiding within themselves great aggression towards the uncle, and if this aggression were to surface, they would lynch the uncle. In the following session he spoke again about the hidden, overall aggression that he felt was aimed at his uncle. He tried to think it through, when suddenly he became very pale, grabbed the table, and said that the entire world was spinning. He asked to leave and return to the ward, insisting on it, even though I said that he had begun feeling bad here, and we would wait together until the dizziness passed. When he refused to remain, I offered to accompany him to the ward. As we walked, he glanced sideways at me, with a kind of wonderment and excitement. Upon arriving at the ward, I bid him farewell and left.

At the next session, Reuben spoke about trivial matters, not mentioning the previous session, but something seemed to be bothering him greatly. Towards the end of the session he said that he wanted to tell me something important—that when home on his last hospital leave, he had wanted to remember the incidents with the girls, that it was as though it was resurfacing; but in spite of everything, he could not remember. He thought that if he were to drive the route he had taken with the girls, he would remember, but was afraid to do so alone. Would I be willing to go the route with him? I thought for a while. I then suggested that we talk about it again and together try to recall the details during the two-and-a-half months left until the end of this year of treatment. And, if we do not manage to remember, I would take the route with him. This was a difficult promise for me to make.

I think of it as an act of faith.

For two months we spoke about the girls—four girls with no face, no shape. In detail, step by step, we reviewed his leaving the house, the clothes he had worn, the route he had taken, but each time we got stuck at the point where he saw a girl on the way, stopped the car with a screech, asked how to find an address, and subsequently remembered nothing except the desolate place where he had taken them, and that afterwards he had taken them home. It seemed that in treatment, too, each time he stopped with a screech at this point.

Little by little, he was able to recall the face of one girl, the clothes of another. During these two months, many things "happened to him." He lost his wallet with his identity card and driving license. He arrived for treatment with a large scratch on his forehead—like the sign of Cain. He also formed an intense relationship with a nurse at the hospital (who, two years later, became his wife).

As we approached the end of this (second) year of treatment, and I was beginning to think that he would not manage to remember in this way, and that it would be necessary to take the ride he had proposed, he inquired towards the end of one session when treatment would end. I began to answer, but he cut me off and asked if it were possible that I might suddenly decide to end the treatment and leave. I answered that I would not. Then, at the beginning of the next session, he immediately said that he had completely remembered the incidents with the girls, and would I like to hear it? And he talked for an hour and a half without a break, describing girl after girl, what he had said, what he had done, "pouring" it all on me; and when he finished speaking, he looked completely drained, and I felt as if I had been run over by a steam-roller. I only said that it had been difficult and that we had taken a big, important step today. The next day he said that yesterday he had feared I would think him a monster and would tell him to leave and never come back, but when I spoke of the importance of what he had told me, he felt I was holding out a hand to him.

Even though difficulties in speaking and shorter lapses into silence still occurred afterwards in treatment, this had been a momentous, real breakthrough in the wall of silence that Reuben had erected around himself. This was the first time he had dared open up and reveal harsh, darkened matter from his hidden, secret world, exposing himself to the most terrifying dread of being rejected, hurt, abandoned, and dominated by another person. I am referring to breaking through the silence and not the non-remembering, because one could perhaps argue that he remembered more than he claimed to remember, and it was only then that he recounted it. But, even so, I feel that it was a precious, profound, and crucial step. For throughout his life Reuben had used disconnectedness, shutting down, and dissociative-autistic encapsulation as his main defensive means for coping with and surviving devastating emotional situations. Loneliness, neglect, and abandonment had been inflicted upon him from an early age, both emotionally and physically, by his mother's narcissistic, rejecting attitude, and by the absence of the protective presence of his father (even when his father was still alive, and certainly after his death). His feelings and needs had always been completely ignored. Consequently, his personality had "to be built round the reorganization of defences following traumata [of being significantly 'let down'], defences that must needs retain primitive features such as personality splitting" (Winnicott, 1969b, p. 260). Over the years, behind a façade of niceness and smiles, he developed a closed emotional world, suspicious, aggressive, hidden, and disconnected. Trusting another person was thus a betrayal of his elemental self-protection and the defense strategies that had been crucial to maintaining his sanity and his very survival. It meant the unraveling of his constantly being on guard against emotional connection and the ensuing alarming experiences of dependence, neediness, loss of power and control, rejection, abandonment, breaking down—the evoking of longing and dread. In addition, remembering and telling me the incidents with the girls was a confession and acknowledgment of guilt in the most concrete way.

The extent of this emerging trust and inner change were further revealed on three occasions when Reuben *chose* to be in treatment. The first was when, after three years of compulsory treatment in the hospital, he was granted amnesty, and was free to leave the hospital and treatment. Continuing treatment clearly expressed his wanting the treatment, as it meant financing it himself from his own savings at a time when his financial state and employment opportunities after being released from the hospital appeared extremely uncertain. He deliberated, but said in his characteristic way that he had to exceed the three-year period in treatment with me, because his relationships with women always broke up after three years. He remained in treatment for another year and ended it after four years, on the eve of his wedding. He said that he now had to invest and concentrate emotionally on his marriage, and I accepted and respected it.

Two-and-a-half years later he returned to treatment because of deliberations over having a child, and treatment lasted three-and-a-half years. After another two-and-a-half-year break (and after a second child had been born), he again returned to treatment because of feelings of distress, restlessness, and a vague sense of problems with himself and in his relationship with his wife, and treatment lasted another three years.

I feel that Reuben's returning to treatment at a time of distress—rather than following his familiar, impulsive, lonely, destructive pattern of behavior—was an enormous change, a venture of trust in the therapeutic relationship. It was something which would have been unimaginable several years earlier, and it was forged during those first difficult years of our living through, t(w)ogether, the depths of long, dark silences and violent inner struggle. Treatment managed to offer an alternative to his rejecting, shattering self-and-other world, and to the breakdown of communication, hope, and sustaining emotional contact.

Discussion

On the "chimeric" quality of interconnectedness

I would now like to consider Reuben's difficult treatment in light of my thinking about the crucial significance of the analyst's "presencing" and withnessing or interconnecting psychically with the difficult-to-reach patient. In particular, I would like to think about the incredible power of—and, at the same time, the complex emotional meaning of—the chimeric element entailed in this kind of difficult treatment.

1. "Presencing" and interconnectedness with the split-off, dark unknown

Reuben's treatment illustrates the processes of the analyst's "presencing" and interconnectedness in a provoking, extreme way. On the one hand, there was Ruben's split-off, impenetrable psychotic state, foreclosed from psychological work, which remained an ominous threat to his sanity and very being. This found massive, harsh expression in his non-remembering and disconnectedness from the "incidents with the girls"—a closed-off, mad, profoundly destructive, and perverse area inside him. On the other hand, my abiding interconnected presence with-in gradually became a great critical force, which bordered on the concrete. Reuben opened his dark world of secrets following my consent to go with him on his drive to reconstruct the "incidents with the girls," a starkly real commitment to his request that, having been made, ultimately did not have to be carried out. This ensued after he tested and verified the reliability of my presence in the course of many hours of total silence and aggressive detachment, session by session. It was only within my sustained and cumulative "presencing" that his mute cry and need for help, which had no means of expression, and his desperate dread of abandonment, could be absorbed and eventually become a new and powerful experience—a critical mass that could overcome the horrors of dependency, emotional connection, and neediness in a person whose emotional environment since early childhood was dominated by a constant disregard of his feelings, massive rejection, and abandonment.

Years later, I read Winnicott's recommendations regarding the necessary holding in the treatment of antisocial tendency and schizoid patients, and I found it fundamentally close to the way I was and felt in Reuben's treatment:

> In treatment of *schizoid* persons the analyst needs to know all about the interpretations that might be made on the material presented, but he must be able to refrain from being sidetracked into doing this work that is inappropriate because the main need is for an unclever ego-support, or a holding. This "holding," like the task of the mother in infant-care, acknowledges tacitly the tendency of the patient *to disintegrate, to cease to exist, to fall for ever*. (1963a, p. 241, author's and my italics, respectively)

In Reuben's case, it was not a tendency; it was a real, devastating fact.

But over the years, I have come to realize that a further profound interconnectedness had taken place between us in this process. I was letting myself *become part* of his emotional reality and mental processes—so as to become the missing functioning part there. It is this more hidden, more complex, more difficult, and more disturbing aspect—indeed, the most chimeric—that I would now like to consider: *my interconnectedness with Reuben's split-off, psychotic parts*. For within Reuben's treatment, and particularly within the battle for Reuben's recall and ability to relate "the incidents with the girls," I was with him, utterly interconnected to his struggle, to his deep inner foreclosure, and the dissociative processes that enable such an inner state, in him-in me; to their breaking through. This interconnectedness gained particularly powerful expression when I told Reuben, in response to his request that I join him on his drive to reconstruct the incidents with the girls, that "we would talk about it again and together try to recall the details during the two-and-a-half months left until the end of this year of treatment. And, if *we do not manage to remember*, I would take the route with him." (I rechecked my old notes to ascertain that I had, indeed, said these spontaneous words of t(w)ogetherness then, as a young therapist, before I had begun to conceive of and formulate this way of thinking.)

It was not merely that "the analyst keeps moral judgment out of the relationship" (Winnicott, 1954a, p. 285). I did not think about nor relate at all to the harrowing experience and anguish of the girls he had hurt, the extent of their hurt, what they had undergone. It was a kind of blind spot, a shared blind spot.[1] Indeed, a "*collapse into being with*" *him* (Eigen, 2006, p. 38).

Would the process that took place in Reuben's treatment have been possible without this profound interconnectedness of mine? I think not. For it is impossible to venture alone into the horrifying, dark, split-off and silenced collapse into madness. Only this joining of the analyst's psyche provides it with a place to be, a place to shatter oneself, to experience[2] the horrid breakdown, to be held and saved. A place that is beyond good and evil. *A chimeric place.*

"Something wicked this way comes"—Bromberg (2006) quotes one of the witches in Shakespeare's *Macbeth*, in relating to dissociation. This "something wicked" has to be met, experienced, and processed within the embrace of the analyst's chimerically interconnected psyche.

Leon Grinberg (1991, 1997), using Bionian terminology, describes a transformation in the analyst that enables him to reach a "state of '*convergence*'" with the patient's unbearable emotions. His strong words, I feel, border on the chimeric:

> The receptive attitude of the analyst reveals itself by his *consent* to be invaded by the projections of the analysand's psychotic anxieties and by his ability to *contain* them so as to be able to *feel, think and share* the emotions contained in such projection, as if they were a part of his

> own self, whatever their nature (murderous hate, fear of death, catastrophic terror, etc.).
>
> (1991, p. 21, italics in original)

For me, the notion of the analyst's "*chimeric*" *becoming and being*[3] gives new understanding of the profound significance of this treatment experience as an elemental mode of transformation.

> Wherever you find yourself with a patient, you have to go. We wish things could be otherwise, could be easier, but we have little choice when light shines through the ruins of injury. I think that is a very Kabbalistic model.
>
> (Eigen, 2005, p. 41)

I think that is also the very essence of a mythical-chimeric model of" presencing" and interconnectedness. Perhaps only a chimeric-enough process could stand a chance.

II. "Presencing" and interconnectedness with nightmares: Into the hidden love

Using Ogden's (2004) categorization of human psychopathology into two (metaphorical) disturbances of dreaming[4]—"undreamt night terrors" and "nightmares"—it could be said that I referred above (in section I.) to the split-off, psychotic or psychically foreclosed states of "undreamt night terrors" in Reuben's treatment. Now, I will relate to the "nightmares"—the dreams and emotional experiences that are interrupted when psychic pain, overwhelming dread, or anxiety about the emotional experience being dreamt do not allow a person to continue dreaming and processing these experiences on his or her own (Ogden's second category, of the neurotic or other non-psychotic phenomena). In this regard, Eigen (2001), too, argues that dreams try to process bits of difficult emotional experiences and may gnaw at impasse points over the course of decades, even a lifetime: "A nightmare, at least, is able to image a bit of the terror that freezes psychic processing" (p. 68).

Ogden emphasizes the need for the analyst's participation in dreaming the undreamt and interrupted emotional experiences that the patient is unable to dream on his or her own. I extend this idea of the analyst's participation to the point where the analyst's *participation becomes interconnectedness*—interconnectedness with the nightmarish, painful, anxiety-racked processes of interrupted dreaming, and with the inability to dream the night terrors involving psychotic phenomena or psychic foreclosure—with those experiences that the psyche recoils from and repels, as they are hard to bear, if not unbearable.

I turn now to Reuben's *interrupted dreaming*, which was blocked and silenced for a long time, and my "presencing" and interconnectedness with it over the years, even before I understood its meaning more fully. This dreaming seems particularly significant since the dreams appeared at especially intense moments in the treatment. Reuben told me the first dream—a nightmare—after he insisted on receiving an injection of Pentothal in order to make him remember the "incidents with the girls" he had molested, and I said that it was not a matter of providing forced information induced by Pentothal, but that we were struggling with inner obstacles to knowing. He then suddenly told me a dream, or rather a memory of a dream he had dreamt in the youth institution when he was 11 to 12 years old.

He was pursued by wolves, and running, fell softly into an abyss ahead of him—an abyss with beautiful, shining stars alongside it.

This was the first time that he *allowed* himself and me to be deeply in touch with his inner emotional reality. The dream captured in a powerful and strange way a dreadful link between catastrophe, falling forever, and beauty.

Pursuing my "presencing" and interconnectedness with Reuben's interrupted dreaming will encompass the years that followed the termination of Reuben's treatment. But it seems that the work of the psyche and the therapeutic relationship, once put into motion, does not cease when the formal treatment is over (Eshel, 1998b, 2009b).

As described earlier, Reuben's treatment with me continued for over ten-and-a-half years, separated by two intervals, which, taken together, spanned a period of more than 15 years. I have not seen Reuben in the 21 years that have elapsed since the treatment terminated. But ever since, he calls me each year before Rosh Hashanah, the Jewish New Year, and tells me in detail about himself, his family life, and his work (which, on the whole, are stable and good), and, before ending, always asks me the same question: "Are you still so beautiful?" The first time he asked it, I was surprised and somewhat embarrassed, mainly because throughout the treatment he had carefully avoided expressing any warm feelings toward me; and he expressed his profound regard for me over the years mainly by referring to other people's high regard for me and his treatment. I first thought that, from a distance, he dared to tell me things he had not allowed himself to say in the intimacy of treatment, and I sought an appropriate response. While this might be true, I then thought that I do, indeed, possess great beauty for him, for we had traveled a long road together, and the treatment with me enabled, and, I daresay salvaged, his hopes and his ability to be in a relationship with himself and with a wife and children. That is a beauty that persists over the years, beyond time and place, and is an expression of feelings that should be accepted.

And so every year since then, when he asks me this question, I simply answer, "I think I am." He smiles and I smile, a good smile, and we end with "Happy New Year" and "Good-bye." (But last time he was ill when he phoned me, and instead of ending with "Good-bye," he poignantly said, "You know I will call you until I die, until death separates us.")

Over the years, I have had further thoughts and encountered relevant ideas regarding his recurring question and my repeated response. Bergstein (2008) has written about "the significant curative effect of the analyst's capacity to bear the patient's love," giving this description of mine as one of his examples.

In two articles, "Mommy, You're Beautiful: Is There a Place for the Concept of Reparenting in Psychoanalytic Treatment?" (Slavin and Pollock, 1996) and "The Innocence of Sexuality" (Slavin, 2002), Slavin describes a four-year-old boy who suddenly says to his mother as she reads him a bedtime story, "Mommy, you're beautiful," and she is happy. Slavin views this "innocent" love and sexual relating as an important outcome of the development process, and in treatment, as representing an important and critical achievement in analytic work—for the sexuality of patients who come to treatment is not innocent, but has become convoluted or lost in earlier parent–child interactions, and has to be retrieved. In his opinion, the analyst's participation in the process, using his or her capacity for "innocent" sexual responsiveness, may be essential to this outcome. This view has important treatment implications. Slavin cites Davies and Frawley (1994), who state that, "when such oedipal experiences begin to emerge in the treatment, such benign flirtation must be receptively met with a mood of innocence and playfulness [by the analyst]" (p. 233).

But it was only more recently, when going over the treatment material, that I—perhaps bearing in mind Ogden's and Eigen's descriptions of interrupted dreams—became acutely aware of the interrupted dreaming that took place here. Reuben's long, massive silence at the start of the second year of treatment began with his agitated and terrified reaction to the dream he had had after my return from a month-long vacation—a month of his great longing for me. He dreamt that he came to my house, where I greeted him joyfully, looking soft and feminine, whilst he knew all the while that he had caused my husband's death in order to get closer to me. A dream—its content, words, fantasies—bringing together, reverberating and entangling, there-here, his "beautiful" mother and me, and the death of the husband and father in his tantalizing, disconcerting childhood, yet before the unfathomable, most destructive, total abandonment in the youth institution had occurred.

Longing, passionate yearning, and dread—at the time too intense and terrifying for us to meet, stay with, make less threatening, and further dream them in treatment. Thus, these powerful emotions that were rekindled and dreamt at that point in treatment, soon became muted and blocked for many years, until the end of the treatment. But suddenly, once again, they opened up and spoke, in a present, vulnerable, response-dependent moment—as is also my recounting of it here—that could be either rejected as provocative, manipulative, perverse, or be allowed to be. And to continue to be dreamt.

Freud (1915a), in unforgettable words on "transference-love," opposed sending back, unmet (by suppressing, renouncing, or sublimating), the moment in which the patient admits erotic transference: "It would be just as though, after summoning up a spirit from the underworld by cunning spells, one were to send him down again without asking him a single question. One would have brought the repressed into consciousness, only to repress it once more in a fright . . . . The patient will feel only the humiliation" (p. 164).

I would add here Ettinger's (2006a) intriguing and relevant conceptualization of the gaze as *fascinance* in contrast to the gaze as *fascinum*. Ettinger draws on Lacan's concept of the gaze as *fascinum*, an unconscious fascinatory element in the image/scene that stops and freezes all movement and life: an anti-life, anti-movement *fascinum*. Alongside it she develops her own concept that offers another possibility for the gaze—a fascinating-fascinated gaze, the gaze as *fascinance* in the primal maternal space ("the matrixial space"). The primordial *fascinance* turns into *fascinum* when abandonment, castration, weaning, or splitting abruptly intervene, thus creating a powerful and permanent unconscious longing to go back and turn the catastrophe-caused *fascinum* into *fascinance* again, with its transforming potential for movement and life. This inner longing consequently invokes endless attempts to reconstruct a similar scene/image in order to break the *fascinum*. I regard Reuben's recurring question and my repeated response as a present moment of interconnectedness (a "matrixial moment," in Ettinger's locution), wherein the horrifying-horrified *fascinum* is allowed to become *fascinance* once more.

I am pleased that I was able to meet Reuben there, in a simple and receptive way, with "presencing," respect, and interconnectedness. "When what we [encounter] catches us off guard and when we [meet] it as openly as possible, it offers *hope*" (Lamott, 1994, p. 101, my italics)—a hope for reflective search and discovery, for *fascinance*, for the becoming of a new possibility, and life.

Tustin's "symbolon," "diabolon," and "metabolon"

Before concluding, I would like to address in this context Tustin's formulation of the "symbolon," "diabolon," and "metabolon," which she introduces in her last book (1990). Tustin offers little clinical elaboration of this formulation, and it has subsequently received little mention in regard to Tustin's ideas. But I feel that it provides me with an intriguing way of grasping and delving into the meaning of the "presencing" and interconnecting aspects of the therapeutic experience with Reuben, and particularly of our annual connection over the years (Eshel, 2013b, and Eaton's 2013 discussion of this paper).

Tustin starts by introducing her formulation of the "symbolon," "diabolon," and "metabolon," with the "symbolon," as described by the Italian psychoanalyst Di Cegli (1987), by means of a compelling Greek metaphor:

> The Greek word *symbolon* means a sign of recognition. It was an object which was broken in two between two parties. Each party retained one half. After a long absence, one party would present his half and if it matched with the other half held by the other party, it would manifest the link between the two parties . . . the symbolon

> was, therefore, a tangible object which, in absence, reminded both parties of their relationships and which, in the tallying of the two-part object, reminded them of their absence from each other. It is, in short, the combination of an experience of presence plus a memory of absence.
>
> (Di Cegli, 1987, quoted in Tustin, 1990, pp. 54–55)

But in situations of early traumatic separateness and frustration, instead of the "symbolon," there is the experience of the "diabolon." The "symbolon" does not become a shared experience between mother and infant; instead of an ecstatic reunion after times of absence and the creative "click" of a satisfying union, there is the experience of a destructive "crash." The Greek word *diabollo* means "to throw through." It is a "diabolic" situation, wherein the child feels that his or her projections of extreme states, such as rapture and tantrums, are "thrown through" a "nothingness," instead of being caught or held by a reflective and caring presence. This absence of help in bearing the explosive feelings in such a traumatic situation is a lack of a "metabolon" experience. The "metabolon" situation is concerned with experiencing and working over extreme states of rage, rupture, and terror, as well as passionate states, modulating but not inhibiting them. "Psychic containment *becomes a fact of existence*" (Tustin, 1990, p. 58, my italics), and thus enables psychic development.

In Tustin's powerful terms, we could say that the "metabolon" existence was slowly created and discovered in the treatment with Reuven. His excessive "diabolon" and split-off, impenetrable state of autistic encapsulation met my sustained and cumulative presence, which gradually became a critical "metabolic" force. I was becoming part of his "diabolic" emotional reality and mental processes—so as to become the missing metabolizing part and experience. A difficult, gradual, and deep shift was taking place in Reuben's emotional world within this new, lived-through emotional reality, thus enabling a quality of experience and change where that possibility had been absent or foreclosed. The "metabolon," in Tustin's words, "*became a fact of existence*" (1990, p. 58, my italics).

I will now relate to the "symbolon" as described by Tustin, especially with regard to the annual connection between Reuben and myself over the years. Here, the idea of the "symbolon" may be very important. The symbolon is compellingly portrayed as an object, broken in two, which suggests *a link*, because each person keeps one half of the broken object. Thus, the symbolon is not so much a reminder of an absent object, as, instead, a potential realization of the relationship in the context of absence. By this felt sense of connection and absence, we can better understand the sense of ecstatic reunion when two parties meet again. By rejoining the broken halves, the intensity of feeling whole through relationship is made tangible.

I experience Reuben's recurring question, "Are you still so beautiful?" as offering me one half of the broken symbolon—an actual, vulnerable moment of longing, yearning, and dread that risks turning toward another person in a truly emotional way; a moment that has to overcome his "diabolon" experiencing of years-long catastrophic, massive rejection and, also, the inability to stay with, meet, and further dream these intense and terrifying emotions previously in the treatment situation. Would I reject his question as provocative, manipulative, or perverse, or would I offer the second half and allow the symbolon match of the two parts, the "click" of an excited reunion after times of absence, that is "a shared experience" (Tustin, 1990, p. 55)? To "click" and continue to be, "modulated but not inhibited" (Tustin, 1990, p. 58)?

And I responded: "I think I am."

****

I have tried to describe here some moments of "presencing" and interconnectedness that seem so intricately chimeric, moments that transform and deepen us, patients and analysts.

Notes

1 But, at the same time, it comes to mind that there is always an inherent blind spot in the creating of vision. It is that area in the human eye in which all the diverticula (nerve fibers) emanating from the retina converge to form the optic nerve, which carries the information detected by the eye to the brain for processing and interpretation. In this spot where the optic nerve is formed and connects eye and brain, there are no photoreceptors, as distinct from other areas of the retina; thus, there is no reception of external stimuli.

2 *Experience* in all its meanings: from the Latin *experiri*—to try, test, prove; and to undergo risk—from the Latin *peritus*, cognate with the word peril, meaning risk, jeopardy, or danger.

3 Again, here I use the words "being" and "becoming" to refer also to Bion's later conception of at-one-ment and the analyst's "being" and "'becoming' O," the unknown and unknowable emotional reality of the patient, that goes beyond the analyst's projective-introjective identification (see footnote 6, chapter 4). The clinical importance of the analyst's "becoming" and "the indivisibility of the transference <-> countertransference in the analyst's reverie" has been elaborated by Grotstein's perceptive writing (2010, p. 25) on infantile trauma and chronic resistance.

4 Ogden's "Dreaming" draws on Bion's conception of dreaming and of being able to dream one's emotional experience (either in sleep or in unconscious waking life) as essential to emotional existence and to the possibility of emotional growth and change.

Chapter 6

Where are you, my beloved?

On absence, loss, and the enigma of telepathic dreams

> If only one accustoms oneself to the idea of telepathy, one can accomplish a great deal with it—for the time being, it is true, only in imagination . . . All this is still uncertain and full of unsolved riddles; but there is no reason to be frightened by it.
>
> (Freud, 1933, p. 55)

> So, touch with both ends at once, touch in the area where science and so-called technical objectivity are now taking hold of it instead of resisting it as they used to . . . touch in the area of our immediate apprehensions, our pathies, our receptions, our apprehensions because we are letting ourselves be approached without taking or comprehending anything and because we are afraid.
>
> (Derrida, 1988, p. 13)

Dream telepathy (especially patients' telepathic dreams) and related telepathic phenomena in the psychoanalytic context, have been a highly controversial, disturbing "foreign body" ever since telepathy was introduced into psychoanalysis by Freud in 1921. Telepathy—suffering (or intense feeling) at a distance (Greek: *pathos* + *tele*)—is the mysterious transfer or communication of thoughts, impressions and information over a distance between two people without the normal operation of the recognized sense organs.

The psychoanalytic literature regarding the vicissitudes of the psychoanalytic encounter with telepathic experiences, from its very beginnings to the present, is complex and thought-provoking, fraught with astonishment and discomfort often verging on a deeper trepidation.

In the present chapter, I will explore the enigma of patients' telepathic dreams, especially from my own analytic experiences with them, in which the telepathic dreams embody an enigmatic "impossible" extreme of patient–analyst deep interconnectedness or analytic oneness, and unconscious communication in the analytic process.

Delving into the profound mystery of telepathy in psychoanalysis

Introduction on a personal note

The way in which this chapter unfolds—beginning with a review of the psychoanalytic literature on telepathic dreams, and moving on to my clinical illustration and a discussion of patients' telepathic dreams in psychoanalytic treatment—is different from the way it was originally conceived and written within me.

I will start by saying that I have long been intrigued by the world of science, rather than by mysticism and the occult. Thus, I could not apply to myself Eisenbud's (1946) description of the difference between indulging ourselves with enthralling stories and films about the occult and the supernatural—with the comfortable assurance that there is no reality behind these dramatic occurrences—and the sense of threat evoked when the occult brushes by us in real life. Under such circumstances, Eisenbud asserts, we maintain our composure by marshaling all our powers of dissociation and disbelief against the unexpected event, minimizing or disregarding it, assuming an exclusively critical approach, especially when these phenomena emerge in a psychoanalytic context.

This was not the case with me. It was only when I was faced in my practice with telepathic occurrences—unusual, surprising, rare, and inexplicable—that my interest in them and my search for an explanation evolved. There were five 'telepathic' dreams by five patients over my 30 years of clinical experience—dreams that 'knew' or occurred in the very place, time, and experiential state that I was in then (as described later). They 'forced' themselves on me and made it absolutely necessary for me—as maintained in "Occam's razor"[1]—to presume the possibility of information-transfer between patient and analyst in another, different way, one that goes beyond ordinary senses and speech. It was thus that I arrived at telepathy (from the Greek: *tele*—far, distant + *pathos*—suffering, intense feeling), a term coined by the English psychologist Frederic Myers in 1882 to "cover all cases of impression received at a distance without the normal operation of the recognized sense organs" (Royle, 1991).

This venturing into less certain realms of exploration was a process which evolved over time: the first two 'telepathic' dreams took me by surprise when my patients recounted them (several years apart), but I then pushed them to some remote corner of my mind (as described by Eisenbud, 1946; Gillespie, 1953). My approach changed only when such dreams recurred three more times, over the years, with other patients—starting from the third dream (presented in detail later). The encounters with the last three dreams over the past eight years remained in my thoughts, seeking to be resolved. Not only was it impossible to ignore five such dreams, but I also believe that there were two critical, wide-ranging factors in those years that facilitated my relating and reflecting upon their telepathic enigmatic nature.

First, over the last two decades (as described in the previous chapters), my thinking regarding the psychoanalytic process has come to emphasize the emergence of patient–analyst interconnectedness in the clinical experience—an interconnectedness at a deep experiential-emotional level, fundamentally inseparable into-its-two-participants, which is generated through the analyst's "presencing" and the often-evolving therapeutic regression.[2]

This patient–analyst deep-level interconnectedness that may grow into at-one-ment is closely linked to the far-reaching changes within science, technology and psychoanalysis in the 20th century, and particularly the quantum mechanics revolution in physics (Mitchel, 1993; Eshel, 2006; Altman, 2007; Tennes, 2007b; also expanded to modern neuroscience and biology by Aragno, 2013, and de Peyer, 2016). The prevailing scientific world view has become one of entanglement and connectedness. Whereas classical physics is based on assumptions of linear causality, determinism, and a sharp separation between observer and observed, quantum mechanics has introduced enigmatic principles of uncertainty and inseparability between observer and observed into the heart of scientific thinking.

In this context, I would add the field of telecommunication or telemedia, since Freud (1933) uses the telephone and wireless telegraph as key images in conveying the idea of telepathy. As regards telecommunication, McLuhan (1994), in his groundbreaking, influential book, viewed the media in the age of electronic technology as a transition from lineal and fragmentary connections in the mechanical age to configurations—to a total, unified global field, to extended human existence in electric technological extensions, which express the "aspiration of our time for wholeness . . . We actually live mythically and integrally, but we continue to think in the old, fragmented space and time patterns of the pre-electric age" (pp. 5, 4).

I think that reflecting upon the enigma of telepathic information-transfer is more feasible from within the post-Einsteinian world view, which is underlain by the enigmatic basic interconnectedness of particles in quantum physics, or the "mythic implosion" of electric age telecommunication, "which eliminates time and space factors in human association, creating involvement in depth" (McLuhan, 1994, p. 9). For now, this mysterious "sort of 'other world' lying beyond the bright world governed by relentless laws which has been constructed for us by science" (Freud, 1933, p. 31) is at the very basis of modern science and technology.

Second, is my growing willingness and ability over the years, through accumulated analytic experience (growing also in theoretical and clinical psychoanalytic thinking), to be given over to the grip of the analytic process with the patient; to learn and think from within the depths of the treatment experience, even when it is harsh, strange, incomprehensible and threatening.

The psychoanalytic process has become, for me, a serendipitous[3] process or journey which arrives, unexpectedly and unpremeditatedly, at a new knowledge, a new possibility. Thus, I went with my patients on a psychoanalytic serendipitous journey through "black holes," through feelings of deadness, sleepiness, dissociation, petrification and silences, yearnings and longings, into the depths of perversion (Eshel, 1998a, 2001, 2004a, 2004b, 2005, 2013b; now chapters 3, 4, 5, 7 here), and on to telepathic dreams.

"Allow ourselves to be touched, wounded, and demolished in our own *being* . . . in order to try to approach what is radically other, what the other feels as being foreign, but from which they cannot escape" (Pontalis, 2003, p. 11). I believe that, over time, I allowed my patients' telepathic dreams to touch and strike me. I let the feelings of incomprehension and discomfort invoked by these dreams, which knew me much better than I knew them, linger in my thoughts, and I tried to psychoanalytically fathom their meaning, essence, and enigmatic emergence in the analytic process.

The attempt to explore and come to grips with telepathic dreams in my own clinical experience, and my ensuing conclusions, have led me to the intriguing psychoanalytic literature written over the years on the vicissitudes of the psychoanalytic encounter with telepathic dreams, from its very beginnings to the present, which serves as extensive background to this chapter.

Psychoanalysis and telepathic dreams

In Laplanche and Pontalis's *The Language of Psychoanalysis* there is no mention of telepathy or related phenomena in the psychoanalytic context. Yet, over the years, sporadic psychoanalytic writings on possibly telepathic experiences, and particularly patients' telepathic dreams, have accumulated and amounted to a body of clinical observations that deserve serious consideration. However, this was met with trepidation, from Freud's first article on this subject (written in 1921 but only published posthumously 20 years later) to Stoller's paper "Telepathic dreams?", written in 1973 but published posthumously 28 years later by Mayer (2001). Even this cursory information brings us directly and intriguingly into the heart of the controversy over and resistance to the idea of telepathy, which forced itself like "a foreign body" into psychoanalysis (Freud, 1933; Major and Miller, 1981; Torok, 1986; Derrida, 1988)—"a crypt that threw psychoanalysis, Freud included, into confusion ever since the 1920s" (Torok, 1986, p. 96). Indeed, a disturbing, "impossible" topic in "the impossible profession" (to use Freud's 1937a locution).

"A momentous, first step": Freud

Occult phenomena, particularly telepathy or thought-transference, were introduced into psychoanalysis by Freud, but his attitude towards the subject was complex, "ambivalent" (Freud, 1921), and went through many vicissitudes (Jones, 1957; Major and Miller, 1981; Farrell, 1983; Derrida, 1988; Gay, 1988; Falzeder, 1994; Roudinesco, 2001; Eshel, 2006: Massicotte, 2014). "The wish to believe fought hard with the warning to disbelieve. They represented two fundamental features in his personality, both indispensable to his achievements. But here he was truly wracked; . . . the topic 'perplexed him to distraction'," wrote Jones (1957, p. 406), a major figure in the controversy.

Telepathy intrigued Freud; for it was profoundly related to his revolutionary ideas and battle over the unconscious, in which "the *Ucs.* of one human being can react upon that of another, without passing through the *Cs.*" (1915b, p. 194). Over a quarter of a century, he oscillated between the enthusiastic Jung and especially Ferenczi (with whom Freud and his daughter Anna conducted experiments on thought-transference), at one extreme, and Abraham and Jones, at the other, who completely opposed any explicit connection of Freud and psychoanalysis to telepathy; in the middle were Eitingon, Rank and Sachs.

The correspondence regarding these struggles between Freud, Ferenczi and Jones reveals astonishing emotional vehemence and upheavals. According to Jones (1957) and Widlöcher (2004), after Freud returned from the USA in 1909, he and Ferenczi visited a famous medium in Berlin and participated in her experiments. Furthermore, in a letter to Ferenczi (15 November 1910), Freud recounted his patient's description of the court astrologer who prophesied events linked to the patient's death wishes towards his brother-in-law (which Freud described later in his 1921 and 1933 articles on telepathy) as "strong evidence for thought-transferences that will certainly be *your* great discovery" (Brabant et al., 1993, pp. 232–233). But soon after, in their subsequent correspondence in November–December 1910, Freud attempted to restrain Ferenczi's growing enthusiasm about reading his patients' thoughts. Alarmed by Ferenczi's "earthshaking communication," he wrote (3 December 1910), "I see destiny approaching and . . . it has designated you to bring to light mysticism. . . . Still, I think we ought to venture to slow it down. I would like to request that you continue to research in secrecy for two full years and don't come out until 1913 . . . . You know my practical reasons against it and my secret painful sensitivities" (pp. 239–240). Ferenczi agreed (19 December 1910). However, 15 years later (20 March 1925), Freud still strongly objected to Ferenczi's presenting an account of the experiments in thought-transference he had conducted with Freud and Anna to the next international congress of psychoanalysis (according to Jones, under his influence): "I advise you against. Don't do it . . . . By it you would be throwing a bomb into the psychoanalytical house which would be certain to explode" (Jones, pp. 393–394). Ferenczi and Anna indeed gave no details of these experiments. Nonetheless, just a year later, it was Freud who refused to continue the imposed silence on his interest in telepathy, and wrote to Jones (7 March 1926):

> My own experiences through tests I made with Ferenczi and my daughter won such a convincing force for me that the diplomatic considerations on the other side had to give way . . . . When anyone adduces my fall into sin, just answer him calmly that conversion to telepathy is my private affair like my Jewishness, my passion for smoking and many other things, and that the theme of telepathy is in essence alien to psychoanalysis.
>
> (Jones, 1957, pp. 395–396; also Major and Miller, 1981; Derrida, 1988; Gay, 1988)

Freud's vicissitudes of attitude towards the possibility of telepathic phenomena found expression in his *four articles* written after World War I (1921, 1922, 1925, 1933), and also in actual enactments where Freud was dissuaded and dissuaded himself from presenting his data and ideas in this regard—"a visible proof of the fact that I discuss the subject of occultism under the pressure of the greatest resistance" (1921, p. 190). These enactments are reviewed in most informative detail by Strachey in his editor's notes in the *Standard Edition* (1955a, 1955b, 1961, 1964), and by Jones (1957) in the chapter on "occultism" in his personal biographical account of Freud. They are also reviewed—very differently—by Derrida (1988) in a strange, searingly intense, and intriguing text, written as a series of fragmentary love letters, in which he focuses on Freud and his attitude to telepathy—he speaks of Freud, he speaks to Freud, he speaks Freud, he criticizes Freud. He writes,

> Until recently I imagined, through ignorance and forgetfulness, that 'telepathic' anxiety was contained in small pockets of Freud. This is not untrue but I am now better able to perceive, after investigation, how numerous, and swollen, these pockets are. And there's a lot going on in them, a great deal, down the legs . . . . An interminable debate between him and himself, him and the others, the other six in the band.
>
> (pp. 14–15)

Derrida calls Freud's articles on telepathy "fake lectures" (p. 18) because, although written for lecturing, they were never delivered, but remained just writings.

These "resistances" to telepathy broke out in a series of dramatic events already surrounding Freud's (1921) first paper on telepathy 'Psychoanalysis and telepathy' (Strachey, 1955a; Jones, 1957; Derrida, 1988): in spite of a prefatory note to the German edition that the paper "was written for the meeting of the General Executive of the International Psycho-Analytical Association in September, 1921," according to Jones (who was then president of the General Executive), there was only a gathering of Freud's innermost circle: Abraham, Eitingon, Ferenczi, Rank, Sachs and Jones, to whom Freud confidentially read the paper—though not all of it. Freud related in his paper (1921) that he had intended to report three cases, but found that he had left the third case material in Vienna out of "the greatest resistance" (the case relating to Dr Forsyth, which, in contrast to the other cases, occurred during an analytic session with Freud) and brought other material instead. This missing third case was recorded 12 years later in Lecture XXX in the *New Introductory Lectures* (1933) (written as lectures, although the 77-year-old Freud knew that he would be unable to deliver them). The original manuscript again disappeared after 1955 (Strachey, 1964, p. 48). Furthermore, Jones added that he and Eitingon dissuaded Freud from presenting the paper at the next Berlin Congress in 1922. Thus, this first paper on telepathy (even without the elusive third case) was never publicly delivered or published in Freud's lifetime, but was published posthumously, 20 years later, in 1941.

A reading of the paper does not at first reveal the reasons behind these trepidations. The two first cases and the case replacing the missing third case describe unfulfilled predictions by fortune tellers, which nonetheless strongly impressed their clients because they involved innermost secret emotional wishes. Thus, Freud infers the existence of thought-transference of most powerful unconscious wishes from one person to another. But the strange, concluding lines of the paper betray the reason and the extent of the trepidation. It is about losing one's head. Freud writes,

> all my material touches only on the single point of thought-transference. I have nothing to say about all the other miracles that are claimed by occultism . . . . But consider *what a momentous step beyond what we have hitherto believed would be involved in this hypothesis alone* [my italics]. What the custodian of [the basilica of] Saint-Denis used to add of the Saint's martyrdom remains true. Saint-Denis is said, after his head was cut off, to have picked it up and walked quite a distance with it under his arm. But the custodian

> used to remark: *"Dans des cas pareils, ce n'est que les premier pas qui coute" ["In such cases, it is only the first step that counts"]*. The rest is easy.
>
> (1921, p. 193, italics in original)

That same year (1921), Freud wrote to the New York psychical researcher H. Carrington that "if I had my life to live over again I should devote myself to psychical research rather than to psychoanalysis." In 1929, Freud denied having made any such statement, but Jones insisted and proved that "in the eight years that had passed Freud had blotted out the memory of that very astonishing and unexpected passage" (Jones, 1957, p. 392). Jones therefore stayed vigilantly on guard to hold back Freud's continuing fascination with occult matters.

However, Freud was not "to be held back altogether." The following year, he published a first article on "Dreams and telepathy" (1922), intended as a lecture for the Vienna Psycho-Analytical Society, but again never delivered, only published in *Imago* (Strachey, 1955b; Derrida, 1988). It is a most cautious, reserved paper, from beginning to end. Freud carefully refrained from taking a stand on telepathy. He opened with the obscure statement, "You will learn nothing from this paper of mine about the enigma of telepathy; indeed, you will not even gather whether I believe in the existence of 'telepathy' or not" (1922, p. 197). He had never had a telepathic dream, he claimed, nor had any of his patients during his 27 years of analytic work. He then brought dreams and detailed background material sent to him by two people "not personally known" to him, and interpreted their telepathic messages as connected with unconscious oedipal emotions, while sleep creates favorable conditions for telepathy. And he ended just as obscurely:

> Have I given you the impression that I am secretly inclined to support the reality of telepathy in the occult sense? If so, I should very much regret that it is so difficult to avoid giving such an impression. For I have been anxious to be strictly impartial. I have every reason to be so, since I have no opinion on the matter and know nothing about it.
>
> (p. 220)

Derrida and Gay react sharply: "So, not a step further in the course of 25 closely-written pages . . . . Everything is constructed so that telepathy be impossible, unthinkable, unknown" (Derrida, 1988, pp. 23, 21); "One wonders why Freud published the paper at all" (Gay, 1988, p. 444).

Nonetheless, three years later, Freud published a three-part article, "Some additional notes on dream-interpretation as a whole" (1925). In the third part, "The occult significance of dreams," Freud returned to the subject with a more definite attitude towards the possibility of thought-transference of strong unconscious wishes [in Jones's alarmed words, "he pretty plainly indicated his acceptance of telepathy" (1957, p. 394)] and concluded,

> In spite of the caution which is prescribed by the importance, novelty and obscurity of the subject, I feel that I should not be justified in holding back any longer these considerations upon the problem of telepathy . . . . It would be satisfactory if with the help of psycho-analysis we could obtain further and better authenticated knowledge of telepathy.
>
> (1925, p. 138)

This evident interest of Freud's led to the omission of this third part of the paper from the German 1930 and 1942 editions, and consequently from the revised English translation of 1932. It was included in the German edition of Freud's works only in 1952, over 20 years later, and in the English translation—in Devereux's *Psychoanalysis and the Occult* (1953), and in Strachey's *Standard Edition* (see Strachey, 1961). Strachey's explanation for this omission suggested that Freud's explicit leaning towards telepathy in that third part provoked strong protests from Jones, and therefore Freud refrained from including this third part in the canon of his famous works.

Indeed, Jones, in his biography of Freud, brings two very sharply worded letters he wrote to Freud regarding this article (1957, pp. 394–395). In particular, Jones's "outburst" at Freud is unusually critical in his second letter (25 February 1926), because of his apprehension over the damage that Freud's "conversion to telepathy" would cause in English scientific circles and public opinion:

> You also forget sometimes in what a special position you are personally. When many things pass under the name of psycho-analysis our answer to inquirers is "psycho-analysis is Freud," so now the

> statement that psycho-analysis leads logically to telepathy, etc., is more difficult to meet. In your private political opinions you might be a Bolshevist, but you would not help the spread of psycho-analysis by announcing it. So when "considerations of external policy" kept you silent before I do not know how the situation should have changed in this respect . . . . At all events it gave me a new and unexpected experience in life, that of reading a paper of yours without a thrill of pleasure and agreement.
>
> (p. 395)

Finally, eight years later, in Lecture XXX, "Dreams and occultism"(1933), the second of the *New Introductory Lectures*, Freud gathered all the ideas and examples he brought in his previous articles of apparently occult occurrences, and added his own, unread and unpublished analytic example of Herr P, which he had left behind in Vienna in 1921.[4] Though initially hesitating to commit himself unequivocally in his views on telepathy ("I have committed myself to no conviction"), he ended the article by saying he must confess that "the scales weigh in favour of thought transference." Supported by Deutsch (1926) and Burlingham's (1932) papers on "experiencing occult events in the analytic situation," he concluded with an intense, personal, poignant and (to me) touching passage that shows how strongly he felt about the subject:

> I am sure you will not feel very well satisfied with my attitude to this problem—with my not being entirely convinced but prepared to be convinced. You may perhaps say to yourselves: "Here's another case of a man who has done honest work as a scientist all through his life and has grown feeble-minded, pious and credulous in his old age." I am aware that a few great names must be included in this class, but you should not reckon me among them. At least I have not become pious, and I hope not credulous . . . . No doubt you would like me to . . . show myself relentless in my rejection of everything occult. But I am incapable of currying favour and I must urge you to have kindlier thoughts on the objective possibility of thought transference and at the same time of telepathy as well.
>
> You will not forget that here I am only treating these problems in so far as it is possible to approach them from the direction of psycho-analysis. When they first came into my range of vision more than ten

> years ago, I too felt a dread of a threat against our scientific Weltanschauung . . . . Today I think otherwise . . . . And particularly so far as thought-transference is concerned . . . . If only one accustoms oneself to the idea of telepathy, one can accomplish a great deal with it—for the time being, it is true, only in imagination . . . . One is led to a suspicion that this is the original, archaic method of communication between individuals and that in the course of phylogenetic evolution it has been replaced by the better method of giving information with the help of signals which are picked up by the sense organs. But the older method might have persisted in the background and still be able to put itself into effect under certain conditions . . . . All this is still uncertain and full of unsolved riddles; but there is no reason to be frightened by it.
>
> (1933, pp. 54–55)

Thus, when Jones (1957) concluded his chapter on Freud's attitude towards occultism, he returned to the strange last lines in Freud's 1921 paper—the French words of the custodian of Saint-Denis regarding his walking beheaded, "*It is only the first step that counts*. [And Freud's:] The rest is easy." And Jones added, "How right was Freud when he wrote [this] about telepathy" (p. 407); his implication seems to be that Freud's step in this direction was too far, too credulous, beyond the pale of reason.

On the other hand, Torok argued in this regard,

> Telepathy would be the name of an ongoing and groping research that—at the moment of its emergence and in the area of its relevance—had not yet grasped either the true scope of its own inquiry or the conceptual rigor necessary for its elaboration.
>
> (1986, p. 86)

For me, Freud's 1933 last words about his anxious yet daring willingness to psychoanalytically explore disturbing and challenging experiences encountered in the psychoanalytic process connect with thoughts that I convey here; and they go with me, like Ariadne's thread, throughout this chapter.

Further steps

In spite of Freud's closing invitation to dare to explore telepathy psychoanalytically, it did not become a subject of mainstream psychoanalytic inquiry.

In the following years, psychoanalysis continued to veer back and forth, from amazement and excitement over enigmatic telepathic experiences (especially telepathic dreams) within the psychoanalytic situation, to ignoring, avoiding, dismissing or silencing them. It can be said that telepathic phenomena have remained a most disturbing and challenging topic in psychoanalysis, related to extreme, enigmatic, striking experiences encountered in the analytic process. It seems that not only the first step, but also every step further counts.

In the 1940s and 1950s, especially in the decade after World War II, there was a resurgence of interest in the subject (which raises the question of its connection with war, as Freud too wrote his four articles on the subject after World War I), followed by a wave of criticism and rejection. Thus, the papers on patients' telepathic dreams by Eisenbud (1946, 1947), a major contributor on the subject, Pederson-Krag (1947), and Fodor (1947) in New York provoked a searing criticism of the "minor epidemic of articles on telepathy and psychoanalysis" (Ellis, 1947, p. 607), subsequent discussions by the three authors, another paper by Eisenbud (1948), and Ellis's (1949) "last" dismissive reply. Further numerous publications—by Ehrenwald (1942, 1944, 1950a, 1950b, 1956, 1957, 1960, 1971, 1972), Servadio (1955, 1956) in Rome, and Gillespie (1953) and Balint (1955) in London—followed, and especially Devereux's (1953) comprehensive collection of 31 key papers. This important volume, and 11 subsequent books (1959–1967) on psychoanalytic or experimental approaches to the paranormal, elicited a most critical review by Löfgren (1968). Brunswick (1957), commenting on Servadio's 1955 paper, also resisted the telepathy hypothesis, typically suggesting an alternative interpretation, which was immediately rebutted by Servadio (1957).

As of the 1970s, the subject of telepathy in the psychoanalytic context largely disappeared. It seems that a major reason was the shift in psychoanalytic thinking towards feeling-transfer and emotional influence between patient and analyst in the analytic process. It began with Paula Heimann's new communicative approach to countertransference, Racker's concepts of concordant and complementary identifications in the countertransference, and Melanie Klein's concept of projective identification, with Bion's (1959) most influential expansion of it to primary communication and containing, as the patient's unbearable experiences are projected-transferred into the analyst's psyche to be modified there. These ideas launched new understandings of patient and analyst's shared emotional experiences and their impact on each other, and became fundamental features in psychoanalytic writing. In addition, the discovery of mirror neurons in the last decade provided possible neurobiological mechanisms for understanding empathic intersubjective resonance with another's emotions, intentions and actions (Wolf et al., 2001; D. N. Stern, 2004). But none included the extreme, enigmatic telepathic phenomena whereby *information* seems to be mysteriously transferred.

Accordingly, in the issue of *Psychoanalytic Inquiry* (2001) devoted to "unconscious communication in psychoanalysis," most of the articles focused on emotional communication and the discovery of mirror neurons. Only Susan Lazar (2001) ventured to consider paranormal phenomena in a comprehensive approach to unconscious communication, and Kantrowitz (2001) related many clinical experiences of uncanny and seemingly magical communication of knowledge to the role of selective attention and preconscious communication in the analytic situation.

During this rather dormant period in the psychoanalytic discourse on telepathy, the subject was still addressed by French psychoanalysts with regard to Freud's legacy (Major and Miller, 1981; Torok, 1986; Derrida, 1988; Widlöcher, 2004). And more recently—very differently and initially not referred to as telepathy—patients' dreams of this nature have been explored by American relational psychoanalysts, as part of their interest in the patient having deep knowledge of the analyst's private life and personality (Crastnopol, 1997; Mitchell, 1988). Such dreams are also described by Symington (1996) in relation to "mimetic patients." Hanna Segal, in an interview with Jean-Michel Quinodoz in 2004, recounts experiences with two patients "which were completely incomprehensible unless it was telepathy" (Quinodoz, 2008, pp. 53–54). And in late Bion's (2005a) Italian seminars (in the sixth seminar held on 16 July 1977—Morning), one of the participants tells about a patient's "dream and the associations. . . that amounted to a perfect description of the event that made me so sad," and Bion evocatively responds to it. His words, I feel, connect powerfully with what I am trying to explore regarding patients' telepathic dreams, and perhaps also with what I am trying to convey in this book regarding the emerging new dimension of analytic process:

> Let me take refuge in the relatively reasonable explanation and say it originates in the relationship between these two people—you can see

> how *rational* that would be, how in accordance with theories of transference and countertransference and so forth. But suppose we are not satisfied with that explanation. Perhaps we should then have to extend our ideas of what is science or our knowledge of the central nervous system and our capacity for receiving information via our peripheral and central nervous system. . . . But the questions that have been raised here may mean that we have to become aware of the possibility that there are other receptor organs of which we are not aware. . . . allow ourselves to recognize *the meaning which lies beyond*. . . . You can hear what these two people say to each other, and you can be aware that you are not satisfied, that there is something that you do not know.
>
> (pp. 64–65, my italics)

At the turn of the 21st century, two American analysts—Ullman (2003) and Mayer (1996a, 1996b, 2001)—introduced extensive experimental research into dream telepathy and "anomalous" processes of information-transfer. Mayer emphasized the specific relevance of this vast research for reconsidering the fundamentally intersubjective nature of the psychoanalytic process. In addition, Mayer (2001) came upon a draft of a paper written by Robert Stoller in 1973, "Telepathic dreams?", and she edited and published it in 2001, ten years after Stoller's sudden death. Stoller had documented 18 (!) striking "telepathic dreams" of four of his psychoanalytic patients from the 1960s, and one dream of his own. But, following his supervisor Ralph Greenson's advice, he did not publish it so as not to jeopardize his career as a young and reputable psychoanalyst, and came back to it only in the years just before his death.

Recently, further telepathic phenomena are described by de Peyer (2016; discussed by me [Eshel, 2016]), and by Reiner (2017), who connected them with Ferenczi's idea of the patient's "astra" fragmentation ("astra" from the Latin word for stars), resulting from massive early trauma and emotional abuse (Ferenczi, 1932, p. 207).[5]

Few analysts apart from Stoller have reported their own telepathic dreams (Farrell, 1983; D. B. Stern, 2002; Ullman, 2003), most of which occurred within difficult, overwhelming treatment situations (Amir, 2000; Bass, 2001; Brenner, 2001), "as though [patient and analyst] were tuned into each other's 'wavelength'" (Brenner,2001, p. 191).

Explanations taken together

Let me now sum up the various explanations of telepathic phenomena in the psychoanalytic literature, especially patients' telepathic dreams during treatment. These explanations may be divided into contributory factors involving patient, patient–analyst relatedness, and analyst. Patient-related factors predominated in the earlier papers and persist to this day, with the focus on the traumatic childhood circumstances of these patients: "suffering people" whose thought-transference is caused by their "being gone" and "astra" kind of fragmentation or "astral fragment" as an extreme response to early trauma and emotional abuse (Ferenczi, 1932, pp. 32–33, 206–207; Reiner, 2017); early deprivation and pervasive separation anxiety (Róheim, 1932); massive early losses (Crastnopol, 1997; Mitchell, 1998); dissociation of severe early trauma (Brenner, 2001); fragile and vulnerable hold on reality and relationships (Ullman, 2003); deprived, narcissistic personality (Strean and Nelson, 1962); hypersensitiveness to emotional states of others (Saul, 1938; Brenner, 2001); strong unconscious wishes (Freud, 1921, 1925, 1933; Hitschmann, 1924, 1953).

From the vantage point of relatedness, telepathy is regarded as a nonverbal, archaic mode of communication between the unconsciouses of patient and analyst, which goes back to primary symbiotic mother–infant communication. In the course of evolution, it is largely replaced by the more developed verbal-symbolic methods of conveying information. But, under the heightened affective circumstances of the analytic process, especially in critical emotionally laden transference-countertransference moments, it becomes activated (Ferenczi, 1932; Freud, 1933; Burlingham, 1935; Meerloo, 1949; Gillespie, 1953; Ehrenwald, 1960, 1971; Strean and Nelson, 1962; Dupont, 1984; Kantrowitz, 2001; Segal, in Quinodoz, 2008; Ettinger, 2006b).

The analyst's role in provoking telepathic phenomena during treatment (Eisenbud, 1946, 1947; Branfman and Bunker, 1952; Balint, 1955; Servadio, 1955, 1956; Shainberg, 1976) was first introduced by Hollós (1933, cited in Eisenbud, 1946). Eisenbud (1946), using many clinical examples, further argued that the telepathic dream features not only the patient's emotionally charged repressed material, but also similar or related emotionally charged material of the analyst's as well. The telepathic dream reveals its pertinence to the analyst in a sudden, affective way. Thus, Eisenbud's patient's dream, that *she met him in Atlantic City and he was wearing a very loud sports jacket*, telepathically exposed highly charged issues of his—of purchasing a conservative jacket and not a brighter one, and regretting it afterwards; and of trying to persuade his wife to join him on a long weekend holiday in Atlantic City, which she refused, and so he dropped the entire idea.

Similarly, Servadio (1955, 1956) argued that the patient's telepathic dream "unmasks" the analyst's hard, concealed feelings towards the patient and also the analyst's own feelings. Thus, Servadio's patient's telepathic dream (1955) exposed not only the analyst's abandonment and neglect of the patient, but also the analyst's feeling of being abandoned by his wife and left to the care of servants.

Balint (1955) is the most radical with regard to the analyst's role and the "unmasking" of the analyst's "professional hypocrisy" (an expression taken from Ferenczi) in the patient's telepathic dream. He related it to an extremely tense emotional situation between analyst and patient, in which the patient is in a state of intense dependent transference, while the analyst is preoccupied at the time with matters external to the analyst–patient situation. The patient resorts to the telepathic dream, which surprises the analyst and thus returns his attention to the patient. Branfman and Bunker (1952) offered a closely related description of two patients' dreams about a "miniature Japanese woman patient" when their therapist was most preoccupied with a young female Japanese patient.

It seems to me that these same elements are also involved in Freud's example of Herr P (the omitted third case described only in Freud's 1933 paper): a patient whose long, unsuccessful, poorly paid treatment "would come to an end"—Freud had warned him—"as soon as foreign pupils and patients returned to Vienna" after years of war; and the three presumably telepathic events during the session relate to three "foreigners" of most prominent professional status and wealth—Dr David Forsyth, Dr Anton von Freund and Dr Ernest Jones—whom Freud enthusiastically met with at the time. Indeed, much suffering and intense feelings over Freud's distance were telepathically encoded there.

Finally, I would briefly add a different explanation for telepathic phenomena based on Jung's idea of "synchronicity," which arises from his notions of archetypes, the collective unconscious and *unus mundus* or "unitary world." Synchronicity means "an acausal connecting principle of meaningful coincidence:" "a coincidence in time of two or more causally unrelated events which have the same or similar meaning" (Jung, *CW* VIII, cited in Stevens, 1994). These ideas were addressed by Schwarz (1969), Spiegelman (2003), Whan (2003) and Tennes (2007). A related explanation is Carington's theory of a common subconscious in which associations formed in one mind automatically become operative in all other minds (1946, cited in Gillespie, 1953).

Having reviewed the psychoanalytic literature, I will now describe my own analytic encounter with my patients' telepathic dreams, and the understanding that has crystallized in me over the years, which found an echo and backing in this literature. This understanding combines specific factors related to the patient, archaic communication, and the analyst, as I will now describe using case material. More generally, it embodies *an extreme, enigmatic "impossible" possibility of the larger drama and mystery of patient–analyst interconnectedness, at-one-ment, and unconscious communication in the analytic process.*

Case illustration: "You alone knew how to wait/search"

Background

Effie (Efrat) came to analysis because of feeling increasingly unreal and detached from her husband, her four-year-old daughter, and her immediate environment; feelings unrelated to external circumstances. She would later add that these feelings had perhaps intensified since her daughter was about six months old.

At the beginning of analysis, Effie recounted the dramatic story of her early childhood. Both her mother and maternal grandmother were Holocaust survivors. They had fled with a neighbor's family from their home in Poland to Russia. Her mother's husband of barely a year, and her mother's father, along with the rest of the family, were due to join them a few days later, but were caught and sent to concentration camps, where they perished.

During the war, Effie's mother and grandmother survived extreme hardship, hunger and mortal terror. At the end of the war, they immigrated to Israel and attempted to rebuild their lives. Not a single relative, close or distant, had survived. Despite exhaustive efforts, they found no one who could provide additional information about what had happened to the rest of the family. They were totally alone; even the neighbor's family with whom they had escaped, had immigrated to a different country.

Effie's mother found work, and a few years later remarried and had two daughters, of which Effie was the younger. During that period, with the help of her mother who lived in close proximity, she stopped working and began studying in university.

Then, a crucial, devastating event occurred in their lives, an event about which Effie had only partial knowledge. When she was about ten months old, her mother's first husband suddenly reappeared. Effie did not know how he had found her mother, whether and how many times they had met, or whether they had only communicated by letters or phone. Apparently, they did meet. He too had remarried and had two young children, although Effie did not know who had remarried first; it seems they had remarried about the same time. He reappeared, and then disappeared forever; Effie did not know whether he lived in some distant part of Israel, or abroad. But he was never seen or heard from again. She did not know whether this had been a joint decision.

Effie's mother then withdrew and shut herself in her room. She would not respond, would not relate, refused to see anybody. Her mother (Effie's grandmother) was called upon to help out, and moved in with the family. She was a caring, devoted woman who mainly attended to meals and the family's other basic needs. Only two sounds cut through the silence in the house: the radio, which all day long and most of the night was tuned to the program *Searching for Lost Relatives*, and the song "Wait for me and I'll come back," which Effie's mother listened to over and over on the record player, alone in her closed room. Effie's father would return from work and sit on the balcony, sucking at his pipe in silence and staring out into the garden; at first, he slept in the sitting room and later the balcony was enclosed so he could sleep there.

After about ten months, Effie's mother came out of her room and switched off the record player, and the song was no longer played. She went back to university, immersed herself in her studies, made up the year she had missed, continued studying and, in time, carved out an impressive academic career in her field. Effie's grandmother, replaced by a nanny, returned to her own home, but continued to be actively involved in their lives at home. The radio continued to broadcast *Searching for Lost Relatives*, but at a reduced volume, and only when Effie's mother or grandmother were home; they both continued to listen to it anxiously.

Only once a year, every year, from the eve of Holocaust Remembrance Day to its end the following evening, would Effie's mother light a memorial candle and play the record once again in her room, and the sounds of the song "Wait for me and I'll come back," by now scratched and worn, would reverberate relentlessly throughout the house, all that night and day. The candle burned, the song played, and Effie's mother remained shut in her room, every year on that day. When Effie quoted me the words of this familiar old song, they suddenly seemed so harsh, poignant, and painful to me:

Wait for me and I'll come back!

Wait for me and I'll come back!
Just you truly wait,
Wait when Autumn's dreary rains
With darkness fill the heart.
Wait when snow is falling fast,
Wait when summer's hot,
Wait when yesterdays are past,
Others are forgot.
Wait though from that far-off place
No letters come to you.
Wait when others cease to wait,
All who waited too.

Wait for me and I'll come back! . . .
Even when my dearest ones
Say that I am lost
Even when my friends give up . . .
Wait, don't give up hope.

Wait for me and I'll come back,
Defying every death!
"What a bit of luck!" they'll say,
Those that did not wait.
They will never understand
How amidst the strife,

By your waiting for me, dear
You have saved my life.

How I made it, we shall know,
Only I and you.
You alone knew how to *search*
As no other knew.
(Konstantin Simonov,
1941)

"You alone knew how to *search* as no other knew," Effie recited the last line. "You alone knew how to *wait*,|" I corrected the word, unable now to recall if silently or out loud, and not yet knowing that she had thus conveyed to me, without my understanding, the very heart of the telepathic occurrence.

Apparently, after that year, family life in Effie's home returned to normal. They talked little of feelings—"but maybe it was also like that before the crisis," said Effie. It was only years later, in late adolescence, that Effie learned from her sister and an elderly relative on her father's side about "the hard year." It began with a comment that Holocaust Remembrance Day was so sad in their house, not just because their grandfather and the rest of the family had perished, but also because of "that man." Effie's efforts to find out more details were in vain; her sister and the elderly relative knew little. Her sister was four years older, but had been only a young child at the time. Effie had never dared ask her mother and father, and they themselves never talked about it, while her grandmother refused to speak of those "old, sad matters." "My little girl" ["*Mein kind*," she would say in Yiddish], "we went through so many terrible things, you know, thank God, we got through it all, there's no point in talking about it, leave it alone, it's over and done with, everything is fine," she would say over and over, kindly but firmly, each time Effie broached the subject, and then fall silent or change the subject.

"Everything was fine" in Effie's life too. She did well in school, went on to university, married an older man and started a family; but the feeling of meaningless in her life grew ever stronger. Her grandmother died and then her father, and she "felt nothing." "I began to feel that my fate would be like that of Hannah in *My Michael* by Amos Oz,"[6] she said. She felt that the book's opening sentences very closely related to her: "I am writing this because people I loved have died. I am writing this because when I was a child I was full of the power of loving, and now that power of loving is dying. *I do not want to die*" (Oz, 1972, p. 1, Effie's emphasis). And so, she came to analysis. She came to me because she had heard that my approach was Winnicottian.

The dream

During the first year of analysis (of four times a week, on the couch), Effie conveyed pervasive feelings of not belonging and heaviness, and particularly had difficulty talking. "Basically, I never talked. I don't really know how to talk about feelings," she said. "I know how to organize, put all sorts of things in order and then . . . a vacuum." She felt "so heavy, not understood, not belonging, not connected to anybody. Once I had such a need to belong, but I got stuck somewhere in the middle." I felt her agonizing loneliness. She was very conscientious about coming to analysis, rarely missing a session or arriving late, but feared and blocked all feelings of connection, neediness and dependence. In the sessions, I often felt that I had to hold her firmly lest she slip away through the empty spaces in her words. Yet, as the year drew to a close, a gradual, subtle shift seemed to occur in her tone of voice and intense feelings of isolation and desperateness.

The dream I describe was recounted at the beginning of the second year of analysis, on a Thursday, the third session of the week (we had no sessions on Wednesdays).

Effie began by saying she was "feeling better now." She was silent for a moment, then continued that she was "coming back" from being detached; she had had two difficult days and everyone said she had been completely detached. She fell silent, then went on. Her husband talked to her but she couldn't hear. It seemed to her that I too had been detached on Tuesday, maybe also on Monday. She was silent again. I asked her whether she thought that her being detached was related to my being detached. She said haltingly, "My body feels weightless. Floating. Not a pleasant feeling. Frightening." She was speaking with great difficulty. I said, "Effie, you were talking about my detachment and you became detached. Come back down to me and tell me what's happening." She slowly began to say that she had slept poorly the previous two nights, on Tuesday and Wednesday. Last night, she awoke very early and remembered a dream, which she then recounted. (As is my habit, I wrote the dream down as she told it, and it is presented here verbatim.)

What I remember is that I am in a different country, hurrying to the place where my father is buried, which I know is about to close at four o'clock. I manage to get there a few minutes before, go into some sort of entrance hall and from there I see that the gate I have to go through is closing. It's no longer possible to go in. I try to persuade the gatekeeper to let me in. I explain to him that I've come from a different place, far away, and I've already come in, and it's very important for me to come in because not being there, and he lets me in. And then I go into some sort of room, with a picture of my father hanging on the left, and next to it several other pictures. Like below the wall, underneath the floor, that is actually where my father is buried, it's not clear to me whether alone or with other people. I don't remember. It's as if the whole way he's buried is so different. And it's as if also in the dream I feel myself different. The entire time I'm someone else, I think. I'm not alone, I think.

She was silent and then continued, "I usually don't manage to explain how important things are for me. I don't feel good about that. I feel myself not understood. That's how it feels to me—people don't understand me, then I become very tense, and then everything gets messed up. But here I said, *'I've already come in. I've come from far away, it's very important for me to go in, let me come in', and he lets me in.*"

"And my father's picture. A beautiful picture. He's smiling. There's a feeling of longing. That's something new, this dream. Up to now my experience with dreams was that they confirm things I've already experienced in life, confirming them through a different world."

I listened in astonishment to the dream and to the things she said. She dreamed the dream on Wednesday night, and Wednesday afternoon I had attended a memorial service in the cemetery for my own father which began at four o'clock. And I had felt intense longing. I had been very attached to my father, and, around the time of the memorial service this year, due to certain family issues, I had especially missed him. I am certain that Effie had no way of knowing where I had been that day. I also realized that I had indeed been detached on the Tuesday, and perhaps also on Monday, without being aware of it.

What encounter with me was Effie struggling for beyond the disconnection, beyond the closed gate, in spite of death and deadness? It was as if she had entered my mind, had been in a place and time I had been in, inside the longing I had felt. *"I've come from a different place, far away, and I've already come in, and it's very important for me to come in because not being there,"* she had said to the gatekeeper, and he let her in. Who was it that was "not there"—her, me? The old deep scar of absence had suddenly reopened, speaking, pleading.

I deliberated whether to tell her all this; I asked questions about the dream and more was said, mostly about her parents', especially her father's years-long emotional distance from her world. Finally, about 10 minutes before the end of the session, I decided to tell her, since so much had not been told to her in her life and had not been talked about with her. I said, "You know, Effie, yesterday I was really in the cemetery for my father's memorial service, at four in the afternoon. And maybe this affected my being detached and your being detached and your dream."

She remained silent until the end of the session and then said, "It is amazing and frightening how much things that happen to you affect me. Do you understand the enormousness of your responsibility?"

"In a forest of frost, in a dawn of cornflowers": the telepathic dream between absence and loss

> O my God, what am I
> That these late mouths should cry open
> In a forest of frost, in a dawn of cornflowers.
> (Sylvia Plath, "Poppies in October," 1962)

In three decades of clinical work, I encountered another four telepathic dreams, aside from Effie's. These five dreams were sporadic occurrences over the years (in the order described below). Yet they always appeared at emotionally charged, significant points in *my* life, and involved the precise details of time, place, sensory impressions, and experiential states that I was in at that time—dumbfounding informational details, not merely experiential-emotional details—that the patients could not have known through ordinary sensory perception and communication. All were connected to matters of life and death in my (the analyst's) world: a young female patient's dream in which *I was telling her that I was pregnant*, which she dreamed on the very day I found out that I was pregnant (with my eldest daughter); a dream of a male patient who "knew" I had miscarried (a different pregnancy) when I cancelled the sessions on those days;

Effie's dream on the night of the memorial service for my father, which was where I was at—in place, hour, and emotional state—on the same day; a detailed cemetery dream by a male patient during the week that both my in-laws died within two days of each other; and a dream about a dying woman that a female patient dreamed three days before my mother's death—during a period when I would leave her deathbed to carry on my analytic work—which depicted very specific details of the situation with my mother on those days, with dumbfounding precision.

All the telepathic elements were unique to these particular dreams, and did not recur in these patients' other dreams (see also Stoller, in Mayer, 2001; Ullman, 2003). The first patient was in psychotherapy, and the other four in analysis; the latter dreams were equally divided between men and women.

In my effort to unravel and understand these enigmatic, abstruse phenomena, a specific set of experiences took on primary importance. Each of these patients, during *early childhood* (aged a few months to almost two years), had *a mother who was absent-within-absence*, that is, a mother physically present yet emotionally absent from her child's early life due to the absence of a significant figure in her own life. In each case, it was the absence of the husband-father (except for Effie's special story)—one case due to sudden death, and the others due to a temporary, but prolonged (over six months) absence of the husband-father. In most of the cases, the mother's experiences of absence and separation were intensified by an earlier absence of one or both of her parents (due to the Holocaust, lengthy separation, or death).

Thus, the silenced cry of this abrupt and critical early catastrophe resides in a world of primal attachment, in a non-verbal or pre-verbal period, with an ensuing fixation on an archaic, symbiotic mode of communication, prior to the formation of boundaries of self and other.

Winnicott, in a memorable passage, describes the formation of x + y + z deprivation:

> The feeling of the mother's existence lasts x minutes. If the mother is away more than x minutes . . . the baby is distressed, but this distress is soon mended because the mother returns in x + y minutes. In x + y minutes the baby has not become altered. But in x + y + z minutes the baby has become traumatized. In x + y + z minutes the mother's return does not mend the baby's altered state. Trauma implies that the baby has experienced a break in life's continuity, so that primitive defences

> now become organized to defend against a repetition of 'unthinkable anxiety' or a return of the acute confusional state that belongs to disintegration of nascent ego structure.
>
> We must assume that the vast majority of babies never experience the x + y + z quantity of deprivation. This means that the majority of children do not carry around with them for life the knowledge from experience of having been mad. Madness here simply means a break-up of whatever may exist at the time of a personal continuity of existence. After 'recovery' from x + y + z deprivation the baby has to start again permanently deprived of the root which would provide continuity with the personal beginning.
>
> (1971a, pp. 114–115)

Does the mother who is absent-within-absence create x + y + z degree of deprivation/absence, or is this even a case of *double absence*—z^2—which is imprinted in the nascent self and in inchoate relating to others?

It is interesting that McLuhan expresses similar thoughts with regard to communication: "In any medium or structure there is a break boundary at which the system suddenly changes into another or passes some point of no return in its dynamic processes. . . . [here] the boundary break had been passed" (1994, pp. 38, 40).

Unlike Balint, who relates telepathic dreams to a patient "in a state of intense positive dependent transference, which however was not fully appreciated and understood by the analyst" (1955, p. 32), I have found that these patients, because of their early traumatic history, defend themselves against any strong and endangering feelings of dependence and becoming attached. Thus, in the treatment process, they struggle to block dependence, and will not allow themselves (and the analyst) to feel their deep regressive yearning for the analyst, except in a buried, hidden way. This abruptly changes when, within this intricate situation, the analyst suddenly becomes emotionally (and sometimes also physically) absent because his or her attention is significantly diverted to other matters, often to absence in the analyst's own world. Under such circumstances, the patient's dread of reliving the deeply traumatic absence, the breaking of personal continuity of existence, now bursts forth—never, never again to return to such devastating absence and abandonment, to that maddening z^2 and the unbearable loss of the early mother.

The telepathic dream is created in *the gap between absence and loss*, between separation and all-out complete absence; it forms a search engine to seek and find the analyst, in order to halt the process of abandonment and prevent a return and collapse into the depths of despair of the early traumatization.

Indeed, if tele-pathy is "suffering at a distance (Greek: *pathos* + *tele*)," the *suffering because of distance, suffering over distance* achieves its critical potential here. The telepathic dream ushers us into the very heart of pathos—the suffering, the intense feeling; the patient's pathos, the analyst's pathos. For whose pathos is it? Whose dream? The dreaming patient clings to the analyst *beyond the boundaries of separateness, separation, time, space, and known processes of sensory perception* in a way that is hitherto not scientifically explicable, yet it occurs. The patient manages to enter the analyst's mind and the analyst's private affairs, experiences, absence—but not fully; that is, in a necessary, uncanny way, to telepathically perceive the most prominent physical and emotionally charged details, which the ordinary senses fail to provide. Yet not fully.

"The gate . . . is closing. It's no longer possible to go in. I try to persuade the gatekeeper to let me in." said Effie in her dream. Only on re-reading these dream words lately, I realized with astonishment how similar they are to the deeply pleading words and the sense of urgency that imbues the final prayer of the Holy Day of Atonement [at-one-ment], the prayer which forms the emotional climax of the pleas that resonate throughout the day—"*Open the gate for us at this time when the gate closes, for the day is fading away*" (Neilah—*The Closing of the Gate*).

"*I have come from a different place, far away, and I've already come in, and it is very important for me to come in because not being there. And the gatekeeper lets me in*," Effie continued in her dream. On those particular days, she detached herself from her world and reached me, while I was in a different, emotionally laden, distant place. "*And it's as if in the dream I feel myself different. The entire time I'm someone else, I think. I'm not alone, I think*" [verbatim].

It can be said that the telepathic dream actualizes the possibility of primary, unmediated patient–analyst interconnectedness or analytic oneness, revealing its power and radical quality:

> Telepathy [is not] an actual transmission of sensory perceptions or of cognitive material from one person to another . . . . We must assume that every telepathic incident involves the temporary fusion of two emotionally linked individuals into one functional unit, re-establishing for a fleeting moment the original mother-child unit as it existed at an early developmental stage.
>
> (Ehrenwald, 1960, p. 53)

At the same time, it implies, in its very name and quality, the ultimately irreducible, irremediable distance between two people.

Ruth's cleaving to Naomi comes to mind to describe the powerful kind of connection embodied-encoded in the telepathic dream. "For wither thou goest, I will go; and where thou lodgest, I will lodge" (Ruth, 1:16). Under the shadow of great loss, Ruth "clave on to" Naomi, her mother-in-law, as she leaves Moab, adamantly following her, refusing any separation or separateness, detaching herself from her own world, crossing boundaries, allowing no room for any further loss.

"A man's reach must exceed his grasp, or what's a metaphor" is McLuhan's (1994, p. 57) paraphrase of Robert Browning's "Oh that a man's reach should exceed his grasp, or what's a heaven for?" In the telepathic dream, the patient's reach exceeds his or her personal boundaries, turns into a paranormal mode of seeking and receiving information, and reaches-grips-holds on to the analyst—"a psychic prothesis, a stretched-out arm, which reaches out mystically towards that which is far off and cannot be approached in actuality by physical means" (Hitschmann, 1924, p. 438).

Indeed, the telepathic dream breaks through the absence and brings the analyst back to the patient, even when it does not make the analyst poignantly aware of his or her emotional absence and the patient's suffering, as Balint (1955) emphatically maintains. And, at its best, the telepathic dream creates *a moment of bare connectedness* of patient and analyst (one with the other and within oneself), thus creating a new observation, a new understanding, a *new possibility*.

Should the analyst—the only one who knows about the telepathic occurrence—tell the patient about it? Opinions are divided on such issues as clinical caution, the analyst's anonymity versus disclosure, and the authenticity of patient–analyst dialog. Thus, Ehrenwald cautioned analysts not to tell patients until a later stage of analysis, when they would be capable of dealing with the burden of such involvement, while that same year Eisenbud maintained that, when analysts are careful, gentle, and wise in their handling of telepathic experiences, they can bring about most helpful and meaningful results. Considering these different approaches, Shainberg (1976) writes of his fear that his patient might be scared by the realization of the extent of his involvement with his analyst, and chose to avoid risk by not telling the patient. Conversely, Mayer (2001) is resolute about the importance of expanding the ability of patient and analyst alike to examine *all* aspects of what the patient knows about the analyst within the analytic intersubjective relationship, including anomalous telepathic knowledge. She sees this as important both in terms of the psychoanalytic situation and clinical psychoanalytic thinking.

Undoubtedly, this is a sensitive, daring, self-revealing moment, which, at times, is no less difficult and delicate for the analyst than it is for the patient. But I feel that it is a meaningful, authentic and unique (intrapsychic and intersubjective) moment, which allows analyst and patient a different kind of exchange—groping and evolving—while facing their intense and enigmatic unconscious interconnection that has now been exposed. It is a powerful connecting moment that both comes into being and is deepened by this exchange. As Derrida writes so evocatively,

> You say "It was me," with a gentle and terrible decision . . . You say "me" the unique addressee and everything starts between us. Starting out from nothing, from no history . . . (committing yourself to it even for eternity) . . . you gather it together without reducing it, without harming it, you let it live and everything starts between us, from you, and what you there give by receiving. Others would conclude: a letter thus finds its addressee, him or her. No, one cannot say of the addressee that s/he exists before the letter['s arrival].
>
> (1988, p. 6)

In concluding, I find that this account did not take me into the domain of occultism, but rather into *the occult of psychoanalysis and the psychoanalytic process*. It ushered me into the heart of the unfathomable *depth, intensity and mystery* of the human psyche and its struggle to survive traumatization and retraumatization, and particularly of patient–analyst deep unconscious interconnectedness in the psychoanalytic situation and its "impossible" extremes, defying space, time and personal boundaries.

Notes

1 The principle known as Occam's razor states, "No more entities should be presumed to exist than are absolutely necessary."

2 Widlöcher (2004) similarly points out with regard to psychoanalytic co-thinking and regression, that "This process [psychoanalytic co-thinking] is more active when, due to regression, the interpersonal interaction between both parties is reduced to a minimum" (pp. 205–206).

3 The term "serendipity" was coined in 1754 by Horace Walpole after an Oriental (Indian or Persian) tale about the "Three Princes of Serendip" (ancient Ceylon) who embarked on a long journey, and made unexpected discoveries by accident, observation and wisdom.

4 According to Torok (1986), Herr P is Sergei Pankeiev, Freud's "Wolf Man."

5 Ferenczi's "astra" is essentially a dissociated state, in which a part of the child's personality leaves his traumatic, painful, emotionally deprived earthly existence and becomes an all-knowing, omniscient "astral" part, "far off in the distance like a star," thereby "being receptive to processes beyond sensory perceptions (clairvoyance, . . . suggestion from a distance)." The pain, as Ferenczi put it, is "displaced to infinite distances" (Ferenczi, 1932, pp. 81, 206–207).

6 *My Michael* by Amos Oz tells of 30-year-old Hannah's growing withdrawal from her husband Michael and her young child, into a private, disconnected fantasy world.

Chapter 7

Pentheus rather than Oedipus

On perversion, survival, and analytic "presencing"

"I have a feeling we're not in Kansas anymore," said Dorothy to Toto.
(L, .Frank Baum, *The Wonderful Wizard of Oz,* 1900)

Contextualizing perversion in psychoanalytic thinking—drive, object-relations, selfobject

The psychoanalytic understanding of perversion[1] has come a long way over the last hundred years, beginning with Freud's early writing (1905) on the subject. I will try to briefly outline its theoretical landmarks and changes over the years, before moving on to my own approach. The understanding of perversion in psychoanalytic thinking may be divided into two major frameworks: the drive model and the object-relations model (Pajaczkowska, 2000; Harding, 2001).

I.

The first framework, historically, is Freud's classical drive model and its vicissitudes. Initially, Freud understood perversion from the economic point of view as a primary fixation of libido at pre-oedipal levels. In "Three essays on the theory of sexuality" (1905), he connects and contrasts neuroses and perversions as the positive and negative sides of one and the same process—the developmental process of infantile sexuality. "*Neuroses are, so to say, the negative of perversions,*" is his famous assertion (p. 165). To Freud, perversions represent unmodified, non-repressed infantile sexuality, whereas its modification through unsuccessful repression gives rise to neuroses. Thus, in perversions, infantile sexuality persists into adult life in the same polymorphous infantile form as in childhood, at the expense of adult genitality.

Several years later (in the context of a growing interest in the ego), Freud began to recognize that perversions may serve as defensive formulations, especially against an Oedipus complex and castration anxiety, rather than simply as pieces of infantile sexuality that had evaded repression. He expresses this explicitly in his essay, "A child is being beaten" (Freud, 1919a). But in neurosis, the repressed phantasy breaks through only as an ego-dystonic symptom, whereas in perversion it remains capable of consciousness, being ego-syntonic and pleasurable (Gillespie, 1995).

In his later writings, especially in "Fetishism" (Freud, 1927) and in his important unfinished essay "Splitting of the ego in the process of defence" (Freud, 1938), Freud postulates other defenses in perversion: the "disavowal" of reality resulting in a "splitting" of the ego. These mechanisms bear significant resemblance to those found in psychoses. Yet, throughout his writing, Freud's theory of sexuality and perversion remains a drive theory, focusing on the Oedipus complex and castration anxiety. "It [the fetish] remains a token of triumph over the threat of castration and protection against it" (Freud, 1927, p. 154).

II.

Toward and during the second half of the twentieth century, a radically new way of understanding perversion evolved by way of attachment and object-relations theories. Rather than emphasizing endogenous drives, this perspective focuses on disturbed early mother–child relations, the mother's pathogenic role, and pathological ego or self-development. Here, perversion is regarded as a primary defense against intolerable, primitive, infantile anxieties and traumas, and a self-induced survival solution to preserve a precarious, crumbling ego or self. This emphasis on primitive, psychotic anxieties rather than on neurotic oedipal and castration anxieties brings perversion closer to psychoses. (As early as 1933, Glover writes that certain perversions have to be regarded as the negative not so much of neuroses but of psychoses, as they help to patch over flaws in the development of reality sense.) This "relocation" of perversion in early disturbed attachment or object-relations greatly affected psychoanalytic thinking, especially in Britain, the U.S., and France, as I shall now briefly review.

In Hungary, Imre Hermann (1936/1976) was the first psychoanalyst to relate sado-masochistic phenomena to traumas in early dependency and the primal desire to cling to the mother's body. In Britain, Khan (1979) emphasizes a specific disturbed early mother–child relationship in all perversions due to the mother's narcissistic idolization of the infant-child as her "created-object" (or "created-thing"), followed by her abrupt withdrawal—perversion being the ego attempt at a self-reparative solution. Glasser (1986) postulates the "core complex," established in the pervert's early infancy, because the longing for complete merging with the object carries with it a threat of annihilation, as the mother was felt to be dangerously engulfing, intrusive, or depriving; the perverse solution thus engages the object in an intense relationship, but sado-masochistically controls annihilating merging and intimacy. More recently, Welldon (1998, 2002) places the emphasis in sado-masochistic perversions on early experiences with a mother who uses her infant to gratify her own primitive needs and fantasies of power.

In American psychoanalysis, most notable are the extensive contributions (with detailed case studies) of Stoller and Socarides. Stoller (1974, 1975, 1991) defines all perversions as "the erotic form of hatred," which convert infantile and early-childhood traumas, especially attacks on the child's gender identity, into adult triumph, and are thereby characterized by hostility, revenge, risk-taking and a dehumanized sex object. Socarides (1959, 1974), drawing on Mahler's concepts, focuses in all perversions on a basic pre-oedipal nuclear desire for and dread of merging with a demonified mother in order to reinstate the primitive mother–child unity, which result from a pre-oedipal failure to pass successfully through the "undifferentiated" symbiotic and separation-individuation phase of early childhood. Perversions ensure ego survival in various perverse practices. Alternating or combining perversions may indicate a greater tendency to avert psychotic breakdown.

Later on, Ogden (1997) describes a form of perversion that derives from a core experience of psychic deadness—as the patient is unconsciously a stillborn infant, born from empty, lifeless parental intercourse. The perversion represents the patient's endless, futile effort to use sexual excitement as a substitute for infusing with life the parental core emptiness, lifelessness, lies and depression that are the source of the patient's inner life. The analysis of perversion fundamentally involves entering into the perverse scene that is being created in the transference-countertransference—namely, in the perversion of analytic intersubjectivity itself.

In France, several different parallel lines of theoretical development extend and shift the understanding of perversions from the area of castration anxieties to the pre-oedipal pathogenic mother and traumatic early experiences. McDougall (1995) writes about "sexual deviation and psychic survival," arguing that besides castration anxieties, sexual deviations are desperate attempts to master anxieties of a much earlier phase, when separation from the mother arouses the terror of bodily disintegration, annihilation, and a sense of inner death. Several French theories of perversion develop around M. de M'Uzan's case of masochistic perversion (which I describe later), primarily because his description of erotogenic masochism disagrees with essential points in Freud's 1924 essay on masochism. De M'Uzan, himself, in his 1973 paper, and particularly in a theoretical paper eleven years later (1984, in English 2003; Simpson, 2003), focuses on excessive quantity of excitation related to fatal irrevocable traumatic situations early in life. Laplanche (1999) shifts from Freud's biologistic endogenous drive theory to primal seduction, which affirms the priority of the other, not the Lacanian Other, but the concrete other—the adult facing the child, introducing "a message to be translated." Anzieu (1989) regards perverse masochism from his notion of "The Skin Ego," as signifying the tearing away and the re-establishment of the infant's shared skin (the symbiotic union) with the mother.

III.

Another important change in the understanding of perversion took place with the development of American Self psychology, and its emphasis on the relation between the self and its selfobject—the primary psychological unit—in the child's early life. For Kohut (1972, 1977) most perversions are desperate attempts to repair the disintegrating self by means of perverse fantasies and activities, as a result of a protracted, traumatic relation with a non-emphatically responding selfobject parent. "The deepest analysis of . . . [perverse] manifestations does not, however, lead to a bedrock of drives, but to narcissistic injury and depression" (Kohut, 1977, p. 173). His followers, particularly Stolorow (1975a, 1975b, 1994) and Goldberg (1975, 1999), further explore the important narcissistic function of perversion, viewing it as an abortive, primitively sexualized attempt to restore and maintain the cohesiveness and stability of a precarious, crumbling self, or to defend against dreaded object situations and affects during the early pre-oedipal era.

Not in Oedipus anymore: perversion—autotomy and survival

Having surveyed the main existing psychoanalytical perspectives on perversion, I would now like to focus on my own psychoanalytic search for understanding perversion and its treatment. (In terms of the theoretical background, my thoughts and ideas belong to the model of disturbed early-childhood relations.)

The following discussion is based on cases of sexual perversion that I have treated over the years—severe cases that, to my mind, do not fall within the debate over whether they are a perversion or a "variance" (Stoller, 1974), or whether "perversion is us" (Dimen, 1997; Stein, 2003). Nor will I be referring to patients whose perversity is expressed only in fantasy, in transference perversion, or in character perversion. The following are cases of actually acted, intense perversions (mostly masochistic) of patients who have undergone years-long psychoanalytic treatment (analysis or intensive psychoanalytic psychotherapy) with me. Their perversions were not first disclosed in the course of the treatment, as usually reported in the literature, but they came to treatment because of those very perversions. These patients actually belong to the type of perverts about whom Laplanche, de M'Uzan, and many other psychoanalysts write: "Doubtless, these patients [erotogenic masochists]—like most perverts—hardly ever consulted the psychoanalyst" (Laplanche, 1999, p. 201), and about whom Stoller adds: "Analysts dislike and fear perversion . . . I have never analyzed an erotically perverse sadomasochist" (1991, p. 53, 4). Yet, the patients presented here are perverts who did come, who stayed, and who underwent a long psychoanalytic treatment with me.

Although it is beyond the scope of this chapter to give a lengthy, detailed description of these treatments, I will nevertheless briefly describe the patients in order to specify the perversions which form the basis of the following discussion.[2] The first patient was a 30-year-old pedophile who underwent intensive psychoanalytic psychotherapy (face-to-face, four times a week) in a psychiatric hospital, following a court order—a coerced treatment, which, after his release three years later, became a voluntary treatment lasting about ten years (chapter 5 in this book). I think that, without this first, most significant, treatment experience with a perverse patient, the rest would not have followed.

The second patient was a young woman who could only have sexual relations with her partner via a blend of fantasies and acts of violence against herself. These practices increasingly escalated, at her own demand, until her partner became fed up with "these disgusting games," as he called them, and told her that, as much as he loved her, he was no longer willing to continue the relationship. After he left her, she went through a long period of loneliness and despair, during which she vacillated between wanting to ask him to come back and attempt to relinquish her violent practices versus thinking that he may have simply grown tired of her and had found an excuse to leave her. But she knew deeply, piercingly, that she was unable to desire or have any sexual relationship with him or with anyone else without that preliminary violence. She attempted suicide. Upon returning home from the hospital, she saw a British film about a girl whose boyfriend also refused to continue a sado-masochistic relationship because of his love for her. This made her think that there may in fact have been love along with trepidation on the part of her own partner, not just rejection, and she decided to seek treatment. She came to me with the request "to put the demon back in the bottle" and turn the practices of violence into mere fantasies so as not to find it necessary to actually enact them—to "let them exist locked up inside." When this indeed happened and the perverse activities ceased three years into the treatment, she asked to continue treatment (analysis four times a week, on the couch) in order to release herself from the grip of the unrelenting, violent fantasies.

The third and the most recent patient (P.), a man in his late thirties, was referred to me by a psychiatrist who had treated him with medication. The psychiatrist told me that his severe sexual perversion had intensified over the last few years to the point of becoming life-threatening. In the year before he came to her for treatment, he had approached several sex therapists who were all so alarmed by the severity of his disturbance that they would not agree to treat him. When he turned to her, she prescribed medication for compulsive disorders, in an attempt to minimize the compulsive nature of his perverse behavior. However, this was unsuccessful and produced harsh physical side-effects, some of which she found rather puzzling. She therefore stopped the medication and told him that, in her opinion, the only treatment which might help him would be psychoanalysis since it is the most profound form of treatment. It should be mentioned that this man had previously never had anything to do with psychology or psychoanalysis, and I do not believe that he had even heard of the word "psychoanalysis" before. His agreeing to her proposal was thus an indication of his despair and hopelessness. After several unsuccessful attempts at finding him a psychoanalyst, she approached me, knowing I take difficult analytic cases. She seemed hesitant to specify the nature and extent of his perverse behavior, lest I, too, would refuse to treat him. However, at the time, I had been crystallizing my thoughts about extending the reach of therapeutic work through the depth and intensity of psychoanalysis, and about analysis as *a unique process of becoming*—drawing on the powerful notions of "a new opportunity for development" (Winnicott, 1954a), "a new beginning [in] the basic fault" (Balint, 1968) and "an area of faith" (Eigen, 1981). If so, I thought, psychoanalysis should be able to offer a veritable treatment option for this person's distress, and I agreed to accept him for analysis.

P. telephoned me the same day. During the first session, he told me that his severe sexual perversion had started as a shoe fetish of licking and kissing shoes "that have a woman's feet inside," along with a masochistic element of wanting them to tread on his fingers, a wish which he recalled having had since kindergarten. It escalated over the years into a masochistic fetish as the "shoe turned into a tool of destruction," and in the past few years had become a particularly severe and violent masochistic perversion. Over the first months of analysis, he gradually presented me with extremely harsh descriptions, told matter-of-factly, of how he frequented prostitutes almost every night, usually a different one each time, to be humiliated and abused by them in increasingly extreme ways with all sorts of torture instruments. He would lie there naked, sometimes he would wear a mask, masturbating until he ejaculated, and would leave the place beaten, trodden upon, wounded, bleeding, and burned by cigarettes that had been put out by the shoes grinding them into his naked body, already yearning for the next abuse. He sought treatment because he knew that, in his own words, "If it goes on like this, it will end in hospital—in a serious injury or in death."

After a few months of analysis (of four times a week, on the couch), when he realized that I would not "throw him out of treatment because of what he told me," he said, "This is the last stop for me. Psychoanalysis. After that—it's the cemetery." Since then he has been clinging to treatment despite some very difficult periods which we have gone through.

In his "ordinary" life, he was a drab accountant in a non-sexual marriage to a woman he knew from work, an accountant like himself, whom he told nothing about his perversion—"a crazy, wild discrepancy" was how he described his split reality in the second year of analysis, as he started thinking about his perverse activities rather than just performing them.

Even more than the previous two cases, perhaps because they did involve sexual relationships, this analysis flooded me with feelings of incomprehension. How can one understand the desire for and the addictive submission to such abuse, to such a violent web of humiliation and physical injury—of a human being? In fact, of any living creature?

It is interesting to note that Freud, too, opens his essay "The economic problem of masochism" (1924) with the incomprehensible, mysterious nature of masochism:

> The existence of a masochistic trend in the instinctual life of human beings may justly be described as *mysterious* from the economic point of view. For if mental processes are governed by the pleasure principle in such a way that their first aim is the avoidance of unpleasure and the obtaining of pleasure, masochism is *incomprehensible*. If pain and unpleasure can be not simply warnings but actually aims, the pleasure principle is paralyzed—it is as though the watchman over our mental life were put out of action by a drug.
>
> Thus masochism appears to us in the light of a *great danger*, which is in no way true of its counterpart, sadism. We are tempted to call the pleasure principle the watchman over our life rather than merely over our mental life.
>
> (p. 159, my italics)

I recall that at the beginning of this analysis, and also later on, I read anything written about severe masochism in an attempt to understand it, make some sense of it. However, nothing I read felt truly relevant or provided me with an unmediated understanding, except for the expression, "the desire for ritualized trauma," coined by Benyamini and Zivoni (2002). Even Ghent's compelling paper, "Masochism, submission, surrender: Masochism as a perversion of surrender" (1990), which views masochism as a perversion of the deep-seated human need for surrender, did not lend meaning to the violent, harsh masochism, described by my patient. Thus, I realized that I would be able to find a tangible, *unmediated understanding* only within and through the treatment itself.

In order to explain my understanding of severe perversion formation, as it evolved within me through the analytic experience with these patients, I will draw on a term from the field of biology—*autotomy*, and introduce a moving poem about it by the Polish poet Wislawa Szymborska (1983). *Autotomy* is a biological term that designates the capacity of some living creatures to waive the wholeness of their body as a means of survival. They divide themselves, in times of great danger, into two disconnected parts—one that is left behind to be devoured by their predator, and another that thus succeeds in escaping and surviving, later regenerating from the part that escapes. The gecko, for instance, saves itself by releasing its tail and leaving it twitching behind for its predator, and the holothurian (sea cucumber) splits itself in two, as described in Szymborska's poem, in words which I find so very accurate and captivating:

Autotomy

In danger the holothurian splits itself in two:
it offers one self to be devoured by the world
and in its second self escapes.

Violently it divides itself into a doom and a salvation
. . . into what was and what will be.

In the middle of the holothurian's body a chasm opens
and its edges immediately become alien to each other.

On the one edge, death, on the other, life.
Here despair, there, hope . . .

To die as much as necessary, without overstepping the bounds.
To grow again from a salvaged remnant.

We, too, know how to split ourselves
but only into the flesh and a broken whisper . . .

Here a heavy heart, there *non omnis moriar*,
three little words only, like three little plumes ascending . . .
(Wislawa Szymborska (1983), translated by
Czeslaw Milosz)

Non omnis moriar (Latin)—Not all of me shall die! Through these words I would like to describe *the perverse solution as profound, massive splitting and dissociation in the service of survival and the preservation of psychic existence*, albeit in a more difficult, complex manner than the holothurian.

A child needs and wants to be loved, protected and admired by its parents. It is my view that at the root of severe forms of perversion lie primary desperate attempts in early childhood to overcome the intrusion of brutal situations, of unbearable psychic or psycho-physical violence and abuse, which could be neither endured nor escaped. In such situations of traumatic destructiveness, the infant-child has to split, dissociate, and remove from within itself the sensations of violence, pain, dread, and annihilation since the significant other on whom it *depends* introduces terror or reacts to him with indifferent, sadistic imperviousness rather than providing protection, holding, containment, and belief in the possibility of repairing these violent situations.

Thus, an *autotomous solution* comes into being—of massive dissociative splitting into two disconnected parts, alien to each other, as a means of psychic survival. One part—the second self that escaped—continues functioning in the world, surviving by inertia, emotionally impaired, lacking and dull, lifeless and alienated from the inner core of its experiences. At times, it seems as if only a husk remains—"That's all there is," says my masochistic patient dryly of his daily life. At times, materialistic success or intellectual functioning somewhat compensates for the splitting and the dissociation from the emotional parts that were left behind to be devoured—"To grow again from a salvaged remnant," in Szymborska's words.

The other part—the one self that was offered to be devoured—is stuck in that devouring state, suicidally attracted to whatever wounds and preys, to whatever embodies and actualizes (at times to the point of total actualization) the dark violence, the devastation, devourment, sadism, and imperviousness—within the psyche and in self–other relations.

Actualizing and not actualizing—the most intense experiences and sensations are invoked here by the attempt to convert an unbearable traumatization that occurred in the past into an exciting perverse scene that takes place in the present. It thus becomes a perverse ritual—frozen, repetitive and violent—an anticipated, self-induced, and stage-managed pain that focuses on the body (rather than the psyche), and therefore offers no real solution, no relief, no cure.

It is a compulsive repetition, an addictive desire for a ritualized trauma, that continually enacts the intrusion of dread, violence, and humiliation—in an effort to gain control over the trauma, to produce it, to appropriate it, to overcome it, and deep down to even yearn to repair it—anything but to leave it as an unbearable, uncontrollable trauma. Thus, the perverse act seizes and clutches, preventing in its corporeality, in its actuality and intensity, a collapse into dread, psychic deadness, and total internal annihilation. Perversion is the pervert's last-ditch attempt to halt the fall into the abyss.

"Physical pain is better than spiritual death," says the patient who repeatedly asks her therapist to hit her, in Stolorow, Atwood and Brantchaft's (1994) article on masochism. My fetishistic-masochistic patient would repeatedly say in the first year of analysis: "It sustains you more than anything else. You won't let anyone or anything take it away from you. If you give it up, it will be unbearable, since there won't be anything else."

Stoller (1975) suggests that perversions may be a defense against psychotic depression, and Louise Kaplan (1993) states:

> What distinguishes perversion is its quality of desperation and fixity. A perversion is performed by a person who has no other choices, a person who would otherwise be overwhelmed by anxieties or depression or psychosis . . . to prevail over these otherwise devastating emotional states. Therefore, the kinky sex . . . is actually an appeasement of personal demons . . . more a trial of survival than a quest for [sexual] pleasure.
>
> (pp. 10, 12)

And, more specifically, Freud, in "Fetishism" (1927), maintains that

> . . . when the fetish is instituted, some process occurs which reminds one of the stopping of memory in traumatic amnesia. As in this latter case, it is as though the last impression before the uncanny and traumatic one *is retained as a fetish.*
>
> (p. 155, my italics)

I am reminded in this context of a story by Jules Verne in which the murderer is discovered because the homicidal incident was frozen in the second just preceding death on the victim's retina, thus becoming the pre-and-post-death moment. The dead eyes register the deadly encounter in a way that the living cannot. In the same way, severe perversion registers and freezes a hemorrhaging traumatic core experience of self-with-significant-other. The perversion embodies the *specific experiential-emotional key quality of the traumatic situation*, and stops at the near-hit, the last impression before reaching the full intensity of dread, annihilation and psychic deadness—*making present the imprint of the past destructive experience*, over and over again, concretely, unremittingly. The perverse scenario exposes the horrors of the dissociated, either as doer or done to. But perversion enables an externalization and a return under the perverse guise to the site of devourment and to an extremely bad object (bad either in its way of relating or not relating), while it sanitizes and obscures the horror, the alarm or the betrayal, the longing for what might have been different, the loss and destruction—the annihilation of life and hope. The attacked, ruptured subject becomes a split object, dissociated from the memory of a past traumatic horror, and perverse—not all of me shall die!

I am linking this to Winnicott's (1974) "Fear of Breakdown," which describes even the most psychotic illness syndromes as a massive *defense organization* against breakdown and unthinkable primitive agonies that have already happened, but since they were so unbearable and dreadful, the patient could not experience them and therefore cannot remember them. Thus, the patient must go on fearing it and compulsively looking for it in the future. The breakdown that has no experiential existence in memory haunts, clutches, and insists on actual realization.

In much the same manner, I regard *perversion, too, as a defense organization—through splitting, externalization, and compulsive sexualization—against a violent, devastating, unbearable, deadening early past situation*. "Desire is the opposite of death," says Blanche when she explains her deviant sexual behavior in Tennessee Williams's (1947) *A Streetcar Named Desire*. Winnicott, in his early essay "The Manic Defence" (1935), writes: "Here the key words are dead and alive" (p. 134). Thus, it can be said that the key quality of perversion is not a sexualized manic "disavowal of castration," but the "disavowal of annihilating destruction."

In my view, the world of severe perversion "is not oedipal anymore." In Greek tragedy, there are three renowned sons whose fates are very different from each other (Verhaeghe, 1999): at the one extreme is (Aeschylus's) Orestes, who murdered his mother, Clytemnestra, to avenge the murder of his father, Agamemnon, and yet is judged to be innocent and escapes the revenge of the Furies, who then become the Eumenides. In the middle is (Sophocles's) Oedipus, who is unable to escape his fate, discovers that he killed his father and slept with his mother, and therefore blinds himself and goes into exile. And at the other extreme, the most tragic and gruesome, is Pentheus, in Euripides's last play, *The Bacchae*, which, like the story of Oedipus, takes place in Thebes. King Pentheus, disguised as a woman, attempts a peek at the Bacchantes' revelry headed by his mother, Agave, and her sisters. He is exposed and caught. Despite his pleas, he is torn to pieces and devoured alive by his mother who in her frenzy sees him as a wild beast, and by the mad devouring Bacchantes or Maenads who savagely celebrate the rite of Bacchus (or Dionysus)—himself a God who dies and is resurrected each year; it is a rite whereby any male creature that passes by is devoured.

Rather than an oedipal world, severe perversion is rooted in the world of *Pentheus*, which has its beginnings in transvestism and voyeurism, continues on to exhibitionism, and goes as far as sado-masochistic violence and cannibalistic murder. It is a world ruled by a mixture of a mother's madness and devourment,[3] derangement, and orgiastic intoxication, and the combination of rituals of desire with destruction and death.

Is perversion treatable?

I will now address the difficult question of the psychoanalytic treatment of perversion and the possibility of change. In presenting my approach, my point of departure will be, rather radically and paradoxically, the famous case of masochistic perversion described by the French psychoanalyst de M'Uzan (1973), who emphasizes the very early, irremediable fatedness of severe perversion.

De M'Uzan's case of masochistic perversion

De M'Uzan (1973) describes a profoundly perverse masochist, Monsieur M. He met him not in treatment but in two consultations, following referral by a radiologist who, during a medical examination, noticed indications of the patient's perverse practices. M. accepted the radiologist's referral without reservation. Yet, writes de M'Uzan, although a case of erotogenic [enacted] masochism—unlike moral masochism, or so-called feminine masochism [in fantasy]—is rarely seen by psychoanalysts, and, therefore, a psychoanalyst, given the chance to study it would be expected to immediately apply himself to its study, it took him ten years to write this paper. Moreover, he did not wish to follow the case further, also postponing the writing of a theoretical discussion of it. In fact, he wrote the theoretical discussion of the case eleven years later (1984/2003 in English), that is, 21 years after the two consultations with M. De M'Uzan thinks that this was because the perverse practices involved in the case were so extreme that at first he did not know what to say, and, similarly, the reader would feel "a mixture of fascination and horrified disbelief, with the acute feeling that all that can be said about it can be nothing apart from more or less successful rationalization" (p. 455). To this, de M'Uzan adds that his reluctance to further study the case was also related to M.'s mocking, provocative attitude, which de M'Uzan sensed behind the "smoke screen" of M.'s apparent friendliness and directness in the two interviews.

Monsieur M. was 65 years old when de M'Uzan met him. At that time, M. had retired from work, having been a highly qualified and respected electronic engineer. He lived in a small house in the suburbs with his adopted daughter and her husband, and appeared to have lead a well-adjusted life, both socially and professionally, unmarked by moral masochism. But when he bared his damaged body, the contrast was overwhelming, and it confirmed his descriptions of his extremely masochistic practices. De M'Uzan gives a detailed, page-long description of the extreme self-inflicted damage to M.'s body, which was covered entirely in tattoos. His navel and rectum were deformed, his right breast was torn off, the little toe of his right foot was amputated by him at the demand of a sadistic partner, and his testicles and penis were extremely distorted by torture.

M., the only son of relatively elderly, "kind" parents, started his masochistic practices at age ten in school, searching for corporal punishment. This escalated in the following years as he became the object of his schoolmates' acts of brutality, and assumed its full development upon marriage at the age of 25 to his 15-year-old cousin. She, too, was a masochist (since age 11, before meeting M.), and their common perversion brought them together. Torture was generally inflicted on the two of them by one or two men, with M. and his wife assuming the role of victim. During the first three years of their marriage they also led a normal sexual life alongside their masochistic practices, and a daughter was born. M. was very attached to his wife, whom he described as sweet and loving, and their eight years of marriage as "eight years of happiness with never a dark cloud" (p. 457). But his wife, exhausted by the extreme torture, died of pulmonary tuberculosis at the age of 23. M. was deeply affected by her death. He entered into a depressed state, and contracted pulmonary tuberculosis, from which he recovered completely after two years in a sanatorium. His masochistic practices then began anew. He married a prostitute in the hope of finding an experienced partner, but divorced her soon afterwards when her involvement in criminal activities rendered him liable to criminal proceedings. De M'Uzan recounts that:

> From this marriage he retained nothing except a young servant girl, whom he had adopted as his daughter. *This was the point at which his perverse practices stopped completely*. . . . Even the content of his dreams, which had been strictly masochistic, became entirely heterosexual and less and less masochistic. . . . From then on his life unfolded within the family milieu which he had created, to which he was very strongly attached, and in which nothing was known of his peculiar past.
>
> (p. 458, my italics)

In explaining this perverse masochism, de M'Uzan focuses on the constitutional factor of "excess of instinctual quantity" (regarding M., his first wife who was his cousin, and his father, after whose death M. discovered from his correspondence that he, too, had been a masochist). This excess leads to an irresistible tendency to discharge tension. According to de M'Uzan, the role of the quantitative instinctual excess is manifested in the chronology of M.'s perverse practices. They began at puberty, and, as he approached the age of 50, "with the approach of old age and biological alternations," all perverse practices disappeared, and the dreams and fantasies finally became entirely free of masochistic representation. To this, de M'Uzan adds that if the excess of quantity becomes associated with an early object-deficiency or primitive, brutal, and precarious "tearing apart" of the "me" from the "other," it threatens the individual capacity for mental integration, particularly when the psychic apparatus has not attained sufficient development. This situation renders the ego much more dependent on elementary experiences at the bodily level, and especially on physical pain, in an effort at reorganization. Thus, the coexistence of the constitutional quantitative factor along with early object-deficiency or brutal separation "puts the seal on the destiny of the subject" (p. 465). Eleven years later (1984/2003), de M'Uzan describes M. as a "slave of quantity" of excitation, which is fatal and irrevocable because of a traumatic situation very early in life that cannot be psychologically elaborated. "Quantity is destiny when it is constituted in actual trauma" (p. 716).

In my view, de M'Uzan's explanation of the sudden, drastic change in the fatedness of M's erotogenic masochism surprisingly lacks any reference to the possibility that this radical change was affected by the changes that took place in M's human environment—mainly his deep, years-long relationship with the girl that he adopted as his daughter. It is here, according to de M'Uzan's description, that he began leading a quiet family life, free of all masochistic activities, and even gradually free of masochistic dreams. Are the excess quantity of excitation and the early object-deficiency or early traumatic separation influenced only by the age factor rather than the formation of significant, very different object-relations? Although not explored any further by de M'Uzan, I find it difficult not to consider the emergence and influence of these different relations as basic experiences that negate the seal of fate of early traumatic situations[4] and enable a new beginning, suggesting that "all is foreseen, and yet freedom of choice is [still] given" (Pirkei Avot, 3:15).

It is in this place—where new, basic experiences and a correction of "failure of early basic environmental provision" (in Winnicott's sense, 1963b, p. 258) come into being within the world of perversion—that I am endeavoring to situate the psychoanalytic treatment of severe perversion, as I will now describe. This approach also embodies—in an essential, broader sense—the search, the striving for, and the possibility of extending the boundaries of psychoanalytic treatment.

"Psychical treatment" and perversion

Let me start with words written very early on, at the threshold of the development of psychoanalysis, in the opening passage of Freud's very early paper, "Psychical (or mental) treatment," which he wrote in 1890. It was believed to be written in 1905 until it was discovered that these astounding arguments actually were written as early as 1890 (Berman and Rolnik, 2002). The young 34-year-old Freud, the neuro-physiologist and soon-to-be psychoanalyst, flooded with nascent ideas, writes,

> "Psyche" is a Greek word which may be translated "mind" ["*Seele*"—see Strachey's translator note[5]]. The term might accordingly be supposed to signify "treatment of the pathological phenomena of mental life". This, however, is *not* its meaning. "Psychical treatment" denotes, rather, treatment taking its start in the mind, treatment (whether of mental or physical disorders) by measures which operate in the first instance and immediately upon the human mind.
>
> Foremost among such measures is the use of words; and words are the essential tool of mental treatment. A layman will no doubt find it hard to understand how pathological disorders of the body and mind can be eliminated by "mere" words. He will feel that he is being asked to believe in magic. And he will not be so very wrong, for the words which we use in our everyday speech are nothing other than watered-down magic. But we shall have to follow a roundabout path in order to explain how science sets about restoring to words at least part of their former magical power.
>
> (1890, p. 283)

It is no small matter to believe—especially when thinking about the treatment of perversion—that "psychical treatment" is not "treatment of the pathological phenomena of mental life" but rather treatment originating in the psyche, treatment by "psychical measures, which operate in the first instance and immediately upon the human psyche." And how much more so, as the analyst's search is for words that are not "watered-down magic," but for words that have regained "a part at least of their former magical power."

In a 2002 lecture, Rolnik argues on this point:

> It is true that Freud would later attempt to close all apertures through which the theological and mystic draft might enter his writing, but he never succeeds in completely sealing them. . . . In any case, it is my view that had that mystic opening chord—*a psyche treating a psyche*—not continued to reverberate in psychoanalytic theory and to nourish it, it would not have lasted a hundred years.

From Freud's (1890) early words in the "Psychical treatment," I move to my own thoughts regarding the therapeutic factor of "a psyche treating a psyche" in terms of the analyst's presence in the treatment of perversion—thoughts that embrace my fundamental, broader assumptions regarding modes of therapeutic action in clinical psychoanalysis—"presenting" and patient–analyst deep interconnectedness.

"Presencing" in treating perversion

I see the analyst's "givenness to being present," or "presencing" as an essential means for treating perversion. As I wrote earlier (chapter 2 in this book), I first developed this approach with regard to massive acting out, acting in, and enactment, arguing that the fate of these acting situations in the therapeutic work is determined largely by the analyst's willingness and ability to give him/herself over to being-in there, staying within the intense impact of the acting situation and communing with it (1998a, 1998b). It thus becomes a way of listening, experiencing, understanding, remembering, and communication. For the acting conveys—in non-verbal ways—inner areas of traumatic experiences which are cut off and lost to words. Furthermore, I emphasized that the analyst's "presencing" in massive acting situations becomes a powerful holding, containing, and protective factor whose existence and cumulative effect changes the self–other field, the inner experience of terror, and of traumatic lack and emotional failure in the patient's world. It thereby enables the breaching, from within, of the repetitive cycle of pathological self–other relations and defenses.

This is markedly so in perversions, wherein the acting—defined as acting out, enactment or performance—is a central element (Goldberg, 1975; Khan, 1979; Kaplan, 1993). From this perspective, I understand the reactions of the psychotic masochistic patient Anna (Stolorow et al., 1994) mentioned earlier, who repeatedly and unceasingly requested of her therapist to hit her, to hit her until eventually she was able to write to him that "physical pain is better than spiritual death." Through her "hit me" request, I think, she was asking her therapist over and over to enter, share, and effect by his presence her lonely and alienated masochistic solution and her dread of psychic deadness.

Moreover, in view of object- and selfobject-relations models of the development of perversions, it seems to me particularly significant in treating perversion to establish this sort of presence—namely, the analyst's basic, functioning "presencing" that focuses on attunement, receptivity, holding and containing rather than proffering interpretations of patient–analyst relationships (object or subject relationships) and especially of patient–analyst separateness.

As described in the theoretical-clinical section of this chapter, object- and selfobject-relations perspectives on perversion formation (including my own and de M'Uzan's) anchor it primarily in disturbed, traumatic core experiences in the early developmental stages. It is viewed as a defense organization of the infantile ego or self in order to survive and control an overwhelming maternal or primary parental environment that is traumatic, engulfing, and annihilating. Therefore, the analyst's givenness to attuned, functioning "presencing" takes on great relevance in the treatment of perversions. This relevance is *ontological-experiential* rather than epistemological. The analyst's "presencing" enables *a new mobilization of the patient's primary and fundamental need for a connected, merged existence with a holding, containing, and protective presence*. At the same time, it also enables the *actual*[6] *becoming of a new, primary interconnectedness* with the analyst—who is "there to be used" (in the Winnicottian sense), steady, sustaining, and experience-near to the patient's needs, fears, and inability to relate. Khan (1979) also writes that the

> formidable therapeutic task in the treatment of the pervert . . . confronts us with the pervert's inaccessibility to influence and change through his object-relations. No human being can do very much in ordinary life for a pervert because he can be as Lewis Carroll's Tweedledee would say, "only a sort of thing in his dream."
>
> (p. 30)

I believe that the sort of analyst's "presencing" described here creates a fundamentally new possibility of seeping into, accessing, and influencing the pervert's inner world.

In Winnicottian terms of regression, the process that I am elaborating upon can be described as the transforming of the patient's withdrawal and dissociative organization—in this context, the perversions—into regression to dependence (Winnicott, 1954b), through the analyst's "presencing." (De Masi, 2003, also has deemed early "sexualized withdrawal [that begins in infancy] to be the nucleus and genesis of perversion—indeed of all perversions" [p. 87]). According to Winnicott, in the withdrawal state, it is the patient who is holding the self. But if the analyst proves himself/herself capable of holding the patient and "*putting a medium around* [the patient's] *withdrawal self*" (p. 257, italics in original), this enables the patient to dare let go of the withdrawn self-defensive organization, thereby converting the withdrawal into regression, which carries with it the opportunity for correction of the failure or inadequate-adaptation-to-need in the patient's past. Thus, a new chance for development ensues. Balint (1968) similarly describes a new beginning as "(a) going back to something 'primitive', to a point before the faulty development started, which could be described as a regression, and (b) at the same time, discovering a new, better-suited, way which amounts to a progression" (p. 132).

I am stressing *terms of regression* in the treatment of perversion because it offers a radical new possibility for the analytic process to influence and correct the patient's past environmental failures in a deep way that goes back to very early developmental processes (chapter 10 in this book). For Winnicott, through regression to dependence in analysis, "the present goes back to the past and *is* the past" (1955–1956, p. 298), and there is a chance for the analytic "present-day environment to make adequate though belated adaptation" and provide good-enough holding and handling that can actually alter the patient's past (1954a, p. 283). "Somehow we have silently communicated reliability and the patient has responded with the growth that might have taken place in the very early stages in the context of human care" (1988a, p. 102).

Patient–analyst interconnectedness in treating perversion

Through "presencing" and regression, patient and analyst enter another realm of experience—of patient–analyst interconnectedness or "withnessing" at a deep, emotional level of contact and impact—a primary and formative two-in-one entity beyond their separate psychic existence. This implies breaching and changing the patient's (and the analyst's) psychic space.[7] Within this deep interconnectedness of their psyches, a new possibility is created and present for getting in touch with, experiencing, containing, and influencing hitherto unknown, most dissociated, or frozen aspects of being and relating that were unbearable and unthinkable to the patient (and the analyst) separately, and could not otherwise be reached or come into being. This new possibility, which becomes part of the actual treatment reality, not only revives the original past situation but is a process of becoming, a transformative process of change by breaching of the limits of the patient's repetition and reconstruction. (In my 2004b paper on the becoming of the fundamentally new experience in psychoanalytic treatment, I have referred to this as "past-present actuality" and the "venture zone" in treatment.)

These are *crucial issues in the treatment of perversion*. Due to its dissociative, secretive nature, due to its being a self-induced survival solution of dissociative splitting and a compulsively driven and exciting ritual that does not truly change the deep inner stalemate, the pervert cannot be extricated from these repetitive cycles on his own. But within and through the analyst's "presencing" within the perversion-laden psychic space, as the patient slowly discloses his secrets, anxieties, feelings, and desires to the analyst, while also slowly and gradually revealing his concealed yearnings, a new inner speech is formed, heard, and evolves, albeit at times wallowing in the darkest burrows. *A present, alternative experiential-emotional reality is created*. It is a difficult treatment; most difficult. The psychic space of treatment and the analyst's interconnected psyche are deluged with the effects of perversion, or with the search for a path in a world of despair, emptiness and losing one's way, especially at the very time when the fierce perverse solution is destabilized and recedes (which is then often compounded when external reality is disorganized by changes in the split perverse structure). At times, the analyst is pushed toward anxious limits of professional and personal abilities (see also Danielle Quinodoz's [2002] poignant description[8]).

But, I believe that the analyst's "presencing" and interconnectedness with the patient within these experiences—which hold together the "autotomous" split parts—slowly, over time, erode the power of the blocked, wordless dread, the secrecy, the dissociation, and the profound loneliness; they struggle "in there" to bear, contain, and mitigate the ferocity of the destructiveness, violence, rage, and desire; to survive the failures, collapses, depression and despair, the intense helplessness, and the patient's feeling of being fundamentally, irreparably flawed. These are all revived, grasping and clinging to the analyst—to the analyst's presence and the connection with him or her—and they are difficult, heavy, and attacking; one may say that their clinging to the analyst and the treatment replaces their clinging to the perverse solution. At the same time, a possibility is created for experiencing and processing them, thus becoming a different way of experiencing, relating, and being. All this enables a profound change in the perverse essence, along with a slow, gradual entry of life, of connectedness, and hope (chapter 8 in this book).

I would like to stress once again that in these treatments, which are based on "presencing," interconnectedness, and regression to dependence and primary experiences, the analyst's actual, sustaining *presence* is immensely important.

Winnicott's (1954–1955) words on "a good breast introjection" in analytic treatment completes the circle begun with Freud's early words (1890) on "psychical treatment" and its "magical power":

> What do we [analysts] want? We want to be eaten, not magically introjected. There is no masochism in this. To be eaten is the wish and indeed the need of a mother at a very early stage in the care of an infant. This means that whoever is not cannibalistically attacked tends to feel outside the range of people's reparative and restitutive activities . . . . *If and only if we have been eaten, worn down, stolen from, can we stand in a minor degree being also magically introjected*, and being placed in the preserve department in someone's inner world.
>
> (Winnicott, 1954–1955, p. 276, my italics)

For me, the magic, the wonder of psychoanalytic treatment, in general, and the treatment of perversion, in particular, is *the magic of the emotional connection created within a profound loneliness*. This connection is difficult, dense, at times daunting, rejected and rejecting, threatening and threatened both when it transpires and also when it does not; as such, it is fragile, woven thread by thread, struggling for its existence, but thereby very powerfully forged. It is this interconnectedness of patient's and analyst's psyches, and consequently within the patient's psyche, that enables—by dint of its ontological-experiential actuality—a breakthrough beyond the harsh and lonely actuality of the perversion. (I believe that of all mental disorders, the existential experience of the pervert is the loneliest, most isolated and alienated—both from the outside world and also within the disconnected parts of his/her internal world.)

These processes transpired slowly and gradually in the treatments of my three perverse patients described at the beginning of the chapter, and manifested themselves concretely in the course of treatment by the cessation of the perverse practices. The "psychical treatment" that takes place through patient–analyst interconnectedness at a deep emotional level of "presencing," contact and impact, the vital neediness and vulnerability involved in this process, and the "Eros" created in it ("Eros" in Racker's sense, 1968[9]) *eventually dissolve the grip of the perversion*. Or, in words taken from Ferenczi (1933), these processes recreate the "passive object-love" and "tenderness" characteristic of early childhood that were distorted and turned into "passion" when, at the early stage of tenderness, an adult's passion or passionate punishment were forced upon the child.

Ghent, too, relates to tenderness in his paper on masochism (1990). He cites the poet Yeats: "Tread softly, because you tread on my dreams," and writes, "We ought to 'tread softly' on patients' masochism and submissiveness. These, too, are often expressing in a disguised and distorted way a deep yearning to be found and recognized" (p. 234).

In order to illustrate the analyst's "presencing" and the critical emotional interconnectedness of patient and analyst in the psychoanalytic treatment of perversion, I will present three vignettes that describe sessions taken from the analysis of perverse patients. The first vignette is from a difficult and critical analytic session with me. The second one is from an analytic session described by Marvin Glasser (1986), which I will contrast with my own. In the third, I return to the analysis of my own patient of the first vignette, more than a year after that session.

Clinical illustration I: Expulsion and return

The fetishistic-masochistic patient whom I described at the beginning of this chapter (pp. 152–154), now in the second year of analysis, arrived at the first session following my holiday break. (The gaps created by the analyst's vacations are most troublesome in these treatments.) As soon as I opened the door, I noticed his swollen face.

He lay on the couch, and after a brief "How are you?" told me quietly and bluntly, in detached detail, that he had gone to a whore that morning, a cheap one who charges only 100 shekels (about $25), a most violent type, who went wild and slapped him and beat him madly, incessantly, for five minutes, and he came very fast and hard, went home, washed up and came to the session.

For the first time in this analysis, I felt great tiredness and disgust, although he had already recounted far more violent and bizarre scenes, perhaps because of this inundating pitiful cheapness. I was thinking to myself, what is the point of all the hard work, of this entire analysis, the great investment of money and years. Better go to a whore every day, get beaten up for five minutes, pay 100 shekels, and be finished.

And I withdraw, fall silent.

Then I noticed that he became very agitated, in sharp contrast to his former quiet and detached manner. As if he'd heard my thoughts, he said:

> Nothing can be done. I ask you: What? What is there to say? When I'm butchered, I exist. It's like the Alien got inside my belly and stayed there, breaking out every time, and that's it. Nothing left to do. There's no solution. Everything just gets worse. I'm finished. I was born and I'll die this way. I'll be dead before I'm forty.

He sat up, shaken, suddenly looking so withered, shapeless and pitiful, with his beaten-up, swollen face. And I realized he sensed and knew that I had *abandoned* him, left him wounded and lost on the battlefield, and had gone off to save myself. Thus, I returned to this despicable, despairing and desperate place, his and mine, and said:

> You are so desperate because you feel that I have given up. And when we both give up there's nothing more to hold on to. It's really very despairing, *but we are going on.*

He lay back quietly, tears in his eyes for the first time in analysis (perhaps in his life), and said, "Death can be so cheap. You should lock me up inside the treatment."

Clinical illustration II: That which was is that which becomes

This vignette is from Glasser's[10] (1986) paper and is quoted here verbatim. He embarks on his own concept of "*the core complex*" in perversions, and illustrates it by describing a session:

> The core complex is a basic, central, coherent structure established in early infancy and made up of the inner-related ingredients of the longing for intimate gratification and security, the anxieties of annihilation and abandonment, with the attendant depression, and the aggression and sado-masochism.

These ingredients can be illustrated by a condensed account of a session with a homosexual[11] patient:

> *He had been complaining about how his mother had been so unforthcoming on her recent visit to him in London. I commented that although he had given me many examples of his mother behaving in this way, I had some doubts about his account because we had seen in many sessions how he couldn't stand her coming close to him and how he was compelled to push her away. He responded by becoming visibly agitated and saying that he found his mother suffocating: she was like a spider on his face (as he said this he placed his spread-out hand over his mouth, nose and eyes and gripped his face). I took up this projection of his "spideriness" on to his mother/me, reminding him of his anger over my absences or late starts, and his bouts of compulsive, greedy chocolate-eating, as well as of his bouts of compulsively visiting public lavatories to carry out fellatio on whatever men he could find. Evidently my comments were too intensive, or too effective, because he went on to say that he felt terrible as I spoke and he felt an extremely strong desire to turn around and seduce me so that I wouldn't go on saying what I was saying.*
>
> The core complex dynamics are well-illustrated: when I challenge his denial of his longings for his mother/me, he feels himself to be invaded and taken over by my comments which, he believes, are aimed at making him be what I want him to be, not himself, and he deals with the conflicting wishes of negating me and keeping me by trying to sexualize our relationship into a sado-masochistic one by carrying out fellatio on me, thus gaining control over me and over what he will or will not take into himself.
>
> (pp. 10–11)

I find myself surprised by the realization that two analysts (in this case—Glasser and myself) can begin with fundamentally compatible theoretical views (i.e., the model of the disturbed early mother–infant relationship for understanding the development of perversion), and yet end up proffering such different actual courses of therapeutic action. For I feel that in the above session, Glasser, who greatly emphasizes the central role of the overbearing mother in perversion formation—the mother whom the child experienced as stifling and annihilating his profound longing for primary merging, intimacy, and security—merely enables in treatment *an experiential repetition* with him of the patient's overbearing relationship with his mother. In this session, which started with the patient's complaint about the mother's distance, Glasser does not offer attuned, empathic reflective listening to what the patient is feeling, which would bring about experience-near understanding, interpretations, and "Eros" (Racker, 1968). Rather, he gives (imposes) interpretations from the position of an analyst who authoritatively knows the truth about the patient and his relationship with his mother. Thus, it seems to me that they do not get beyond the patient's sexualization, and do not reach his lonely, deep-rooted distress.

Analyst, "tread softly," for you tread upon the dreams, deep yearnings, and "core emotional needs" (in Glasser's own words) that were crushed and distorted at an early age and are waiting to be found, recognized and met.

Returning to my clinical illustration: can the warp be smoothed out?

I will now go back to my fetishistic-masochistic patient, in order to illustrate the turbulent nature of the analysis when the perverse practices ceased, the struggle (and yearning) to break through beyond his split world to a new possibility, and the significance of *holding on to treatment instead of to the perversion*. It is difficult, however, to describe the analyst's tacit "presencing" through a verbatim report. For the sense of connection and understanding in "presencing" is achieved mainly by letting the patient's intensity speak to us, and listening to and communing with the experience, its voices, imagery and enactments—feeling and evolving with their impact.

The vignettes are taken from two successive sessions that took place into the third year of analysis, over a year after the session I described earlier, and several months after the cessation of the perverse activities:

The patient began,

> You wanted me to bring myself here. So I am bringing my inner me, my madness, my depression. I'm saying what I said yesterday, although I'm less depressed and sad. In the past, I almost never had any deliberations. I led a very particular life, going for fetish and brutal sado, hiding from my surroundings. I'd come home, kiss the wife on the cheek, everything would be fine. Here, too, I'd come and talk logically, and then go on to some brutal fetish. Now I'm telling you everything is shit, it's all nothing, and I leave here and put up a hell of

> a struggle not to do fetish. It's tearing me to pieces. Now I can't find an opening in all the shit. When I talk to you, it's a relatively good moment, but when I leave here . . .
>
> It's all ups and downs, nothing steady in my behavior and feelings. So even when I tell myself, at the end of the day, "You're calmer now," I remind myself this is just until the next downer; it's an illusion. My entire development has been sucked into a whole complex of devious things. It all boils down to feeling like a great big nothing, that I am one big nothing. In the film Pulp Fiction, John Travolta takes risks, and eventually dies like a dog. So, what nice words will you make up now . . .

I said,

> At those moments, when you take risks and feel so insecure, and when you become desperate, my words are needed. [Note that I said, "my words are needed" and not "you need my words," in order to stress patient–analyst interconnected being in the process, and not I–you separate experiences.]

P said, in an urgent voice,

> And if you won't understand . . . It's not just the perversion. It's my whole conduct. It's a different world. My whole essence is different, the essence of a world where you don't really exist in normal reality, you're not really there, ever. You're not real; it's all one big show. And the fetish—that's real. But the fact that now I'm not spending money on fetish and brutal sado, that's real and makes me feel good. That's great. Really. But that's just so little. And it shakes you, and upsets everyone around you. It's easier to go to a brutal fetish, kiss the wife on the cheek, and shut up.
>
> And what if you say, "Why did I take on such a case?" I think that if the treatment, if psychoanalysis, has the slightest chance of taking a person whose development is so perverted from a very early age, and lead him to a normal way of life, if such a chance exists—and, frankly, I think chances are there's no chance at all—then I believe the treatment will be long. Whether it succeeds or not, it will clearly take years. The treatment is so . . . I think about it all the time—except for the few

> hours I sleep at night, it's with me all the time. Because I think that, if there is such a thing as moving from one track to another, it seems so very difficult. My inner world is something, Heaven help me, it's something else entirely, a world that in order to penetrate or change it—it's an atomic bomb. My inner world, it's a world where you can't grasp what's going on there inside me. I don't say this in desperation. You're the closest to understanding me. Maybe it can't change, and that's the conclusion we'll come to in the end, that it can't change. It's so different. Maybe it's impossible. My inside is such a totally different world. If I won't get cured, I'll die. Better to die.
>
> I had no idea where things would go, and no thoughts about the things I think about now. Over the last months, I've been bringing to the sessions the madness that happens all the time, that at the moment I'm alone in the struggle, there's no God, I get into an absolute panic, all's lost, total despair, everything is just shit. In a real sense, it's the real me. But if I come to you desperate and claim there's no point in the treatment and nothing good is ever going to happen, you are getting exactly what's happening to me. So, now, in contrast to the past, you know almost everything—that every day I'm in a state of excitation and my soul is devastated, very sick.

In the next session he said,

> I'm tied to the fetish to the very core of my being, but something has happened . . . I want to choose from the start, clean and pure, if such a thing is possible . . . I very much want a girlfriend or wife, a partner. I can't see how I even get there. It seems too far away to get. It's hard when you start out so low, from the bottom. It's like Mount Everest for me.

Concluding remarks

I began with a term from biology ("autotomy"), and I would like to conclude, as well, with a further reference to biology (also influenced, perhaps, by de M'Uzan's biologistic thinking), quoting Darwin in his writing on evolution: "The structure of every organic being is related, in the most essential manner, to that of all other organic beings with which it comes into competition, from which it has to escape, or on which it preys" (*On the Origin of the Species*, 1859).

Furthermore, Jonathan Weiner (1995), in his book *The Beak of the Finch: A Story of Evolution in Our Time*, follows the discoveries of two scientists, Peter and Rosemary Grant, who spent some 20 years, beginning in the 1970s, in the heart of the Galapagos Archipelago—where Darwin received his first inklings of the theory of evolution—proving to their surprise that Darwin did not fully recognize the strength of his own theory. Weiner demonstrates that evolution is neither rare nor slow, taking place by the hour, and we can watch it. Chapter 19 in the book, "A Partner in the Process," opens with a quote from Theodosius Dobzhansky: "Creation is not an act but a process; it . . . is going on before our eyes. Man is not compelled to be a mere spectator; he may become an assistant, a collaborator, a partner in the process of creation" (Dobzhansky, quoted in Weiner, 1995, p. 267).

I would like to apply the biological-factual words of Darwin and his followers—about evolution and the partnership in the process of creation—to personal evolution as well. I believe that in psychoanalytic treatment, in general, and in that of the pervert, in particular, if sufficient time is given to "presencing" and analyst-patient interconnectedness and impact, *the psychic structure of the patient is influenced and changes, in the most essential manner, within the abiding, deep, and sustaining connection with the analyst's psyche*.

Notes

1 Throughout the chapter, "perversion" refers to actual sexual perversion (cf. *DSM IV-TR* under Paraphilias) and not to the psychoanalytic expansion of the term over the last decades to perversion of the transference relationship and character perversion (especially in Kleinian thinking).

2 I find it necessary to specify the cases that have led to my ideas on severe perversion; one might metaphorically say, "Which part of the large elephant's body do I take hold of in order to know the elephant?" Here, as Winnicott writes: "It is not my aim in this paper to give a description of this case since one must choose whether to be clinical or theoretical . . . Nevertheless I have this case all the time in mind" (1954a, p. 280).

3 It is interesting to note that, as regards female sexuality, Freud could write: "Our insight into this early, pre-Oedipus phase in girls comes to us as a surprise, like the discovery, in another field, of the Minoan-Mycenean civilization behind the civilization of Greece. Everything in the Sphere of this first attachment to the mother seemed to me so difficult to grasp in analysis—so

grey with age and shadowy and almost impossible to revivify—that it was as if it had succumbed to an especially inexorable repression. . . . It does indeed appear that women analysts . . . have been able to perceive these facts more easily and clearly . . . for this appears to be the surprising, yet regular, *fear of being killed (? devoured) by the mother*" (1931, pp. 226–227, my italics).

4 I am reminded here of Winnicott's emphasis (1963b) on the significance of the correction of "failure of early basic environmental provision" in severe mental disorders: "It is in the psychoses—not in the psycho-neuroses—that we must expect to find examples of self-cure. Some environmental happening, perhaps a friendship, may provide a correction of a failure of basic provision, and may unhitch the catch that prevented maturation in some respect or other" (p. 258). According to Winnicott, this corrective provision is not enough in the analytic process, and should be supplemented by a correction of the early traumatic failure—now relived through the analyst's failure ("failing the patient's way")—in the treatment.

5 According to Strachey's translator note, "'*Seele*' is a word which is in fact nearer to the Greek 'psyche' than is the English 'mind'" (Freud, 1890, p. 283). The Greek word *psukhé* is indeed translated "soul, breath" (*Collins Dictionary*).

6 "*Actual*" is intended here in its two meanings: "In the present and in the process of actualization, that is, trying to bring into existence what didn't happen" (Pontalis, 2003, p. 45).

7 Danielle Quinodoz (2002), in a paper summarizing a transsexual patient's analysis, writes of the change in the patient's psychic space from a two-dimensional, flat, concrete reality to a volumetric, three-dimensional internal space when the dimension of psychic reality is added. To my way of thinking, this change is the consequence of the "presencing" and interconnectedness with the analyst's psyche, which establishes the new dimension.

8 In this context, I would like to relate to Danielle Quinodoz's (2002) account, in a subsection entitled "An earthquake prior to the establishment of order," describing the extremely strong feelings of dismay, disappointment, collapse, and abandonment that she experienced when her transsexual patient informed her after approximately five-and-a-half years of analysis (which lasted seven years) that s/he plans to go ahead with a series of sex-change operations. She writes: "For a moment I felt that everything was collapsing; Simone was abandoning me, slapping me in the face, administering the most violent aggression ever: there she was putting everything back on the concrete level, on that of external appearances, whereas I had thought that she was now in search of a more internal, psychic, sense of identity" (p. 787). Quinodoz then describes the way she processed these feelings.

Such difficult sessions surrounding a violent return to the perverse solution (also described in the first clinical example that I will present here) are familiar to analysts and therapists of severe perversions, and they usually follow a revival in treatment of feelings and experiences of the core traumatic failure.

9 Racker (1968) powerfully states, "The analytic transformation process depends, to a large extent, on the quantity and quality of *Eros* the analyst is able to put into action for his patient. *It is a specific form of Eros, it is the Eros called understanding*, and it is, too, a specific form of understanding. It is, above all, the understanding of what is rejected, of what is feared and hated in the human being, and this thanks to a greater fighting strength" (p. 32, my italics). "To understand is to overcome the division into two . . . *To understand, to unite with another, and hence also to love*, prove to be basically one and the same" (p. 174, my italics).

10 I am grateful to the late Dr Mervin Glasser, whose words I borrowed to illustrate my (different) approach.

11 I am quoting this account, even though homosexuality has been expunged from paraphilias (perversions) in *DSM-IV*, because this account visibly illustrates the therapeutic action of the session.

Part II

The "voice" of breakdown

Part II delves into unbearably painful, silenced, and buried traumatic screams and the immensity of the brokenness of a human psyche, beyond sexuality, beyond perversion, beyond massive dissociation, and deadness. I will continue to explore how working within the dimension of analytic presence and patient–analyst deep interconnectedness or "withnessing" that grows into at-one-ment, may enable us to meet, reach, and transform the patient's most unknown, unrepresented states, mainly of core catastrophe (Bion) and unthinkable, unexperienced breakdown and madness (Winnicott).

Prologue

The annihilated last scream

A Talmudic story

I will begin this part with an ancient story from the Babylonian Talmud:[1] Yoma 69b (a story about the time of Ezra and Nechemya—approx. 500–400 BCE—upon the return of Jews from exile in Babylon to the land of Israel to rebuild the second Temple):

> "And [they] cried with a great [loud] voice unto their God" (Nechemya 9:4). What did they cry? "Woe, woe, it is the one who has destroyed the Sanctuary, burnt the Temple, killed all the righteous ones, driven all Israel into exile, and is still dancing among us!". . .
>
> They sat in fast for three days and three nights, and he was given over to them. He came forth from the Holy of Holies like a fiery lion-cub. Thereupon the Prophet said to Israel: "This is the evil desire of idolatry, as it is said, 'This is the evil'" [Zechariah. 5:7].
>
> While they were capturing him, a hair was torn out from his mane. He cried out and it went [was audible] four hundred *parsaot* [miles]. Thereupon they said: "What shall we do? Perhaps, God forbid, they might have mercy upon him from heaven!"
>
> The Prophet said unto them: "Cast him into a leaden pot and stop up his mouth with lead, because lead absorbs sound, for it says, "This is the evil, and he threw the leaden stone into its mouth" [Zechariah. 5:8].
>
> They said: "Since this is a time of [God's] grace, let us pray for mercy [to eliminate] the [evil] desire of sex". They prayed for mercy, and he too was handed over to them. He said to them: "Realize that if you kill that one, the world ends." They imprisoned him for three

> days, then looked in the whole land of Israel for a fresh egg and could not find one. Thereupon they said: "What shall we do? If we kill him, the world would end. Shall we beg for half-mercy? They do not grant 'halves' in heaven." They put out his eyes and let him go. It helped inasmuch as he no longer excites desire toward relatives [incest].
>
> (Babylonian Talmud Yoma 69b)

This mythical, intriguing, somewhat enigmatic, dark story about *Yetzer ha'ra*—usually translated as the "Evil Inclination" of Idolatry and Sex—brings out a crucial difference between the mercilessly cruel fate of the little, abused, and vulnerable cub, who was savagely executed and silenced, and the desire for sexual transgression. The sexual desire warns them that he is necessary for the continuation of life. Prudently, they imprison him for three days. And, indeed, when realizing that nothing can be done, for halfway prayers are not answered, they blind him and let him go. The blinding only reduces the desire for incest with close relatives.

I find myself wondering why this Talmudic story, where the Rabbis of the Talmud expressed their deepest thoughts and understanding on the complex human psychology, evil inclination and desire (Boyarin, 1993), chooses to bring into the scene a little, terrified and screaming cub. It feels to me like an enigmatic message (Laplanche, 1987), that somewhere beneath the cloak of the collective verdict, and beyond "productive" sexuality, there lies—buried, silenced, annihilated—*an infant's last scream.*

Looking for the fiery

Bion (2005b) in his Tavistock seminar on 3 July 1978, given at the age of 81, a year before his death, returns to the dreadful imagery of the "debris" of the patient's psyche caused by catastrophic emotional explosion (trauma), which he described earlier (1970, p. 13), and movingly says:

> To sum up: we are presented with the debris, the vestiges of what was once a patient and what still could be analogous to blowing on the dying embers of a fire so that some spark communicates itself to others; the fire is built up again, although it appeared to be nothing but dead ash. Can we look at all this debris and detect in it some little spark of life?
>
> (2005b, pp. 44–45)

The "vital spark, this urge towards life and growth and development," and the struggle with deadness and annihilation are abiding concerns in Winnicott's work and writing (Winnicott, 1964b, p. 27; Goldman, 2012). Here, I would also add Homer's riveting expression of the firebrand in the black ash, hidden there to save the "fire-seed" (*Odyssey*, 5:490) when struggling to survive a great, terrifying loneliness.

Can I look and find in the debris of my patient's psyche some hidden little fire-seed of life and love?

Chapter 8

"For You have returned my soul within me with compassion"

"Presencing," passion, and compassion in the depths of perversion, breakdown, despair, and deadness

> Not passion but compassion.
> *Com*—means "with."
> What kind of withness would that be?
> Translate it.
>
> (Anne Carson, "The Truth about God," 1992)

The lines of Carson's poem beautifully capture the main theme of this chapter. Compassion here is the analyst's "withness" or interconnectedness with the patient's agonizing states of deep distress, annihilation, and despair. I will describe the way in which I have come to view the move from passion to com-passion within the terms of the psychoanalytic work grounded in the analytic presence and patient–analyst "withnessing" or interconnectedness; and in particular, the analyst's crucial struggle to be able and willing to be-with-in the patient's reliving of unbearable overwhelming early breakdown and madness.

Compassion

A theoretical-clinical context

Compassion, from the Latin *com*—with, *pati*—to suffer, means to suffer-with (and I would add—to suffer-with-in; to be present within another's suffering and be-with it). It is different etymologically from words that are often regarded as synonymous, such as pity (from the Latin *pietas*, meaning duty) or mercy (from the Latin *merces*, meaning recompense).[2] In addition, the word "patient" is derived from the same Latin word *pati*—to suffer.

Hence, as the etymology of the word suggests, compassion is being-with the patient and being the patient.

Thus, the *withness of compassion* is what distinguishes it from other feelings of sorrow for the suffering of others, such as pity and mercy (and also from such feelings as kindness and generosity). Compassion involves and shares, while pity and mercy are often considered more distinct, more distant and impersonal, and may include aloofness, feelings of superiority, and condescension toward another's suffering. The distance and impersonal nature of pity and mercy are defiantly expressed by Yehuda Amichai, one of Israel's leading contemporary poets, in his poems "God Has Pity on Kindergarten Children" and "God Full of Mercy" (1962, quoted below):

> God-Full-of-Mercy, the prayer for the dead.
> If God was not full of mercy,
> Mercy would have been in the world,
> Not just in Him.

According to Hannah Arendt (1965), pity is concern for the misery of another, unprompted by intimacy with, or love for, the sufferer; while compassion is a love directed "towards specific suffering" of "particular persons." Pity "may be the perversion of compassion" because the person who pities "is not stricken in the flesh" and keeps a "sentimental distance." Arendt maintains:

> For *compassion*, to be stricken with the suffering of someone else as though it were contagious, and *pity*, to be sorry without being touched in the flesh, are not only not the same, they may not even be related. Compassion, by its very nature, cannot be touched off by the sufferings of a whole class or a people, or, least of all, mankind as a whole. It cannot reach out farther than what is suffered by one person and still remain what it is supposed to be, co-suffering. Its strength hinges on the strength of passion itself, which, in contrast to reason, can comprehend only the particular, but has no notion of the general and no capacity for generalization.
>
> (p. 85, italics in original)

Compassion has hardly been addressed in the psychoanalytic literature. The few papers on compassion—five that I located, most of them written in the last decade—display great variance with regard to the essence and meaning of compassion in the context of the psychoanalytic treatment, although all take a very humane stance.

Bernstein (2001) attributes this avoidance of compassion in psychoanalytic work to "the fear of compassion" or of "being human, though a psychoanalyst" (p. 209). He argues that a misreading of Freud has perpetuated two compelling shibboleths: the fear of countertransference and the abstinence rule, which deprived psychoanalysts of the privilege of having the use of all of their feelings, especially the feeling of compassion and of behaving compassionately with their patients. He briefly describes two difficult treatments of disturbed female patients, arguing that the early one failed because he was then unprepared to allow himself to act as a compassionate human therapist; while, in the second case 15 years later, he was able and willing to assume compassionate responsibility.

Feiner (1993) attributes this inhibition of psychoanalytic compassion to the dialectic between compassion and standards. In this regard, Nacht had already suggested in 1965, in his paper on "Criteria and technique for the termination of analysis," that in every case the analyst's attitude of benevolent neutrality has to gradually change and be replaced by a new *presence* (a *deep-down goodness*, described in his previous papers). But with patients whose ego functions have been disturbed by real severe trauma and much suffering, it has to include a truly authentic "attitude of gratification" on the part of the analyst (in certain aspects of the analytic relationship), stemming from genuine compassion for the misery that underlies the patient's incessant and outrageous aggression and demanding-ness.

Young-Eisendrath (2001) views the amelioration of suffering during and after treatment and increased compassion for self and others as the main objectives of a successful psychoanalytic treatment. She posits that the two means by which compassion is cultivated are an "unobjectionable, idealizing transference" (p. 276) that is filled with hope of transcending the suffering, and the investigation of the patient's suffering within patient and analyst's "interdependent relationship of discovery."

In the tradition of Self psychology, Kohut (1978, 1984) deals with compassion in relation to empathy. Orange (2006) relies on Kohut and Feiner (1993) for psychoanalytic thinking about compassion, as well as on the implications of complexity theory. In her view, compassion is that part of empathy that makes the analyst willing and able to descend into the patient's realms of suffering and shattered life. This enables emotional understanding and integration of the patient's suffering as opposed to dissociation and fragmentation, and affirms the human dignity of the patient.

The above articles, however, relate to compassion from interactive, relational two-person psychology perspectives. Even Orange's paper on compassion is, as she herself writes, "a more relational version of what I once [in her 1995 book] called the psychoanalytic function of witness" (2006, p. 7). But, while the term *witness* applies to an interaction between two subjectivities (Stern, 2012; Reis's attempt to broaden the conception of witnessing, 2009a, 2009b), I have proposed the notion of *psychoanalytic "withness"*—the being there, with-in the experience of suffering, in deep patient–analyst interconnectedness, that may become at-one-with the patient's innermost experience.

The unique conceptual space opened up by Bion's writing, especially his later writing, has facilitated my thinking on passion and compassion and the movement from one to the other—although, as Sandler (2005) writes, "The words compassion and passion are used by Bion in some seminal texts. Nevertheless, they do not attain the status of concepts. Bion uses the word 'compassion' in its vernacular, colloquial sense" (p. 146).

First, I encountered Bion's (1963) remarkable words on passion:

> I mean the term to represent an emotion experienced with intensity and warmth though without any suggestion of violence . . . . Passion is evidence that two minds are linked and that there cannot possibly be fewer than two minds if passion is present.
>
> (pp. 12–13)

Later on, Bion goes further and presents his profound conception of at-one-ment and the analyst's being and becoming O, the unknown and unknowable ultimate emotional reality of the patient (although Bion does not relate it to compassion): "With this [O] the analyst cannot be identified; he must *be* it" (1970, p. 27, italics in original). This "becoming" of the analyst has been elaborated in Grotstein's (2010) writing on infantile trauma and chronic resistance (particularly negative therapeutic reaction), as involving "the necessity for the analyst . . . to '*become*' the analysand's anguish and agony" (Grotstein, 2010, p. 25, italics in original).

Lastly, there are Bion's (1991) compassionate, touching words: "I do not think we could tolerate our work—painful as it often is for both us and our patients—without compassion" (p. 522).

All these ideas of Bion's have infused themselves into my thinking of compassion as patient–analyst "withnessing" within the violence of the suffering—*com-passion* that incorporates passion experienced with intensity and warmth, though without any suggestion of violence, that goes beyond the analyst's projective-introjective identification, and that is the analyst's "being" and "becoming" at-one with the patient's inmost emotional reality.

Despite the paucity of psychoanalytic writing on compassion, psychoanalysts in Israel have, over the last few years, produced some intriguing writing on this subject and in particular on compassion as a patient–analyst interconnected occurrence.

Kulka (2008a, 2008b), linking Self psychology and Buddhism, views compassion as "the repeal of the *individuality partition* between subject and subject." Thus, "compassion is not an interpersonal state, but a suprapersonal state; not a feeling, but an ethical decision for non-dual interconnectedness, an existential transcendence that turns man into pure presence" (2008a, pp. 118–119, italics in original). "Compassion, that which infuses foundational parts of Eastern cultures, is the abolition of duality, repealing the separation between water and fish . . . between one human and another, between humans and the world" (2008b, p. 1).

Ettinger (2006), artist and psychoanalyst, relates compassion to the primary maternal connectedness in the *matrixial borderspace*. She distinguishes between *empathy-within-compassion* and *empathy-without-compassion*. "Empathy-within-compassion" means empathy (to the patient) within compassion (also toward the patient's significant primary figures), and this is in contrast to "empathy-without-compassion"—an empathy to the patient only. In Ettinger's view, empathy to the patient without compassion also to the patient's archaic and actual significant primary objects creates internal splitting, "endangers the matrixial sphere itself," and ". . . leads to a fixation in a 'basic fault' positioning" (2010, pp. 2, 4).

I, however, would like to move back from these inclusive views of compassion as interconnectedness of all beings and compassion towards the patient's significant objects, and focus on compassion only in *patient–analyst interconnectedness*. I will concentrate on the analyst's difficult, sometimes even exceedingly difficult, struggle to give him/herself over—with all one's might, mind, heart, soul (Eigen, 1981)—to being and staying within the painful, annihilated-annihilating realness of the patient's suffering, in deep interconnectedness, in patient–analyst suffering.

One last note on compassion: perhaps another reason for the avoidance of the subject of compassion in the psychoanalytic literature is that the word has become saturated with religious connotations, especially Christian and Buddhist. Yet I venture to mention the compassion that is in the Jewish morning prayer that a religious Jew recites every morning immediately upon awakening—thanking God "*for You have returned my soul within me with compassion; great is Your faithfulness*." Though I am not a religious person, I relate deeply to this wondrous intertwining of God's great faithfulness and the compassion of returning the soul each morning, each day, after the terrors of the night of "*troubling thoughts, evil dreams and evil fancies . . . lest I sleep the sleep of death*" (words from the prayer recited before sleeping). It is even enigmatic—God's need for great faithfulness and faith in returning the soul with compassion. This compassion that is interwoven with faithfulness and faith in the process reverberates in my analytic use of compassion.

Case illustration

"For You have returned my soul within me with compassion"

The clinical material presented here is taken from a four-times-a-week analysis of a patient with severe fetishistic-masochistic perversion, which I described in the previous chapter on perversion up to the cessation of his perverse practices in the third year of analysis (Eshel, 2005; chapter 7 in this book). I will now proceed to later periods in this analysis.

P. started analysis when he was in his late thirties because of severe perversion that had intensified over the last few years, to the point of becoming life-threatening. As I described earlier, he was referred to me by a psychiatrist following an unsuccessful attempt to treat him with medication, which produced harsh physical side-effects. Therefore, the psychiatrist told him that psychoanalysis would be the only treatment that might help him since it is the most profound form of treatment. His agreeing to her proposal was an indication of his despair and hopelessness. The psychiatrist referred him to me, knowing I take difficult cases, although she feared that I might also refuse to accept him once I learned about the extent of his perversion. However, at the time, I had been crystallizing my thoughts about extending the reach of therapeutic work through the depth and intensity of psychoanalysis; and therefore, thinking that psychoanalysis should be able to offer a real treatment option for this person's distress, I agreed to accept him for analysis.

P. telephoned me the same day. During the initial session, he told me that his severe perversion had started as a shoe fetish of licking and kissing shoes, along with a masochistic element of wanting them to trample on his fingers, a wish which he recalled having had since kindergarten. It escalated over the years into a masochistic fetish, and in the past few years it had become a particularly severe and violent masochistic perversion. Over the first months of analysis, he gradually presented me with extremely harsh descriptions of his almost nightly visits to prostitutes, usually a different one each time, to be humiliated and abused by them in increasingly extreme ways with all sorts of instruments of torture. He sought treatment because he knew that "If it goes on like this, it will end in hospital—in a serious injury, or in death."

After a few months of analysis, when he realized that I would not "throw him out of treatment because of what he told me," he said, "This is the last stop for me. Psychoanalysis. After that—it's the graveyard." Since then he has clung to treatment despite some very difficult periods which we have gone through.

In his "ordinary" life, he was a dreary accountant, in a non-sexual marriage with a woman he knew from work, whom he told nothing about his perversion. At the end of the first year of analysis he told her the "truth" about himself and his secret life. She reacted with shock and repulsion, and decided that they should separate, and they were divorced.

During the first years of analysis, up to the cessation of the perverse practices into the third year, I came to know how essential to the analytic work was the analyst's (my) abiding "presencing" and interconnecting with the perverse patient, thus *being with-in* and listening to the perversion beyond its pathology, for its survival function and for the profound loneliness and despair it carries. I drew on the fundamental function of the evolving process of therapeutic regression in Balint's and especially Winnicott's terms in the analysis of the perverse patient—namely, to understand it primarily as a situation of need resulting from an early, most traumatic, maternal-environmental failure (rather than manipulative acting out), with the ensuing treatment priorities of holding, reliability, and attentiveness to the patient's need states and dependence. This analytic work, in Winnicottian terms of regression, enables the transformation of the patient's withdrawal and massive self-defensive organization—for this patient, of the perversion—into regression to dependence in treatment, which carries with it a new opportunity for correcting the patient's past experiences and for emotional development (Winnicott, 1954a, b; 1964a; 1988a, b).

Toward the end of the third year, after the perverse practices had ceased, analysis was filled with great agitation and confusion, and with massive holding on to the treatment and to me instead of the perversion. It led to a deeper regression in the analysis. In the sessions, he would speak feverishly, addressing his words to me, frequently calling me by my first name, Ofra—which he had never done previously—in the sessions and also in voice-mail messages that he now began leave. I will present some detailed vignettes, using his own words, as I feel that they most closely depict the actual experience, and convey the turbulent nature of the analytic situation at that time.

It was a Monday session—always a particularly difficult session after the weekend break.

He began: "Don't remember a period in my life like this, don't know what's happening to me, mentally and physically exhausted. Don't know what's happening. [Sighed, and remained silent]. My entire old world is collapsing, dissolving and disappearing, the whole world of evil, and I'm facing a new world, don't know what to do. I don't have the tools to cope with it."

I said: "Tools need time to develop." But my words remained suspended in space.

He went on: "Don't know, don't know what's happening . . . . Don't know, Ofra, just don't know what's happening to me, how all at once this thing that I used to fall into has disappeared—where has it gone to? All sorts of strange things, don't know, don't know what's happening in my head [he put his hands on his forehead]. Don't know, don't know, not anything I know, all sorts of things are flying in the air. Maybe I'm going mad, don't know, it's as if my brain is emptying out, as if things are flying in the air, like in a hurricane, as if something is making things fly out of my brain. In the last few days things are unclear to me, I'm not in control of what's happening to me, it's as if I'm falling apart, the first time in my life, falling apart completely. Don't know what to do—I'm going mad."

I said: "You're not going mad. You're changing, changing a lot."

He said: "I've never had thoughts like these, never in my life. The very element of violence has disappeared. I'm standing at the entrance to a new world, and I don't know how to behave. What to do with my brain and my dick. Don't know what I want from myself. We talked so much, Ofra, and all of a sudden something big collapsed all at once, not gradually. What a huge jolt."

He became silent, and lay quietly, as if sleeping, until the end of the session.

After about eight turbulent months, his confusion diminished. "Apparently, I have to get used to this new situation, that I'm not so much of a fetishist any more, and I need to calm down a bit," he said. He continued to abstain from his perverse activities. He frequented the cinema, listened to a lot of music, started exercising on the days that he was not in analysis, and began to look for and date women through internet dating sites. He called this period "the age of uncertainty" because previously everything had been familiar to him and under his control. He said: "I've never been out with a woman, I've never touched or been touched by a woman. I've never slept with a woman. I'm very scared of it, it's new. It's hard to get out of the gutter." (He said this even though, in fact, he had been married for years. Here, I would like to add that this was a man who could not bear to be touched. In the first year of treatment, when I asked him about his descriptions of the cruel fetishistic-masochistic practices, why the whores had to dig their high heels into him and extinguish their cigarettes on his body with their shoes rather than with their hands, he replied that he could not bear to be touched by a human hand.)

Nonetheless, despite his deep misgivings and fear, he now proceeded from telephone calls to dates, and began meeting an increasing number of women. These meetings were usually for no more than a single evening. In the course of time it became easier for him to meet women; some of these dates were even enjoyable. And still, deep inside, he felt cut off and vulnerable, and an immense inner emptiness was growing and taking hold of him. It seemed that the fetish that had disappeared had left behind a vacuum and profound emptiness.

Was this what he had foreseen when he spoke repeatedly about his perversion during the first year of analysis?—"It sustains you more than anything else. You won't let anyone or anything take it away from you. If you give it up, it will be unbearable, since there won't be anything else."

Now, in the fourth year, he was saying: "It's amazing, amazing, how the fetish took over my entire life, and now there's nothing, nothing. Don't know what's going on here. With women, it doesn't seem real; I don't really want it. Last night I talked to that woman who approached me—don't know, it seemed pointless like, what, what, for what, suddenly everything seemed pointless, strange, strange . . . . Don't know what to do, Ofra, altogether feel completely cut off. Don't know where everything I've fantasized till now is, where everything that filled me all those years has gone. . . . Everything hurls me into a world that has no center. I'm so empty inside . . . . Feel so unreal, so unable to exist in the world of the living—and mainly, so ill."

He gave himself time until his birthday, which was very close to the end of the fourth year of analysis, to try it out. "The transition between worlds is a tremendous jolt. Ilan Ramon[3] didn't survive the transition between worlds. I'm going through a jolt that is just as great. It will end either in death or in a different life."

Into the breakdown

But after his birthday, throughout the fifth year of analysis, profound despair, unfathomable emptiness and death seemed to possess him and to have become the only reality—dreadful and absolute. This was a terrible, excruciating year in analysis. He reverted to searching the internet for the most ferocious fetishistic-masochistic websites with "extreme violence and self-destruction." He masturbated to horrendous fantasies, even though he did not revert to actually performing perverse activities. He said: "It's a kind of total self-destruction, without any brakes, as if I don't have a drop of self-love in me, a drop of compassion [*compassion* here is his word], a drop of self-pity, a drop of anything, anything. It's unbelievable, Ofra, unbelievable—only dread, hatred, violence, feelings of inferiority and fear of criticism."

He requested a year's unpaid leave from work because he could not live with the huge disparity between his internal world and his external "normal, false" painstaking functioning. "I'm normal there, that's what doesn't let me get better. My death is the normal life which I built all those years around the fetish." He lived on his savings, and his entire existence was drawn into the treatment, collapsed into the treatment. He wanted to be "hospitalized in treatment," and to *be*. To exist. To feel real.

But now it seemed that the defensive shield of the perversion had been totally breached. "Fetishistic energy isn't an energy of life; it's energy that repairs death. It's between life and death—dead-alive, more dead than alive; death-in-life," he said. Indeed, I, too, had written on perversion as an "autotomous" massive splitting defense in the service of psychic survival so that "not all of me shall die": "The perverse act seizes and clutches, preventing in its corporeality, in its actuality and intensity, a collapse into dread, psychic deadness and total internal annihilation. Perversion is the pervert's last-ditch attempt to halt the fall into the abyss" (Eshel, 2005, pp. 1078–1079).

But now this last-ditch attempt to halt the fall into the abyss had collapsed. Perversion no longer repaired death, no longer secured survival. Throughout this year, death was the very heart of his existence. It was everywhere, all the time, invading every hour with menacing forcefulness.

He came to every session, never late, never asking for any change of time, arriving psychically and physically ill—"the fetish and violence are destroying every bit of goodness in me"—or lifeless, empty, without the strength and will to live. Frequently, he would sleep during the sessions—a still, motionless and soundless sleep. He would leave me many telephone messages, at least one message a day, and on Wednesdays and weekend breaks, when we did not meet, he would leave several messages. His words in the sessions and in the messages were full of despair, harrowing emptiness, and death, and no attempt on my part to understand and interpret had any significance, meaning, or impact. He would say over and over again, "I have nothing to say to you, Ofra; I simply have nothing to say to you. Everything is one huge nothing. I'd rather be sucked into a black hole. Everything's a load of bullshit, everything's empty words, it's better to be sucked into the nothingness, Ofra, and finished—to disappear completely. I just don't have any plans, I don't want any plans, anything—just nothing, Ofra, nothing, I have nothing to say. Everything is so pointless, including your words . . . . They're so meaningless, there's nothing in them, Ofra, nothing, nothing."

Suddenly, unexpectedly (and perhaps not so unexpectedly) during this period, harsh details of his very early childhood were revealed. Until now, whenever he had asked his mother about his childhood, she had answered, "Everything was fine." But now when he asked, she said, "It was very hard," and told him about the dead baby. It turns out that his mother had had six pregnancies. Two of them ended in miscarriages before the birth of his brother, who was 18 months older than he. As a result, she was prescribed total bed rest during that pregnancy. She did not work at all during those years, since she was pregnant most of the time, and the pregnancies were difficult. He thought that his father wanted a lot of children. When his mother was pregnant with him, she fell while carrying his brother in her arms, and thought that she was going to miscarry again. But he was born, a year and a half after his brother, with a heart defect—persistent truncus arteriosis—for which he was operated on at the age of seven with only his father present. His mother did not come to the hospital.

In the year after his birth, "when I was very small," he said—his mother did not remember exactly when—she gave birth to another son in her sixth month of pregnancy, and the baby died twelve days later. She remembered only that they had told her something was wrong with it. She did not remember whether she ever saw it, did not remember whether she stayed in the hospital for the twelve days until the infant died. It did not have a name. She did not remember whether they buried it, "but somewhere inside [his] head," he remembered that she had once told him that his father and his grandmother (her mother) had taken care of the matter, and buried it. When he was 20 months old, his mother became pregnant with his next brother, who was born when he was two-and-a-half years old, and she almost died in childbirth.

I suggested that we were beginning to understand that during those early years his mother had undergone dreadful experiences, misery, suffering, depression and death. I said that a baby is born into the psyche-and-body of its mother and comes into being and grows there. And he was born to a mother who became distraught, alive-dead, and his yearning as an infant and small child to attach to and grow within her psyche and body had overwhelmed and filled him with her agonized feelings—with depression, death, a dead baby.

At first it seemed that these words held meaning for him. "I'm a tiny baby that terrible things have happened to," he said. Two-and-a-half years later he would say: "I went mad when I was a baby," but now this emergent understanding very quickly turned into a terrible, lethal attack on my capacity to really meet, take in and feel the desperation of the fundamental nothingness and death within him. It became something which came from without, illusory, "as if"—too far from that baby and small child overwhelmed by traumatic, annihilating impacts. The more there were words and the greater the understanding, the wider yawned the gap he felt was between us; and there was no real contact with death and dying.[4] He said repeatedly: "I'm a dead baby and a perverse adult. All day I've been thinking that I want to die tonight, don't want to get to tomorrow. And that's it. I hope I'll die tonight. Simply feel completely redundant, Ofra, completely redundant. You're so healthy, Ofra, and I'm so sick. There's no point of connection between us. There are big words, and a big illusion, and big lies, but nothing apart from that. After the session with you, I hope I'll go to sleep and won't wake up. Won't wake up."

I said: "Then your body-psyche will decide whether we will be able to go on." And at the end of each session I did not know whether he would survive and come to the next session. There no longer seemed to be even the fragile reminder of his sense of life and hope; only a state of devastating despair.

Analysis was now a meeting place with a terminal object (in Bollas's sense, 1995, p. 76)—indeed, a terminal and annihilating[5] object—and the despair of his first year of life. Was this his way of making me meet and experience the terminal, annihilating, invasive presence of a depressed, dead-alive m/other in the grip of depression and death, who induced depression and death, and who could not be extricated from death? Or might it be that damage that begins so early cannot be repaired—as he repeated over and over—except in death? To die, and then perchance, to begin anew?

I was reminded at that point of the last words of Otto Weininger, a brilliant young thinker, imbued with self-hatred, hatred of his Jewish ancestry and hatred of women. A year after he published his book *Sex and Character* and converted to Protestantism, at the age of 23, he wrote in his final notes: "An honest man, when he feels that he is irreparably deformed, goes willingly towards death" (Sobol, 1982, p. 121). He wrote this and then killed himself. I was becoming exceedingly worried.

I suggested, for the first time in my clinical work, that he should go back to the psychiatrist who had referred him to me and get some medication that would afford him temporary relief from this terrible suffering. But he replied angrily and bitterly, "How can you say that to me? I thought you were holding the hope, you and psychoanalysis. I don't need anything else to keep my body alive; for that there's the fetish, big time, and familiar for so many years. But I don't exist. I'm not. There's nothing here. I'm dead. That's the fundamental thing—I'm dead." His words, I felt, cried out the very real ongoing desperation of his being . . .

"In the very ill person there is but little hope of new opportunity" (Winnicott, 1954a, p. 281). Inwardly, I struggled to find some hope while faced with this overwhelming, immense desperation. I seized upon Winnicott's writings on "Fear of breakdown" (published posthumously in 1974), and its continuation in "The psychology of madness" (1965a), which are of great importance to me. Winnicott relates to the disastrous impact of being broken down in infancy, at the time when "the ego-organization is threatened. But the ego cannot organize against environmental failure in so far as dependence is a living fact" (1974, p. 103). The extreme agony of early breakdown, which Winnicott also calls Madness X (1965a), is so unthinkable and "indescribably painful" that it cannot be experienced; and a massive defense organization, which the patient displays as an illness syndrome, must be organized against it. In my patient's case, it was the ferocious fetishistic-masochistic perversion that turned him from a passive victim of unbearable early damage and destruction into an active "doer" of them, over and over again, while beneath it there yawned an abyss of inner death and emptiness.

I reminded myself that, according to Winnicott, in those depths of annihilation and the agony of early breakdown or Madness, a profound inner struggle arises between the buried, unexperienced past agony, and a "*basic urge*" to experience it and thus have it "be recovered in experience . . . remembered in the reliving of it" (1965a, p. 126) in treatment. This evokes the fear of breakdown or of the return of the original madness, but also the patient's great need to reach to this original, unthinkable state of breakdown, to risk reliving and experiencing the early agony—this time in treatment, with the analyst and his or her different holding and "auxiliary ego-supporting function" (1974, p. 105) that will make recovery possible.

I thought that we were now within this process, touching the core breakdown, madness, and profound devastation. But I was not sure whether he would be able to survive the extreme horror of it. Can one survive contact with such excruciating breakdown and annihilation? In "Fear of breakdown," Winnicott refers to his patient whose suicide he did not manage to prevent—a patient who wanted to die because of her deep feeling of inner death that had already happened to her psyche in early infancy, although her body continued to live. She killed herself in despair of finding a solution, thus consigning her body to the death which had already happened to the psyche (1974, p. 106).

In the face of these relentless death threats, I tried to extract a promise from him that he would not commit suicide during the next six months.

I said, "I won't continue the treatment unless you promise not to kill yourself." He replied, "What, you'll abandon me just like that, after five years like this?"

I said, "You'll always have a place in my thoughts, I'll always care about you, and I'll always think about what's happening to you and how you feel—whether you are alive or dead. And I think that that's the way you'll feel about me. But I won't continue the treatment if you don't promise that you won't kill yourself. There's no point to it if you've already chosen death."

He said: "And if I promise and don't keep the promise?"

I said: "I trust your promise."

He did not promise. But, he did stop threatening to kill himself. Yet, both in the sessions (he never failed to attend each session) and in the many phone messages that he left me, he wished every night that he would not wake up in the morning. He repeatedly said: "I felt sick looking at the internet sites of violence and evil last night. I wished that I wouldn't wake up in the morning. Nothing's happening, I'm completely dead. I've completely despaired of you, of the treatment. Two years without actually engaging in fetishistic activities, and the fetish in my brain is winning, is taking over. And I'm dead, Ofra, simply dead. I'm simply dead. That's it."

I would reply: "These are very troubled words. Thank you for not despairing of sharing these feelings with me." But I felt that my words were also an attempt to protect myself from the intensity of this violent, repetitive desperation to which I had no answer.

The breakthrough

I now come to the point at which something different transpired. It was a Monday session, after the weekend break. At the beginning of the session he said that he was dead. True, for more than two years he had not engaged in any more fetishistic activity, and this month he was not even entering the internet sites, but he was dead. Nothing was happening inside him. Over the weekend he had tried meeting women again, but these meetings did nothing for him. "Nothing's happening. I'm dead, just dead," he said, and fell silent. His words reached deeply within me. Is death really victorious? I no longer tried to extricate us from this state with agreements and promises or with interpretations.

I said: "We've done things. Things have happened. We're trying to do the best we can in this fateful encounter of ours, but we really don't know whether we'll succeed in crossing this huge dead place. It's like sailing on a tiny boat in an ocean of death . . ."

He remained silent, collapsing into a sleep-like state, until the end of the session.

I sat behind him, and Ansky's play *The Dybbuk* came to my mind—how the possessing spirit, the dybbuk, was exorcized from Leah, but then she died. And here, the fetish has gone, but will he live? And I saw a sort of *pieta*—not Michelangelo's well-known, frontal, seated *Pieta*, but a figure of a woman walking with a dead body in her arms. I saw her from the side, did not see her face, and she was wandering about. I felt terrible distress, which changed to acceptance, and then I felt sorrow—very quiet, profound, pure sorrow; without words, even to myself; it was as if this sorrow had become all being. I sat within this immense sorrow, in silence, until the session was over. At the end of the session I woke him up, and he went away, heavily, stooped. Outside, it was dark. Was it the end?

Late that night (more than two hours after he left) he called me, sounding excited. He said,

> When I left you I wandered around. Eventually I got to the gutter district. I went to the same place where that prostitute had been [a prostitute who three years earlier, after an act of sado-masochistic fetishism, had kissed him and said, "Why are you like this?"]. She wasn't there. There was someone else, someone I think I did fetishistic acts with a long time ago.
>
> "I paid her a reasonably small sum, and she agreed to a kiss and to do it with her hand. [As I mentioned earlier, this was a man who had not been able to bear the touch of a hand, particularly a non-violent touch, and certainly not on his sexual organ.] She had high heels, but it made no difference, and she had breasts, and a mouth like that. It went very quickly and very smoothly, perhaps too much so. When I finished I trembled terribly, and I burst out laughing. I said, "Wow, it went so easily." She didn't understand what I was talking about, or why I was trembling. So that's it, it wasn't like other times, it was nice to get it out like that, it's a shame that I have to pay for it and do it in the gutter. But perhaps it's a stage, I don't know, perhaps it's a stage. I'm still talking to you from the gutter district of Tel-Aviv.

I said, "You sound excited." "Yes," he replied, "I'm happy, it's so strange."

The next morning, he left me a long phone message: "I had to tell you how I *feel* this morning. I came home tired last night and went to sleep. I think that a lot of tiredness had accumulated inside me last night. What happened this morning, there were many times that I wanted very much to come to treatment or to hide there. But this morning I got up, and I don't remember such a real feeling or one so intense as this feeling. I think the only thing in the world I wanted when I opened my eyes this morning was to come and hide in treatment. Don't know whether it was to hide in you or with you—it's all the same. It's unbelievable how much *I wanted to come to you* [laughs]. Then I said to myself, it's not so terrifying, in any case it'll be several hours until you get there, and it'll be different then. But that's it, that's it. I wanted to tell you, but I didn't want to disturb you early in the morning. So I waited a couple of hours, telling myself 'She said that I could call.' OK, we'll meet at two."

We met at two.

From that point onward, although there were other difficult periods, there was a beginning of new movement, and a new sense of aliveness, at first hidden, but gradually becoming more apparent. I think about Winnicott's unforgettable words in "Fear of breakdown:" "But, alas, there is no end unless the bottom of the trough has been reached, unless *the thing feared has been experienced*" (1974, p. 105, italics in original). And I add: "Unless the bottom of the trough has been reached, *unless the thing feared has been experienced*" in a compassionate holding, within the analyst's "presencing" and interconnecting with the patient's gripping unbearable agony, devastation and death. Analyst-and-patient t(w)ogether there, with-in. For me, it was a very deep moment of *com-passion* and *at-one-ment* with the patient's innermost emotional reality.

P. called the year that followed "a mad race of hope and illusion." Now, suddenly, he no longer masturbated at night to the fetishistic-masochistic fantasy: "What amazed me was that I had within me some amazing inner strength which I'd never before experienced—I'm sure I'll still pay for it—something which stopped me from performing a fetish. Strange things are really happening. The shoe in the fantasy has disappeared, as if something has blotted it out. I don't know what to say."

He began relationships with two women (he was still afraid of a relationship with only one). He met them, ate with them, listened and talked to them, related to them, entered their houses and their beds. "They are surrogates for learning to live with a woman," he said. The dreadful emptiness gradually faded, but when he tried having sex with them his penis was dead. Yet, although he was extremely embarrassed by these repeated experiences with both women, he refused to imagine a fetish fantasy with them, though he was sure that by doing so he would have had an erection. He repeated over and over, determinedly, "I want different sex. In those moments with them, I *felt*. I was deeply depressed, I was sad, but I was there. I really *was*. I existed."

It was also when masturbating that he "bamboozled the automaton" and "created an alternative parallel track." He would now say repeatedly, "We'll live and we'll see." He also began to dream.

One of the two women left him because he refused her suggestion to take Viagra. He met another woman named Doreen, beautiful, and several years older than himself. He felt that "something real is beginning to bud there," and she became his only partner. After three months of "feelings of terror—terror, not simply fear—in bed," his penis began to function. At the session in analysis, exactly two years after the session described earlier in which the "bottom" of psychic death had been reached (I was surprised to see that it was on exactly the same date—January 21), he said to me: "I'm waiting for the stage that my search will find myself. As for the tiny boat in the huge ocean, I'm relying on you, and perhaps on myself. It's hard to believe that things change so much." I was surprised to hear that he had retained within himself the memory of the tiny boat in the ocean.

After nine months of the relationship with Doreen, during which he told her about the perverse fetishistic-masochistic world he had been in, and she stayed with him, he said to me in our Monday session, after the weekend break:

"It's seventy-three hours since we met. We've given me a brainwashing. Now I need a heart-washing—I want to learn to love. I want to connect, heart and soul. Inside me, in a sort of bizarre quantum leap, things have been happening that I don't know where they come from and where they're going to, but, fuck it, I'm not complaining. Every time I say, wow! things have been happening, I don't know from where; I also think I'm not trying to destroy them—but even if I did want to destroy them, I doubt whether I would succeed. And all weekend long I've been saying to you, '*Houston, we have a problem.*' Once a spacecraft caught fire, and once a spacecraft was saved. I intend to be saved. Just as once I used to say, 'There's nothing inside me and I have nothing,' this time I *want*, this time there is inside me, and I *have*. I want to feel more . . . I think that what I'm missing now is love. My brain's racing like mad, my dick is already here, but it's not happening yet in my heart. Still deep-deep-deep-deep, it's not happening yet. Houston, we have a problem here. You have to reply."

And I replied: "Houston hears, Houston's thinking. It's really a distant and dangerous journey, opening up like that and wanting so much to feel."

He said: "All weekend long I said to myself and to you, 'I'm on a journey that began without me, but will end with me.'"

Concluding thoughts: unless the bottom has been reached

This difficult treatment demanded of me to descend-with the patient into breakdown and total sense of devastation, deadness, despair, and hopelessness. My patient's dedication to the analysis, and Winnicott's unique words on experiencing the patient's early breakdown were there with me.

According to Winnicott (1974), the breakdown that has already happened cannot be accessed due to the extreme defense of not-yet-experienced terrifying core agony, and the collapse of temporality. Thus,

> The only way to 'remember' in this case is *for the patient to experience* this past thing for the first time in the present, that is to say, in the transference. This past and future thing then becomes a matter of the here and now, and *becomes experienced by the patient for the first time*.
>
> (p. 105, my italics)

This also applies to emptiness: "Emptiness occurring in the treatment is a state that the patient is trying to experience, a past state that cannot be remembered except by being experienced for the first time now" (p. 106). I emphasize that in order *for the patient to be there and experience* these agonizing feelings, *the analyst must be there*, with-in. Only then, can the deadly breakdown that has already happened be experienced and lived out t(w)ogether in the treatment.

I think of my patient and what transpired during the analysis in terms of the distinction between *suffering* and *feeling pain*, where in *feeling pain* the pain-inducing event cannot be endured and worked through within the bounds of the psyche, but merely touches upon its border, affecting it painfully and traumatically with every recurrence (Federn, 1952; Bion, 1965; Mitrani, 1995; Eshel, 2013a). Pain, catastrophe, despair and dying—bombarding experiences that the mother could not take into herself and thus suffer her baby's agony and contain and mitigate it—were now relived, powerfully and desperately bombarding the boundary of my psyche. Bion's (1959) powerful words achieved critical emotional realness here:

> From the infant's point of view she should have taken into her, and thus experienced, the fear that the child was dying. It was this fear that the child could not contain . . . This patient had had to deal with a mother who could not tolerate experiencing such feelings.
>
> (p. 104)

But worse than that, my patient, as a baby, had had to deal with a mother who was herself overwhelmed by unbearable traumatic feelings, thus overwhelming him, violently, fatally, with the deadening impacts of her psychic reality. She was not the "dead mother" described by Green (1986; also Eshel, 1998a, 2016a—chapter 3 in this book), whom the child must find a way to enliven. Rather, she was a mother who inflicted devastating catastrophic feelings, depression, death, a dead baby, which possessed and threatened the child's psychic existence, thus rendering him a traumatized, ravaged, near-death infant-child.[6]

Bollas (1995) similarly notes:

> The sadomasochists are still trapped by their need continuously to remaster an early trauma, although they have converted the anxiety of annihilation into the excitement of its representation . . . . These sadomasochistic alliances enact the near-death of the self, in which the child self avoids its killing but forever feels the near-hit as a kind of narrow escape . . . . That the self did indeed once nearly meet its end, that there *was* something awful in the environment that caused such mental intensities is an unexamined feature of the sadomasochist's life.
>
> (pp. 209–210)

I would say, in keeping with Winnicott's ideas of *fear of breakdown* (1974), that the advances of the third and fourth year of the analysis "ended in destruction" (p. 105) because there was *no reconnecting to the full intensity of the patient's breakdown and annihilation.* But these unbearable core experiences could not be escaped. Therefore, over the entire fifth year, all these menacing, unbearable, uncontained and unsuffered feelings were overwhelmingly relived in the treatment, bombarding the boundaries of his psyche and mine, in a desperate plea to be taken in, suffered, and transformed. I was there with these feelings, speaking about them and speaking them, thinking and understanding them, struggling to ensure survival; more and more in the grip of these feelings, but not yet there, in the patient's inmost devastation, not "unless the bottom of the trough ha[d] been reached, unless *the thing feared ha[d] been experienced*" (Winnicott, 1974, p. 105).

I was experiencing the *terror* of breakdown, suicide, and death, but not yet death itself. Until the time that I starkly took them into myself and *was with the dying child-man, holding the dead body in the arms of my psyche*—thinking, feeling, and "dreaming" the death (Bion, 1992, p. 216; Ogden, 2004; Eigen, 2001; Grotstein, 2007, 2009). Thereby, this desperate attacking plea turned into suffering and profound immense sorrow within me. It became a wordless, deep psyche-to-psyche interconnectedness and com-passion; and the death that was taken in and *became experienced and suffered for the first time* by me-with-him-in-oneness, was transformed, and could then become, within him, a different new possibility of being and experiencing.

Epilogue

Go with me to an end with love

Six years have passed since "the call to Houston." It can clearly be said that the descent in analysis into the realness of annihilating breakdown, devastation, emptiness, psychic death, and suicidal despair—and reliving them patient-with-analyst t(w)ogether, enabled the fundamental possibility of being-in there and experiencing the catastrophic impact, and coming through it differently.

Indeed, P. has lived during the last years in a satisfactory relationship with a woman, and has attained a higher level of functioning in life, even enjoying it. Yet, he refuses categorically to end analysis. The only attempt, three years ago, to end the analysis after a year of working through the imminent separation, came to an end when in the last month he suffered a bout of depression and then had a serious accident on the very day that was supposed to be the last day of the analysis.

He cannot leave analysis, he has told me sadly and repeatedly, because he is still unable to love. "Still deep-deep-deep-deep inside, love is not happening yet," neither to his spouse, nor to himself. He does have a relationship, a solid and good relationship, but this is not love; the love he longs for is still missing. In spite of the great change that has occurred, he still cannot experience or convey real love. This longing was accompanied by a powerful regressive urge in analysis to go backwards, earlier and earlier, to have a chance to relive and feel what he had missed when he was very little.

Was psychoanalysis able to relive this very basic love? And could I? I came to know, indeed to live, a deep, unyielding devotion in this analysis; but love? In the language of the Talmudic story (pp. 181–182), it is as if the little lion-cub has been rescued and released, but he is no longer alive and fiery; and he desperately wants to become fierily alive again.

One evening after P.'s session, sitting immersed in these thoughts, I heard from far away Leonard Cohen singing "Suzanne," a song that I had not heard for many years, and I recalled the words:

> And just when you mean to tell her that you have no love to give her
> Then she gets you on her wavelength
> And she lets the river answer that you've always been her lover
> And you want to travel with her, and you want to travel blind
> And you know that she will trust you
> For you've touched her perfect body with your mind.

These words brought my thoughts full circle, and the turmoil within me was stilled. I was certain that P. had "got me on his wavelength," and we have traveled t(w)ogether with-in his emotional reality for many years. And this journey, with love, unknowing, withnessing, trust, and hope deeply woven into the fabric of its being, still goes on and has not reached an end. The quest for the fiery vital spark of life and love continues.

Notes

1 The Talmud (Hebrew תַּלְמוּד *talmūd* "instruction, learning," from a root *LMD* "teach, study") is a central text of Rabbinic Judaism. The term "Talmud" primarily refers to the collection of post-biblical writings named specifically the Babylonian

Talmud (*Talmud Bavli*), although there is also an earlier collection known as the Jerusalem Talmud (*Talmud Yerushalmi*).

2 *Collins Dictionary: 21st Century Edition* (2002, pp. 690 and 561, respectively).

3 Israeli astronaut, killed when the space shuttle *Columbia* was destroyed upon re-entering the Earth's atmosphere in 2003.

4 It felt very similar to the impenetrable "catastrophic loneliness" of the severely traumatized patients and the ineluctable separation between analyst and patient, that Grand (2000) powerfully described: "The trauma survivor remains solitary in the moment of h[is] own extinction. No one knew h[im] in the moment when he died without dying; no one knows h[im] now, in h[is] lived memory of annihilation. This place where he cannot be known is one of catastrophic loneliness . . .. Death has possessed h[im] in its impenetrable solitude" (p. 4).

5 I would like to add an intense description by Eigen (2010) of annihilation, which is closely related to the agonizing experience expressed here: "Annihilation is not a static state. It goes on and on and on. It's electrifying. I don't have the words for it. It's like being in an electric chair with the current continuously on, or being suffocated but you never die. You keep getting more and more suffocated . . . . I felt that this is partly what babies must feel, in their own way . . . . Screaming and screaming and then the scream fades away" (pp. 26–27).

6 The new concept of "epigenetic transmission" is rooted in such traumatic environmental conditions or traumatic attachment in early life (Jacobson, 2009; cited in Zulueta, 2012). This may explain Boris's (1987) fateful words: "Some infants, more than others, may have an idea that they ought to die, if not now, soon, if not acutely, chronically. . . . But as analysis shows, primal programmatic urgencies continue throughout life" (pp. 353–354). Gonzalez (2010) similarly describes the foundational, deadening impacts of a profound condensation of life with death that began in early childhood.

Chapter 9

The "voice" of breakdown

On facing the unbearable traumatic experience in psychoanalytic work

How can the "voice" of trauma and breakdown be imagined?

In this chapter I will be addressing the "voice" of trauma and breakdown from theoretical and clinical perspectives—in particular, the profound difficulty of hearing this silenced, crying "voice;" the critical importance of experiencing the unbearable and the unexperienced *with* the analyst; and the immensity of the terror and hope that lie at the heart of reaching to the original unbearable traumatization in psychoanalytic work.

The "voice" of trauma and breakdown

At the beginning of his far-reaching, seventh and last chapter of *The Interpretation of Dreams* (1900), Freud introduces an unexpected proposal. It comes just after he describes the "moving dream" of the burning dead child *who was standing beside his sleeping father's bed, caught him by the arm and whispered: "Father, don't you see I'm burning"* (p. 509)—a dream explained by Freud (simply, if enigmatically) as a wish-fulfillment dream that transforms the dead child into a living one; the dream thus fulfills the father's wish that the child still be alive. But this dream has also been reinterpreted as though Freud's later theory of trauma in "Beyond the pleasure principle" (1920)—of traumatic repetition, especially regarding traumatic nightmares—is already whispering here, pleadingly, from within the very theory of wish-fulfillment (Lacan, "Tuchè and Automaton," in Caruth, 1996).

It is then, following this startling crying dream, that Freud proposes that after "the work of interpretation" we veer to a new path—not "towards the light, elucidation and fuller understanding" of all the earlier paths, but *into "darkness."* He writes:

> It is only after we have disposed of everything that has to do with the work of interpretation that we can begin to realize the incompleteness of our psychology of dreams . . . . For it must be clearly understood that the easy and agreeable portion of our journey lies behind us. Hitherto, unless I am greatly mistaken, all the paths along which we have travelled have led us *towards the light*—towards elucidation and fuller understanding. But as soon as we endeavour to penetrate more deeply into the mental process involved, every path will end *in darkness*.
>
> (pp. 510–511, my italics)

Twenty years later, Freud (1920) encounters and grapples with the notion of trauma in his seminal and complex essay "Beyond the pleasure principle," often regarded as one of his most intriguing and provocative essays. Although he begins with the dominance of the pleasure principle in psychoanalytic theory, he goes *beyond* the pleasure principle to the compulsion to repeat traumatic experiences and traumatic dreams that "disregard the pleasure principle in every way" (p. 36). This leads him, throughout the essay, to a radical reformulation of his metapsychological theory founded on the primacy of the pleasure principle.

Freud first addresses the change in the aims of psychoanalytic technique after 25 years of intense work. At first, the focus was on

> discover[ing] the unconscious material . . . psychoanalysis was then first and foremost an art of interpreting. Since this did not solve the therapeutic problem . . . the chief emphasis lay upon the patient's resistances . . . . But it became ever clearer that the aim which had been set up—the aim that what was unconscious should become conscious—is not completely attainable by that method. The patient cannot remember the whole of what is repressed in him, and what he cannot remember may be precisely the essential part of it . . . . He is obliged to *repeat* the repressed material as a contemporary experience instead of, as the physician would prefer to see, *remembering* it as something belonging to the past.
>
> (p. 18, italics in original)

Freud then elaborates the concept of trauma, which necessarily implies "a breach in an otherwise efficacious barrier against stimuli" (p. 29), provoking the compulsion to repeat which is "more primitive, more elementary, more instinctual than the pleasure principle which it over-rides" (p. 23). It is the vital task of the compulsion to repeat, to master or to bind the excessive stream of excitations. Only after this task has been accomplished, is it possible for the dominance of the pleasure principle (and its modification, the reality principle) to proceed unhindered.

Freud notes that in some people these repetitions are particularly striking. "They give the impression of being pursued by a malignant fate or possessed by some 'daemonic' power" (p. 21). He illustrates this with a strange, dramatic story:

> The most moving poetic picture of a fate such as this is given by Tasso in his romantic epic *Gerusalemme Liberata*. Its hero, Tancred, unwittingly kills his beloved Clorinda in a duel while she is disguised in the armour of an enemy knight. After her burial he makes his way into a strange magic forest which strikes the Crusaders' army with terror. He slashes with his sword at a tall tree; but blood streams from the cut and the voice of Clorinda, whose soul is imprisoned in the tree, is heard complaining that he has wounded his beloved once again.
>
> (p. 22)

The disastrous actions of Tancred, mortally wounding his disguised beloved in a battle and then, unknowingly, seemingly by chance, wounding her again, powerfully represent for Freud the way that the experience of a trauma repeats itself, unwittingly and unremittingly, through a person's unknowing acts. This repetition, at the heart of the trauma, which overrides any principle of pleasure and reality, thus also created "an extensive breach" (Freud, 1920, p. 31) in Freud's theoretical and clinical thinking.

Cathy Caruth, who writes extensively on trauma, bases her intriguing book *Unclaimed Experience: Trauma, Narrative, and History* (1996) on this particular point in Freud's article, and elaborates the notion of "the wound and the voice"—the crying wound. She evocatively suggests that

> The resonance of Freud's example goes beyond this dramatic illustration of repetition compulsion and exceeds, perhaps, the limits of Freud's conceptual or conscious theory of trauma. For what seems to me particularly striking in the example of Tasso is not just the unconscious act of the infliction of the injury and its inadvertent and

> unwished-for repetition, but the moving and sorrowful *voice* that cries out, a voice that is paradoxically *released through the wound.* Tancred does not only repeat his act but, in repeating it, he for the first time hears a voice that cries out to him to see what he has done . . . . Tancred's story thus represents traumatic experience not only as the enigma of a human agent's repeated and unknowing acts, but also as the enigma of the otherness of a human voice that cries out from the wound, a voice that witnesses a truth that Tancred himself cannot fully know.
>
> (pp. 2–3, italics in original)

For Caruth, the moving quality of this story is its striking juxtaposition of the unknowing, injurious repetition and the witness of the crying voice. This is a "double wound" because the wound-trauma of the psyche, unlike the wound of the body, is an event that *is originally experienced too unexpectedly and overwhelmingly to be fully known*, and is therefore not available to consciousness until it imposes itself again, in the repetitive actions and nightmares of the survivor. It is its very unassimilated nature—the way it was precisely *not known* in the first instance—that returns to haunt the survivor later.

Therefore, according to Caruth,

> what the parable of the wound and the voice thus tells us, and what is at the heart of Freud's writing on trauma, both in what it says and in the stories it unwittingly tells, is that trauma seems to be much more than a pathology, or the simple illness of a wounded psyche: *it is always the story of a wound that cries out, that addresses us in the attempt to tell us of a reality or truth that is not otherwise available.*
>
> (1996, p. 4, my italics)

This "voice," in its delayed emergence and its belated address that stubbornly insists on bearing witness to a disconnected, silenced, hidden wound, brings us to the need for analytic hearing of ear, mind, and heart—a "hearing heart," as I have earlier suggested (Eshel, 1996, 2004a, 2015a; chapter 1 in this book).

But what is the necessary, correct, or even feasible way of hearing trauma when faced with its enigmatic, tantalizing appearance of muteness, repetition and a strange cry, of a pleading demand to know along with inaccessibility, of a disguised, mortally wounded woman and a tree that streams blood—especially in a situation of massive dissociation? What is the meaning of this repeated "double wound" crying in the clinical situation?

Caruth begins her book with a citation from Tasso:

> Though chilled with horror,
> with a second blow
> He struck it, and decided then to look
> (Tasso, Jerusalem Liberated,
> quoted in Caruth, p. 1)

What then is the meaning, to the patient, to the analyst/therapist, of being "chilled with horror" when the traumatic experience threatens to emerge, and how is this horror to be faced in treatment?

Into the breakdown

"[I]t is so difficult for us to believe that Freud has left us to carry on with the researches that his invention of psycho-analysis makes possible, and yet he cannot participate when we make a step forward," writes Winnicott, late in his life (1969c, p. 241). In my view, Freud's extraordinary theory of trauma in "Beyond the pleasure principle" (1920) has germinated later innovative ideas, research, and unknown future developments relating to trauma and traumatic memory in psychoanalytic theory and practice. And yet,Freud came to an abrupt halt with regard to understanding the critical meaning of actual childhood trauma and its complex and harsh implications in the clinical experience of psychoanalytic treatment.

Freud abandoned the seduction theory as early as 1897, in a sharp and enigmatic shift, since the seduction theory—that neuroses are the consequence of a child's sexual abuse by an adult, usually the father—had been so central to his original formulations of hysteria in the two preceding years (1895, 1896).[1] Consequently, the study of trauma in psychoanalytic thought and practice since Freud was considerably delayed, and evolved significantly, for the most part, in the last few decades and in terms of dissociation rather than repression. It can be said that the psychoanalytic exploration of trauma itself followed a *traumatic course* and therefore also needed a double, belated emergence to find a "voice." This traumatic course had its stormy inception in the early period of psychoanalysis. The work of Sandor Ferenczi (1873–1933), especially in his last years, brought to the fore the importance of actual childhood trauma and its impact on personality and on the analytic treatment. It created a growing, tragic and irreconcilable rift between Freud and him, particularly over Ferenczi's final innovative clinical thinking and the presentation of his last, seminal paper "Confusion of tongues" (1933), which led to allegations that that he had become mentally ill, and to his subsequent ostracism from the psychoanalytic community (Haynal, 1988; Stanton, 1990; Aron and Harris, 1993; Aron, 1996; Berman, 2004; Eshel, 2016a, d).

Whereas Freud abandoned the seduction theory and replaced it with the intrapsychic drive model, infantile fantasies and repression, Ferenczi strongly emphasized the realities of childhood traumas of sexual and physical abuse and the subsequent dissociation, fragmentation, and even atomization of the personality. He maintained that dissociation, unlike repression, defends against overwhelming memories of traumatic experiences. These claims were a daring contradiction of Freud's view that memories of sexual abuse are based on instinct-driven fantasies. Furthermore, Ferenczi investigated daring therapeutic methods for coping with the reliving of traumatic overstimulation, terror and dissociation in treatment, with the analyst serving as an important reparative force.

> "[E]ither Ferenczi was seeing patients [Freud] had not seen before or, more likely, that Ferenczi was seeing what Freud could not allow himself to experience and therefore to see", suggests Bollas (2011); Ferenczi "could follow psychoanalysis in ways that [Freud] could not bear".
>
> (pp. xv, xvi)

After Ferenczi's untimely death and the ostracism of his later ideas by the psychoanalytic community, it took many years for the issues of childhood trauma, dissociation and the possibility of accessing memories of childhood abuse to be readdressed in psychoanalytic theoretical and clinical thinking. In the British psychoanalytic literature, these ideas were developed mainly by psychoanalysts of the Independent (Middle) group with regard to object-relations theories, traumatic early relationships and therapeutic regression. This group included Balint, Ferenczi's analysand and disciple, who attempted a conciliatory gesture toward Freudian "classical" theory and technique (1968); Winnicott (1945, 1965a, 1965b, 1974); Khan

(1963, 1964, 1971); and Fairbairn (1952) in Edinburgh. In the American literature this area was addressed by Sullivan (1954); Shengold (1989); Modell, who wrote extensively about the effect of trauma on memory (1990, 2005, 2006, 2009); Levine (1990a, 1990b, 1997, 2014); and Herman (1992). From the end of the 1980s and the early 1990s this subject was frequently discussed by relational psychoanalysts: Davies and Frawly, who focused on the treatment of adult survivors of childhood sexual abuse (1991, 1992, 1994; Davies, 1996); Bromberg (1998, 2006, 2011); Donnel Stern (1997, 2003, 2004, 2009, 2010, 2012); and Howell (2005), who defines trauma as the "event(s) that cause dissociation" (p. ix). In France, Davoine and Gaudillière (2004) have produced groundbreaking work on madness and trauma.

The exploration of trauma in the clinical situation revolves around the profoundly complex relation between the silenced, dissociated wound and the voice that cries out; the knowing–not-knowing of the unbearable traumatic experience, at once demanding and inaccessible. It is a kind of unbearable double telling—the story of the unbearable nature of the traumatic experience and the story of the ongoing unbearable nature of its survival (Caruth, 1996). "Traumatic experiences do not produce memories but actualities" (Hernandez, 1998), and the horror of reaching to the original trauma, which both defies and demands going there.

For me, the most inspiring psychoanalytic writings in this regard are Winnicott's posthumous papers "Fear of breakdown" (thought to have been written in 1963, but published posthumously in 1974), and its continuation in "The psychology of madness" (1965a), and "The concept of clinical regression compared with that of defence organization" (1967a). Winnicott describes the disastrous impact of breakdown at the beginning of one's life. The extreme primitive agony of this early breakdown, which Winnicott also calls madness X, is so unthinkable and "indescribably painful" that it cannot be experienced. Therefore, a new massive defense organization of a psychotic nature, displayed as the patient's illness syndrome, must be constructed immediately against it, in order to shut down and decimate this threat of unthinkable agony. Consequently, the individual becomes imprisoned in an extremely dissociated, ever-present "unthinkable state of affairs that underlies the defence organization" (p. 103), which has already happened, but since it has not yet been experienced, it cannot get into the past tense, and is feared and compulsively sought after in the future. It is thus a timeless, ongoing catastrophe, then, now, about to happen—never and forever;[2]

an endless impact on one’s being that will continue until and unless it is relived and experienced.

Winnicott describes a profound inner struggle in those depths of unthinkable agony of early breakdown or madness—a struggle between the buried, unexperienced, dreadful past agony and a “*basic urge*” to experience it and thus “to be recovered in experience because it cannot be recovered in memory . . . madness can only be remembered in the reliving of it” (1965a, p. 126, 125, italics in original). It is to be relived in treatment, with the analyst, “in reaction to the analyst’s failures and mistakes,” but at the same time, and more importantly, with the analyst’s different holding and “auxiliary ego-supporting function,” which will make recovery possible. Thus, the crux of the analytic work that this thinking entails, relates to the crucial question of how this reliving of the devastating past is to happen this time—will it be in the same unthinkable, unexperienced way, or can it happen and be lived through and experienced even though it has not been experienced and could not have been experienced before? Could there be a “hope of getting at something here in the analysis that had never been before” (Winnicott, 1986a, p. 32)?

The strength of Winnicott’s (1974) words—“‘breakdown’ to describe the unthinkable state of affairs,” “primitive agonies (anxiety is not a strong enough word here),” and “these traumatic events carry with them unthinkable anxiety, or maximal pain” (1967a)—captures what is so difficult and crucial in this reliving, experiencing and recovering of early breakdown in treatment.

Thus, using Caruth’s words, it is the treatment that will be the venue of the “double wounding”—through the belated emergence of the trauma and the possibility of hearing the voice that cries out from the wound. And with the addition of Winnicott—the treatment will actualize both the cry of the belated traumatic reactivation and a new opportunity, never before experienced, for reliving, experiencing, and correcting it.

The great clinical significance of Winnicott’s ideas relating to fear of breakdown is powerfully emphasized by Winnicott himself, from the very beginning of his paper: “My *clinical experiences* have brought me recently to a new understanding, as I believe, of the meaning of fear of breakdown . . . which is new for me and which perhaps is new for others who work in psychotherapy” (Winnicott, 1974, p. 103, my italics; cf. Ogden, 2014).

Clare Winnicott (1980) also underscores this crucial clinical importance in strong words: “The moment at which I connected what was happening in the treatment with the theoretical formulation in Winnicott’s paper 'Fear of breakdown' was for me one of those cumulative experiences when everything adds up and comes together. At that moment I saw the *possibility* of a favourable outcome for my patient" (1980, p. 351, italics in original).

Indeed, Winnicott's vision opens new possibilities of understanding and working analytically with the more deeply disturbed aspects of patients' personalities and experiences. Max Hernandez, an eminent Peruvian psychoanalyst, writes in this regard:

> Winnicott's notion, in a way, could be considered a radical reworking of one of Freud's last clinical comments—a reworking of vast consequences. Freud (1937b) wrote, "Often enough, when a neurotic is led by an anxiety-state to expect the occurrence of some terrible event, he is in fact merely under the influence of a repressed memory (which is seeking to enter consciousness but cannot become conscious) that something which was at that time terrifying did really happen. I believe that we should gain a great deal of valuable knowledge from work of this kind upon psychotics even if it led to no therapeutic success" (p. 268). But for Winnicott (1974) [regarding more psychotic phenomena], "the original experience of primitive agony cannot get into the past tense unless the ego can first gather it into its own present time experience and into omnipotent control now (assuming the auxiliary ego-supporting function of the mother (analyst))" (p. 105). In the analytic process, the patient may stop looking for or to the past event not yet experienced only if s/he gathers the original environmental failure into the area of her/his omnipotence within the transferential experience.
>
> (Hernandez, 1998, p. 137)

The emphasis thus lies in allowing the unbearable agony to be gradually experienced and lived out with the analyst in the treatment situation.

"All this is very difficult, time-consuming and painful," writes Winnicott, "but alas, there is no end unless the bottom of the trough has been reached, unless *the thing feared has been experienced*" (1974, p. 105, italics in original).

Thus, the cardinal question here, and in my opinion one of the most difficult questions at the heart of psychoanalytic work, is how willing are we, analysts and therapists, to reach to the unbearable realness of the patient's most traumatic experience, breakdown and madness; to face the chilling horror and pain in hearing the voice that cries out from the bleeding wound; "a voice from the crypt" in Grotstein's words (2010, p. 10). When the patient in treatment repeatedly points to the ongoing wounding, without the ability to go through it, how do we stay within and go through these devastated-devastating states of catastrophic change—*in statu nascendi*—until patient-with-analyst "t(w)ogether" become able to experience, tolerate and cope with the anxieties that were unthinkable in their original setting.

"Someone must feel it in order for us to embrace it as reality" (Eigen, 2004, p. 65). I believe that it is only by *being within* the patient's deepest feeling states and their emotional impact, within the gripping pull toward breakdown and recovery until "*the thing feared has been experienced*"—that the catastrophic impact turns into a catastrophic change (Bion, 1965) and can *become a catastrophic chance*.

In the previous chapter (chapter 8), I described this approach by using a clinical example of a very difficult analysis with a severely fetishistic-masochistic patient. The cessation of perverse practices in the third year of analysis led to an extreme collapse, especially during the entire fifth year, into profound devastation, emptiness, psychic death and violent suicidal despair. Working within this collapse in analysis enabled the deep reason for the patient's breakdown in early life to unfold. And most importantly, it engendered the crucial possibility that had never been experienced before, of reliving the patient's unbearable breakdown and deadness—this time t(w)ogether with the analyst—and experientially coming through it differently.

I will now further illustrate this thinking with three detailed clinical examples from psychoanalytic writings by Hernandez, Guntrip, and Guttieres-Green, and from an autobiographical essay by Virginia Woolf. All of them bear the inscription of an early breakdown, in which a massive defense organization has shut down and decimated the experience of unthinkable agony. It thus lurks within the psyche as an unexperienced, unlived and dead part, deeply woven into the psychological fabric of their living. Hence, the critical importance in the treatment of *experiencing the unexperienced*, rather than uncovering a particular trauma; that is, the fundamental possibility of being-there, patient-with-analyst, to undergo the annihilated-annihilating experience that made it impossible for the patient to be there and experience it alone.

Case illustrations

Hernandez: the breakdown that was heard[3]

Hernandez, in his perceptive theoretical-clinical paper (1998), expands Winnicott's conception of early breakdown to a theory of trauma in general: the unbearable traumatic reality that has already happened cannot be accessed and experienced due to its massive defense organization and temporal displacement, thus producing an ever-present sense of both imminence and avoidance of the traumatic experience. Hence, Hernandez emphasizes the critical importance of being with the patient in the full impact of the "unthinkable state of affairs" and the secondary traumatization that takes place in the clinical situation, without imposing meaning on "the unthinkable void, that emptiness full of pain of primitive agonies" (p. 140). This necessitates the analyst's adaptation to the patient's ego needs, so as to provide holding, and ensure that the recurring experiences of anticipatory fear of breakdown gradually fall within the range of the patient's growing capacity.

Hernandez illustrates this way of working with the unbearable traumatic experience using clinical material taken from a long analysis of a 30-year-old man who sought treatment for the anxiety he felt whenever he was at work or with friends—feeling that his boss "picked on him," and that his friends laughed at him. There were moments, he said, when this anxiety was intolerable. In such moments, he feared he would fall to pieces or worse. He had twice been hospitalized for attacks of unmanageable anxiety, and knew it was bound to happen again. Toward the end of the first session he told Hernandez that he had to entrust something to him but he had better wait for an appropriate moment. He was trembling and did not shake hands with Hernandez because he was sweating. During the treatment, he spoke about his life and family. He had been a lonely, sad, withdrawn boy. He was a very good soccer player, and that had been his only solace. During puberty he had felt extremely self-conscious. It was "hell" to get changed before and after the matches. The boys laughed behind his back, and that prevented him from becoming a professional player. He finished his studies and continued living with his parents. His mother had recurrent bouts of depression, and had been hospitalized several times when he was a small child.

> On one occasion, toward the end of the session, he said, in an almost inaudible tone, that he was worried about "being followed." He could

not explain this feeling, but he urged me to believe him. He did not pursue the point for some time. He spoke about how uncomfortable the sweating and tremor in his hands were for him. People realized he was nervous and were either condescending or would make jokes about him. Life was very difficult. He had bouts of insomnia, and he would wake up in the middle of the night sweating, without being able to recall what he had dreamt. After some time, he said he had to tell me what he had intimated in the first meeting. He became even more tense and nervous, and he told me that he had been raped by a group of boys. It had happened during a school outing, when he was eight years old. Afterward they had mocked him. He remained silent for the rest of the session. For some time, he spoke in an almost obsessive manner about a friend who had betrayed him with a girl. Perhaps this friend knew what had happened to him. At times he imagines, or "kind of sees, like in a film," the whole episode. Then suddenly he questioned me as to why I had not asked him about what had happened to him. While I remained silent, he grew tense and anxious. I said that he might be feeling that I did not realize how painful the whole experience was for him, and that I did not care about it at all. In the next sessions, he referred to the moments that preceded the rape and to what had occurred when he went back home: no one paid any attention to him in spite of the fact that his underwear had bloodstains on it. I told him that he might be feeling my silence as he had felt his parents' lack of response in the past.

At that period in the analysis he was worried about losing his job: he was going to end up in the psychiatric ward again. He kept referring to "that which happened to me." I noticed that, without having a very clear explanation for it, whenever I referred to this point I said, "that which you said happened to you." On one occasion, immediately after I had said this, he stood up very angrily and said, staring at me: "You don't believe me? Are you saying that I'm a liar?" He was trembling and sweating copiously. I told him: "It seems it hasn't happened, it is still happening." He wept all through the session. At the end I accompanied him and indicated that he could wash his face, and I waited by the door until he left. During the following weeks he went into the rape episode, exploring with great diffidence the reasons for his submission, his passivity, and his bewildering emotional tie to the gang leader. He tried to be precise about the circumstances. Yet the exercise

> seemed to lead nowhere. But then in one particular session his manner of speaking changed. He spoke in a grave, somber manner of his having felt himself to be outside of his body, as though he was not himself, as if he were emptied, lifeless. While pointing very slowly and with great effort to the lamp plug, he said, in a low voice, "as if someone had disconnected me from life itself." It seemed as if he had been able to face the naked, terrible experience that lay under the anxiety, the fears, and the "flashbacks" of the violation itself.
>
> (pp. 138–139)

I feel that the treatment experience here gradually, carefully, and with much sensitivity and patience carved out a place through the patient's "paranoid" reactions; a place where the inaudible voice that erupted from the depths of the trauma could be heard—the stifled crying from the bleeding double wound-trauma of the rape and the overwhelming parental neglect that he had suffered as a child prior to the rape. And this thoroughgoing way enabled the unfolding of the traumatization until the growing terror of the annihilated-annihilating innermost core was reached. The catastrophic reactivation, undergone *with* the analyst, became a *catastrophic chance*.

Guntrip: the deadly breakdown

I will now proceed to another more complex clinical illustration, in which the information about the trauma was known, but was a totally unremembered, not-yet-experienced breakdown—an early breakdown that "has already happened" but "has not happened yet" (in Winnicott's words). It is Guntrip's own case described in his autobiographical paper, "My experience of analysis with Fairbairn and Winnicott: (How complete a result does psychoanalytic therapy achieve?)." According to the *Collins Dictionary,* "complete" means "absolute, perfect, finished, having all the necessary parts, [Latin—*complere*, to fill up]," and all these meanings are correct here.

The paper (1975), written towards the end of Guntrip's life, addresses the question in the subtitle from the outset, as regards Guntrip's psychoanalytic treatments with Fairbairn and Winnicott, two outstanding psychoanalytic figures:

> The question 'How complete a result is possible?' had compelling importance for me because it is bound up with an unusual factor; a total amnesia

> for a severe trauma at the age of three and a half years, over the death of a younger brother. Two analyses failed to break through that amnesia, but it was resolved unexpectedly after they had ended . . . and yet each in different ways prepared for its resolution as a post-analytic development.
> (pp. 145–146)

Guntrip's account centers on his mother's failure in mothering him, and is based on what she told him in his teens and as an adult. Guntrip's mother was an overburdened "little mother" before she married, because her mother, "a feather-brained beauty queen," left her to manage her eleven siblings, even as a schoolgirl. This responsibility for her widowed mother and younger siblings impressed Guntrip's father, a Methodist preacher who established and led a Mission Hall. They married, but he did not know that she had already had her fill of mothering babies and did not want any more. She breastfed Guntrip because she believed it would prevent another pregnancy; but she refused to breastfeed his brother Percy who was born when Guntrip was two years old and died when Guntrip was three and a half, after which she refused further intimacy. When Guntrip was one year old, she opened a business which lost money steadily for seven years, and left him to the care of an invalid aunt who lived with them.

Guntrip's total amnesia revolved around the trauma of Percy's death and all that lay behind it:

> [Mother] told me that at three and a half years I walked into a room and saw Percy lying naked and dead on her lap. I rushed up and grabbed him and said: "Don't let him go. You'll never get him back!" She sent me out of the room and I fell mysteriously ill and was thought to be dying. Her doctor said: "He's dying of grief for his brother. If your mother wit can't save him, I can't", so she took me to a maternal aunt who had a family, and there I recovered. Both Fairbairn and Winnicott thought I would have died if she had not sent me away from herself. All memory of that was totally repressed.
> (p. 149)

After Percy's death and his return home, Guntrip began four years of an active battle to force his mother into mothering him: from age three-and-a-half to five, with repeated psychosomatic illnesses and dramatic, sudden high temperatures; and from age five to seven, with disobedience, as he began school and became more independent. His mother would fly into violent rages and beat him cruelly. At the age of seven he attended a larger school and steadily developed a life of his own outside his home. When he was eight, his mother's new shop became an outstanding success. She became less depressed, giving him all the money he needed for various hobbies and activities. In her old age, his mother would say, "I ought never to have married and had children. Nature did not make me to be a wife and mother, but a business woman" (p. 149). "When your father and Aunt Mary died and I was alone, I tried keeping a dog but I had to give it up. I couldn't stop beating it" (p. 150).

Guntrip felt that his experiences of schizoid isolation and unreality, and especially the mysterious exhaustion illnesses triggered by abrupt separations from "Percy-substitute" friends, were caused by the unremembered severe trauma of his brother's death, his own subsequent illness, and the earliest relations with his mother. These exercised on him "an unconscious pull out of life into collapse and apparent dying" (p. 149). Therefore, in spite of his apparent success as minister of a church in Leeds, a psychotherapist and a family man, he sought psychoanalytic treatment.

But the amnesia persisted throughout the rest of Guntrip's life and two analyses, until he turned seventy. His analysis with Fairbairn began at age 48 and continued for 11 years, up to age 59—over 1,000 sessions (1949–1960). Fairbairn focused, according to his theory, on an oedipal analysis of the "internal closed system" of internalized libidinal and anti-libidinal bad-object relations in Guntrip's post-Percy period. However, after three or four years of analysis, Guntrip felt that his real problem was not oedipal three-person bad-object relations and conflicts, but his mother's failure, from the start, to relate to him, and his deeper schizoid problem. The crunch came after eight years of analysis, when the sudden death of Guntrip's long-time friend resulted in another terrifying eruption of "Percy illness." However, at that time, Fairbairn was seriously ill and unable to work for six months, interpreting, upon resuming work, that in his illness he had become Guntrip's dying brother in the transference. Guntrip, afraid that due to Fairbairn's frail state of health, he would have no one to help him with the intense reactivation of the Percy-trauma and afraid of Fairbairn's dying on him, resolved to seek analysis with Winnicott before Fairbairn died.

Guntrip went to Winnicott from Leeds once a month for several sessions, and had 150 sessions from age 61 to 67 (1962–1968). He felt that Winnicott's profound intuitive contact with infancy enabled him to reach back to an ultimate good mother at the very beginning of his life and recreate her in Winnicott in the transference. Winnicott thus entered into the emptiness of Guntrip's earliest traumatic years left by a non-relating mother, which the Percy-trauma embodied. It was not just the loss of Percy, but a double trauma of both Percy's death and being left alone with a mother who could not keep him alive that caused Guntrip's collapse into apparent dying; but now, he felt he was no longer alone with a non-relating mother.

Guntrip last saw Winnicott in 1969 (Winnicott returned ill from New York at that time, but Guntrip does not mention this). On New Year's Day in 1971 he heard that Winnicott was ill, and about two weeks later he was informed that Winnicott had passed away. That same night Guntrip had a startling dream. He *saw his mother, black, immobilized, staring fixedly into space, totally ignoring him as he stood at one side staring at her and feeling himself frozen into immobility*. It was the first time he had ever dreamt of her like that; previously she had always attacked him. His first thought was, "I've lost Winnicott and am left alone with mother, sunk in depression, ignoring me. That's how I felt when Percy died" (p. 154). He was afraid that the loss of Winnicott was becoming a repetition of the Percy-trauma. But eventually he realized that this time it was different. He had not dreamt of his mother in other abrupt separations and death—Then he fell ill, as after Percy's death. This time a compelling dream sequence began, which continued, night after night, taking him back in chronological order through every house he had lived in, until the house of the bad first seven years. Family figures appeared, his father and mother kept recurring—his father always supportive, his mother always hostile, but no sign of Percy; he was trying to stay in the post-Percy period of battles with mother. Then, some two months later, two dreams finally broke through the amnesia over Percy's life and death. Guntrip *saw himself in a dream clearly aged three, holding a pram containing his one-year-old brother. He was strained, looking anxiously over to the left at his mother, to see if she would take any notice of them. But she was staring fixedly into the distance, ignoring them, as in the first dream of that series.*

The next night the dream was even more startling:

> *I was standing with another man, the double of myself, both reaching out to get hold of a dead object. Suddenly the other man collapsed in a heap. Immediately the dream changed to a lighted room, where I saw Percy again. I knew it was him, sitting on the lap of a woman who had no face, arms or breasts. She was merely a lap to sit on, not a person. He looked deeply depressed, with the corners of his mouth turned down, and I was trying to make him smile.*
>
> (p. 154)

In this dream, Guntrip felt he had retrieved the memory of collapsing when seeing the dead Percy, and trying to grab him. But it was more. He had actually gone back in both dreams to the earlier time before Percy died, to see the "faceless" depersonalized mother, and the black depressed mother, who totally failed to relate to both of them—a contention similarly and powerfully expressed in Ogden's (2014) paper, which expands on Winnicott's "Fear of breakdown" (1974). For Ogden, the breakdown of the mother–infant tie in infancy is the unthinkable agony that could not be experienced; thus, the driving force of the patient's need to find the source of this fear is the feeling that unexperienced critical parts of himself are missing, lost and unlived, and that he must reclaim them. Guntrip was criticized over the years for controlling his treatment primarily by structuring the overall therapeutic situation by means of a self-determined goal of lifting his amnesia (Glatzer and Evans, 1977; Padel, 1996; Markillie, 1996). But, in my view, Guntrip's claim is greatly supported by Ogden's paper.

This dream-series made Guntrip re-examine all of his analysis records, until he realized that although Winnicott's death had reminded him of Percy's, the situation was entirely different. He had not dreamt of Winnicott's death, but of Percy's death and his mother's total failure to relate to them. He compellingly concludes:

> What gave me strength in my deep unconscious to face again that basic trauma? It must have been because Winnicott was not, and could not be, dead for me, nor certainly for many others . . .. Winnicott had come into living relation with precisely that earlier lost part of me that fell ill because mother failed me. *He has taken her place and made it possible and safe to remember her in an actual dream-reliving of her*

> *paralysing schizoid aloofness*. Slowly that became a firm conviction growing in me, and I recovered from the volcanic upheaval of that autonomously regressing compelling dream-series, feeling that I had at last reaped the gains I had sought in analysis over some twenty years. After all . . . had been worked through, one thing remained: *the quality of the over-all atmosphere of the personal relations that made up our family life in those first seven years*. It lingers as a mood of sadness for my mother who was so damaged in childhood that she could neither be, nor enable me to be, our "true selves". I cannot have had a different set of memories. But . . . what is psychoanalytic psychotherapy? It is, as I see it, the provision of a reliable and understanding human relationship of a kind that makes contact with the deeply repressed traumatized child in a way that enables one to become steadily more able to live, in the security of a new real relationship, with the traumatic legacy of the earliest formative years, as it seeps through or erupts into consciousness.
>
> (pp. 154–155, italics in original)

Thus, Guntrip ends on this sad-happy note about breaking through the amnesia and finally being more able to live. When Guntrip wrote this article, he was 73 years old. But by the time the article was published, about a year later, Guntrip was no longer alive (this was announced in a special note on the article's first page). He died before he turned seventy-four, following an operation for cancer of the esophagus; both his analysts had died at about the same age, Winnicott at seventy-four and Fairbairn at seventy-five.

The death of Guntrip, who so wanted to live, leaves me with an uneasy feeling and questions. Guntrip begins the article with the question: "How complete a result does psycho-analytic therapy achieve?" (p. 145). And I ask, "How complete a result *should* psycho-analytic therapy achieve?"

Could it be that Guntrip's body–psyche, frail and aging, was unable to tolerate the breaking through of the dissociation and the return of the early trauma along with the devastating "double wounding" (Caruth, 1996) of Winnicott's death, even though he desperately longed and struggled to break through his amnesia?

Is there a survival wisdom underlying the dissociative defense organization which should be taken into account, despite its cost? Or does being *alone* with these traumatic impacts evoke a return of the overwhelming breakdown, thus reactivating the traumatic memories but not the ability to withstand and live through the immensity of death, abandonment and emotional wounding that erupted once more? Guntrip was "left with the full scale eruption of that traumatic event, and no one to help [him] with it" (p. 151), as he himself wrote before he left the treatment with Fairbairn, fearing that Fairbairn would die as Percy had died.

Further reflections on loneliness, being-with and being without

Over the years, I have come to regard the story of Oedipus primarily as the tragic story of a person who attempts to break through massive early dissociation all alone, and is destroyed by his uncompromising lonely struggle to reach to the underlying unknown and fatal breakdown in his early childhood.

In particular, I am reminded here of Virginia Woolf's posthumously published autobiographical "Sketch of the Past" (1976/2002), which closely resonates with Guntrip's writing and was also written in the last two years of her life. Like Guntrip, she expresses a deep yearning to be attached once again to her past experiences and to relive her entire life more fully, with more "moments of being":

> Is it not possible—I often wonder—that things we have felt with great intensity have an existence independent of our minds; are in fact still in existence? . . . Instead of remembering here a scene and there a sound, I shall fit a plug into the wall; and listen in to the past . . . I feel that strong emotion must leave its trace; and it is only a question of discovering how we can get ourselves again attached to it, so that we shall be able to live our lives through from the start.
>
> (p. 81)

Woolf, too, describes struggling with a sudden sense of unreality and "non-being": "There was the moment . . . when for no reason I could discover, everything suddenly became unreal; I was suspended; I could not step across the puddle; I tried to touch something . . . the whole world became unreal" (p. 90). "As a child then, my days, just as they do now, contained a large proportion of this cotton wool, this non-being . . . Then, for no reason that I know about, there was a sudden violent shock" (p. 84).

Woolf's "Sketch of the Past" describes her life under the shadow of a series of traumas and the deaths of her mother, her half-sister Stella (her mother's oldest daughter from her first marriage who replaced the dead mother), her father and her brother Thoby. Even her parents' marriage was a second marriage for both after the deaths of their beloved first spouses. Woolf writes,

> My mother's death had been a latent sorrow—at thirteen one could not master it, envision it, deal with it. But Stella's death two years later fell on a different substance; a mind stuff and being stuff that was extraordinarily unprotected, unformed, unshielded, apprehensive, receptive, anticipatory . . . . But beneath the surface of this particular mind and body lay sunk the other death . . . when once more unbelievably—incredibly—as if one had been violently cheated of some promise; more than that, brutally told not to be such a fool as to hope for things; I remember saying to myself after she [Stella] died: "but this is impossible, things aren't, can't be, like this"—the blow, the second blow of death, struck on me; tremulous, filmy eyed as I was . . . sitting there on the edge of my broken chrysalis.
>
> (p. 130)

In addition, as a young child Woolf had been sexually abused by her adult half-brother, Gerald Duckworth.

Four months after she ceased writing "Sketch of the Past," Virginia Woolf committed suicide by drowning herself in the River Ouse (leaving a loving and grateful letter to her husband, just as Guntrip had left a grateful last letter to his family).

Is this once again the "trance of horror" brought on by *experiencing all alone* the reactivation and the overwhelming destructiveness of these unbearable traumatic memories? In Woolf's words: "that collapse . . . as if I were passive under some sledge-hammer blow; exposed to a whole avalanche of meaning that had heaped up and discharged itself upon me, unprotected, with nothing to ward it off" (p. 90).

Oedipus, Guntrip, Virginia Woolf—for me, they embody the unprotected excruciating *loneliness* of the encounter with innermost traumas that are too terrifying to experience.

What I am trying to say regarding the clinical work goes beyond the analyst's death (in Guntrip's account), to the *analyst's not-being there*—whether literally or emotionally absent. I believe that in order to reach to the very heart of the traumatic dissociated state and its terror, the analyst has to be-there, within the patient's world, in a way I describe as the analyst's "presencing" within and the ensuing deep patient–analyst interconnectedness or "withnessing" in going through the process (Eshel, 1998a,b, 2001, 2004a,b, 2005, 2006, 2007a 2009, 2010, 2012b, 2013a,b; 2014, 2016, 2017b, chapters 1–8 of this book).

The patient–analyst "*withness*" or deep interconnectedness of patient-*with*-analyst—carries still further the concept of "witness" that has increasingly gained currency in psychoanalytic thinking, particularly in cases of trauma (Caruth, 1995; Donnel Stern, 2012; Reis, 2009a). It is this very fundamental quality of the analyst's "withnessing" presence that engenders a different possibility within the traumatic zone, where that possibility had been previously absent and foreclosed. In Eigen's rendering of Winnicott's notion of not-yet-experienced breakdown, "Winnicott points to a terror too terrifying to experience as a moment searching for someone to endure it, if only a little, or a little at a time" (2004, p. 26).

This being with-in the terrifying reactivation of the traumatic experience evokes Ogden's (2001b) spontaneous statement to his patient, "I won't let that happen," at the height of the patient's state of overwhelming anxiety and feelings of impending disintegration when recalling his childhood neglect and his molestation by a neighbor. "I was aware that I was promising a lot," writes Ogden (p. 166), and in a telling footnote adds: "I do not believe that I could spontaneously have said [that] to the patient, had I not spent many years reading and rereading Winnicott's papers on the psyche-soma and the role of regression in the analytic process" (p. 171). "I won't let that happen"—now the analyst's presence with-in, interconnected-to-the-patient, won't let that happen . . .. And in Ogden's later words on Winnicott's "Fear of breakdown": "The patient is not alone when he is with an analyst who is able to bear the patient's and his own experiences of breakdown and primitive agony" (Ogden, 2014).

However, it is difficult and daunting to undergo the traumatic experience, whether as witnessing or as "withnessing" that may grow into at-one-ment with the patient's innermost experience, for the trauma destroys and distorts the psyche. Even in the modern mythology of Harry Potter, who as a baby survived Voldemort's murderous assault because his mother sacrificed her life to protect him, the last book reveals that at that time a fragment of Voldemort's evil soul inadvertently latched onto

Harry's soul (*Harry Potter and the Deathly Hallows*, Rowling, 2007). The reliving of the trauma floods the treatment with the unbearable that needs experiencing—with breakdown, madness, loss, destruction, psychic death, agonizing despair and helplessness, distortion and "identification with the aggressor" (Ferenczi, 1933), mounting psychological and physical risk. They permeate, impact, attack, and desecrate the analyst psyche when he or she is being-there, within. Various descriptions have been given to this traumatic impact: traumatic countertransference (Herman, 1992), "contagion" of trauma (Terr, 1985), vicarious traumatization (McCann and Pearlman, 1990), secondary traumatic stress (Baird and Kracen, 2006), eight patterns of transference-countertransference in survivors of childhood sexual abuse (Davies and Frawley, 1994), and "countertrauma" (Gartner, 2014). According to Davoine and Gaudillière (2004), the analyst must become the "horrified other" who allows the impact of the trauma to break down the boundaries of analyst and analysand, of past and present.

I would like to illustrate this way of thinking with an agonizing clinical example.

Guttieres-Green: the abandoned breakdown

This clinical example is taken from André Green's last book, *Illusions and Disillusions of Psychoanalytic Work* (2011), published several months before his death. The book explores, theoretically and clinically, disappointing and sometimes tragic processes in psychoanalytic treatments. The clinical section presents a dozen disappointing or failed cases drawn from Green's analytic work and from the clinical experience of his colleagues, followed by a short commentary by Green on the difficult essential points or characteristics of the case. This is interesting because Green rarely presented clinical examples in his writings. It can be said that here Green goes beyond himself, "goes beyond a comfortable position concerning clinical practice and introduces a deep approach to failures in psychoanalytic treatment" (Fiorini, 2011, p. ix).

I will relate to the case reported by analyst Litza Guttieres-Green, entitled "Ariane: an unresolvable transference." This is a difficult analysis of a 41-old woman, Ariane, which took place over 20 years ago. Ariane was referred to treatment because of severe anxiety attacks, accompanied by a feeling that she did not exist, alcohol abuse, disappointing love affairs and suicide attempts. She spoke of a void, a black hole that both terrified and attracted her.

Ariane's mother was ill from her birth and died when Ariane was six; the child suffered very early in life from feelings of terror and hostility. She remembered nothing of her childhood. Her only recollection related to her mother's burial: she had been left at home, and, from the window, saw a crowd of people and her family dressed "in black." She had been afraid and had hidden under the table. In spite of her difficult childhood, she had successfully completed a university degree, was highly regarded, married a fellow student, and had two children. But she saw all this as a "frantic headlong flight" during which she did her best to "fill holes," without managing to avoid depressive episodes.

Due to political events, Ariane and her husband were forced to go into exile with their two very young children, and Ariane became severely depressed. She went through failed psychotherapies, and risked her marriage by leaving her husband and returning to him several times. She lost her job. She underwent short-term psychiatric hospitalizations because of suicide threats, panic attacks and alcohol abuse, and was treated with psychotropic medications, all to little avail. When first consulting Guttieres-Green, Ariane maintained that she had no more hope and that "death would be a liberation."

In spite of this difficult clinical picture, Guttieres-Green accepted her for treatment, and the relationship between them became at once difficult and fragile. A constant sense of emergency prevailed, with treatment occasionally interrupted by hospitalizations. Guttieres-Green experienced feelings of helplessness and thought she was going through something akin to what her patient was describing. It was difficult to follow the flow of associations, to memorize, understand, think about and interpret the confused material. Sometimes Guttieres-Green was overcome by extreme sleepiness during the sessions, barely managing to keep her eyes open. She tried to maintain a setting that was capable of containing and protecting the patient—and herself—against the patient's destructiveness. She read Freud, Ferenczi, Winnicott, Tustin, Green, in search of answers to problems the patient was confronting her with. She came to believe that Ariane's mother had been unable to establish ties with her daughter that could survive her own death and give her daughter a sufficiently secure basis. Ariane had not acquired confidence in a lasting and reliable relationship; she withdrew behind a mask of narcissistic indifference, while the grudge and hatred against her deceased mother were being relived in the transference.

Gradually, however, Ariane's acting out decreased, more elaborate material appeared, and real analytic work began. Ariane came regularly and no longer spoke of discontinuing treatment. She acknowledged her dependence and attachment, and she also took care of her children. She now brought many dreams to treatment. Although she was not free of anxiety, her capacity for insight led her analyst to hope that matters would develop favorably.

The *hole*, the *void*, which Guttieres-Green and Ariane's previous therapists interpreted as representing Ariane's mother's tomb in which she had taken refuge, were now linked by Ariane to *a lack at the origin of her life*. "I would like to find a sense of continuity again to fill this void," she said. She had always connected it with her mother's death because her therapists, Guttieres-Green included, had made this link for her, and because she did not know how to interpret it.

> I think that it was before [mother's death], something that did not happen left a hole. I've never been able—or known how—to speak about it. I began to understand when I told you that I did not know my mother. (p. 125)

Here Guttieres-Green said to herself that the loss of memory hid a breakdown that had already happened (according to Winnicott, "Fear of breakdown").

Buried memories and unconscious fantasies gradually became accessible, although they retained particular characteristics. While Ariane was able to render her fantasies into images and communicate them to her analyst, she pointed out that in all her dreams the characters "spoke" in French, the language of the analysis, and not in her mother tongue. It was in the course of the analytic work that she learnt to look at them directly, in her analyst's presence; even if they remained frightening, she was able to find the words to represent them. She said, "I have learnt to speak with you" (p. 127). However, these representations had a massive, repetitive character, as if there was a link that she could not make, so that she was unable to get beyond them. Something remained unrepresentable.

Was it not the "voice" of the core catastrophe that happened long ago and still goes on, unmet, *not-yet-experienced*? According to Guttieres-Green's description, different interpretations of the void, the black hole, the deadly tomb, did not succeed in creating hope in a more stable way. For Ariane, what was empty and missing was always more important than what was full; hate triumphed over love. She said:

> I am desperate because in spite of the changes, I continue to feel alone and empty. My life has no meaning even though I cannot say why. What we have understood and reconstituted together surrounds a hole. What is in this hole, I will never know; it did not take place, quite simply, and that is what is lacking. So I cannot know what I am lacking, nor can I have any hope of filling this void.
>
> (p. 127)

Guttieres-Green consoled herself with the symptomatic improvements: Ariane seemed calmer, and less self-centered; she spoke about those around her, and not just about her own terrors.

The following summer, the patient decided to end the treatment and return to her country of origin with her children and husband. The treatment ended after the summer vacation. Ariane would telephone from time to time; gradually, the telephone calls became less regular—Guttieres-Green thought that Ariane only wanted to make sure that she was alive—and then they stopped altogether.

I quote the final paragraph, verbatim:

> She came back; several years had gone by, and I was horrified by her appearance: she had grown older, of course, but she seemed degraded; her husband had left her and remarried; her children had gone away to study, and had started to work. They were doing well, but she did not see them much. They had their own lives. "Everyone has abandoned me, I am alone," she said with a little smile. She was not looking after herself, and had no money; she showed me her ruined teeth: "I've aged, you can see!" I asked her if she was in therapy. "No, I would like to come back to you." I refused. She understood, but she had hoped it might be possible, she said, with her little resigned smile. Staring into space, she seemed to be dreaming . . . about what? I will never know. She left again, leaving me with the feeling of having witnessed a disaster and of having been partly responsible for it.
>
> (p. 128)

I think that this is a tragic and disastrous ending[4]. In what I am about to say I am not being critical or condescending towards Guttieres-Green. I appreciate her frankness and courage in presenting this difficult case. All of us, analysts and therapists, have been faced with moments, places, individuals in treatment—hopefully not many—that render us unable, or unwilling, to go on treating. And a severely disturbed patient, who arrives without any money, without a husband, all alone, wretched and degraded, with rotting teeth, does not generate a willingness to take her back into treatment again.

But let me reconsider this case in the light of Caruth's and Winnicott's ideas with regard to hearing the crying "voice" of devastating early trauma and breakdown. I would rely here particularly on Winnicott's radical ideas of "fear of breakdown" where, as Clare Winnicot commented, "something surfaced from the depths of clinical involvement into conscious grasp and produced *a new orientation to a whole area of clinical practice*" (1974, p. 103, my italics). And Winnicott himself maintains, from the very beginning of the paper, that this new clinical understanding of the meaning of a fear of breakdown leads to a restatement of "problems *that puzzle us as we fail to do as well clinically as we would wish to do*" (p. 103, my italics).

It seems to me, given my understanding of Winnicott's notions of "fear of breakdown" and "The psychology of madness," that this was not an untreatable patient with "obstinate and insurmountable resistance to recovery" as André Green concludes in his commentary on this case (p. 131). Nor was she, in Green's words, "a gaping hole that the psychic work cannot fill, the content of which even she is unable to imagine," with "transference, which resisted analysis, . . . without any possibility of evolving . . . she continues to be like an open wound" (pp. 130–131). Rather, her return was a fateful moment in which a real *breakdown* was being conveyed. The patient was confronting her analyst with the essence of her catastrophe, her being lonely, lost, empty, her collapsing to the very lowest level. In this concrete and terrifying way, she was handing over to her analyst the relentless imprint of an early disaster on her ruined psyche and life, the true, actual meaning of devastation, desolation and nothingness. Indeed, "*the last scream just before hope was abandoned*" (Winnicott, 1969a, p. 117, italics in the original) cried out from the depths of her inconsolable "open wound."

Moreover, in keeping with Winnicott's (1974) ideas of "Fear of breakdown," I would add that the previous "so-called advances [in the analysis] ended in destruction" (Winnicott, 1974, p. 105) because there was not yet a reconnecting to the full, painful immensity of the patient's breakdown, which was actualized in her return. I believe that this could have become the place-time in the treatment in which "the bottom has been reached" and "*the thing feared*" could be met and experienced (Winnicott, 1974, p. 105). It opened up the possibility of facing the overwhelming nature and extent of the inaccessible underlying catastrophic state, which was waiting to be heard; a possibility not-yet-experienced because from the very beginning of her life, this patient had had an unavailable, seriously ill mother, with whom the matrix experience of "mother and child *live an experience together*" (Winnicott, 1945, p. 152, italics in original) could not take place. This left a "void," a "gaping hole," which the patient became able to feel and convey in treatment, saying "I think that it was before [mother's death], something that did not happen left a hole" (Green, 2011, p. 125). Thus, it now became possible for the first time, in a "past-present actuality" (Eshel, 2004b) for the analyst to be with her with-in the realness of the breakdown, and go through it, patient-with-analyst "t(w)ogether"; the analyst thus bears and experiences with the patient and for the patient the relived breakdown that had already happened but was not-yet-experienced.

André Green ends his book by stating: "It is meaning that provides real holding, and not the object" (2011, p. 190). In my opinion, the emergence of meaning that provides real holding necessitates the analyst's being-with-in the patient's descent into breakdown and total sense of devastation. Eigen writes similarly and poignantly: "More is involved than the capacity to know. . . . A capacity as deep or deeper than the sense of catastrophe must be called forth if healing or profound change is to occur" (1993, p. 219).

I would like to conclude with Bion's powerful words, which I feel are most relevant and important in this regard—one quote is from the Los Angeles third seminar (on 17 April 1967), relating to his patient. The second is from the Tavistock seminar (on 3 July 1978), when Bion was 81 years old, and also, like André Green, an eminent psychoanalytic author after 50 years of psychoanalytic practice.

Bion (2013/1967) relates to his patient:

> [A]ll this goes on in such a way that one is invited to dismiss it as not being of much consequence, he's not getting on with his analysis, or

> something of that sort, and that the experience cannot be as painful as that. Until something happens to your attention to him, and you see the expression on his face, which is quite unmistakable, and which shows *intense suffering*, . . . something of that kind, which is extremely painful to him. So painful indeed . . .
>
> (p. 71, my italics)

And eleven years later, at Tavistock, 1978:

> I don't want to appear to be criticizing or running down my colleagues, but I have recently become more and more convinced that psychiatrists and psychoanalysts *don't believe in mental suffering, and they don't believe in any treatment of it* . . .. Fundamentally they never get to the point of feeling that the person who comes to the consulting room is actually suffering and that there is an approach to it that is on the right lines. Even psychoanalysis may be close enough to be on the right track, to be worth pursuing further. But not, "yes, I know" . . . a technical facility, very easily acquired, tends to produce a barrier against the real thing.
>
> (2005b, p. 48, my italics)

I feel that Lindner (1976) in *The Fifty-Minute Hour*, very early in my therapeutic career, and in later years Caruth (1996), Bion, especially his late writings (1970, 2005a, b; 2013), Eigen's elaboration on "the area of Faith" (1981, 2004), and particularly Winnicott's writings on regression and fear of breakdown, have inspired me to be more daring and have greater faith in the powerful possibility of being-with the patient in experiencing breakdown and trauma; or perhaps they have enabled me to uncover and embrace the daring and the faith that are inside me. And they have also provided me with words to convey the immensity of terror and hope at the heart of this difficult psychoanalytic work.

Notes

1 This was, indeed, a sharp and enigmatic shift. A year earlier, on April 21, 1896, lecturing to the local Society for Psychiatry and Neurology on "The Aetiology of Hysteria," Freud was still committed to the seduction theory before this select professional audience. The great Richard von Krafft-Ebing was presiding. Freud's lecture "was a lively, highly skillful forensic performance . . .

[in an] effort to persuade his incredulous listeners that they must seek the origin of hysteria in the sexual abuse of children. All eighteen of the cases he had treated, Freud noted, invited this conclusion." But the lecture, he wrote irritably to Fliess a few days later, "had an icy reception from the donkeys and, on Krafft-Ebing's part, the odd judgment: 'It sounds like a scientific fairy tale.' And this, after one has shown them *the solution of a thousands-years-old problem, a source of the Nile!*" Well, Freud added rudely, "they can all, euphemistically expressed, go to hell." He perceived the atmosphere around him to be chillier than ever and was certain that his lecture made him an object of ostracism (Gay, 1988, p. 93, my italics). The lecture and the publication of the paper "The Aetiology of Hysteria" (1896) marked the end of this line of Freud's theory of the traumatic origins of hysteria.

2 In T.S. Eliot's words it is "Never and always." "Here, the intersection of the timeless moment/ . . . Never and always" (Little Gidding, p. 215).

3 I am grateful to Dr. Max Hernandez for his generous permission to use this clinical example.

4 I wonder whether the name which Guttieres-Green chose for her patient—Ariane—reveal her own complex feelings over abandoning her patient. Ariane is a French translation of the Greek name Ariadne, a name mostly associated with a woman in love, ruthlessly abandoned. Ariadne, in Greek mythology, was the daughter of Minos, King of Crete, who fell in love with Theseus, the son of King Aegeus of Athens, who came to Crete to be sacrificed to the Minotaur in the labyrinth, but instead intended to kill it. Ariadne helped him by giving him a sword and a ball of thread, so that he could slay the Minotaur and find his way out of the labyrinth. She eloped with Theseus after he succeeded in killing the Minotaur, but Theseus abandoned her, sleeping, on the island of Naxos. Ariadne was desolate and wanted to die, but she was discovered by Dionysus who married her, and they had two children. In the end, however, Ariadne dies a tragic death (in some myths, she was killed, and in others, she committed suicide).

Chapter 10

From extension to revolutionary change in clinical psychoanalysis

The radical influence of Bion and Winnicott

Wilfred R. Bion and Donald W. Winnicott have exerted a profound influence on the theory and practice of clinical psychoanalysis over the past sixty years. Their groundbreaking ideas have been widely investigated by psychoanalysts and psychotherapists around the world, and have turned into a vibrant wave in psychoanalysis that challenges traditional theory and practice. Yet it seems to me that the revolutionary meaning of their most radical ideas has, in certain ways, been evaded, underestimated, or criticized and rejected (also Reiner 2012; Symington and Symington 1996). This is especially true with regard to the radical departure of their clinical ideas from conventional psychoanalytic work. In this chapter, I will attempt to examine the evolution of their clinical ideas into the launching of what I consider a revolutionary approach in clinical psychoanalysis—a transition from *extension* to *scientific revolution* and *paradigm shift* (or *paradigm change*) in psychoanalysis, to use terms derived from Thomas Kuhn's account of the nature of the evolution of science.[1]

In his seminal theory of the evolution of science, Kuhn (1962) argues that scientific theory and knowledge undergo alternating "normal" and "revolutionary" phases rather than progressing in a linear, cumulative acquisition of knowledge. During long periods of "normal science," scientists work to enlarge the central prevailing paradigm by "puzzle-solving activity" that is guided by the paradigm, thus significantly increasing knowledge and accumulating a growing body of puzzle solutions within this paradigm. However, over time, findings or observations that cannot be explained or solved within the context of the central paradigm accrue and pose a serious problem to the existing paradigm. This leads to a "crisis" that triggers revolutionary research. Eventually, a new paradigm emerges, which opens up new approaches to understanding and practice in that field.

Kuhn (1962) writes:

> The transition from a paradigm in crisis to a new one from which a new tradition of normal science can emerge is far from a cumulative process, one achieved by an *articulation or extension* of the old paradigm. Rather *it is a reconstruction of the field from new fundamentals, a reconstruction that changes some of the field's most elementary theoretical generalizations as well as many of its paradigm methods and applications*. During the transition period, there will be a large but never complete overlap between the problems that can be solved by the old and by the new paradigm. But there will also be a decisive difference in the modes of solution . . . . *The resulting transition to a new paradigm is scientific revolution.*
>
> (pp. 84–85, 90, my italics)

The emerging new paradigm gains its own followers, and often an "ensuing battle over its acceptance" takes place between the followers of the new paradigm and the holdouts of the old, normal paradigm. According to Kuhn, this process is followed by a "communication breakdown," and there is a need for "translation" from the language of one paradigm into that of the other in order to "allow the participants in the communication breakdown to experience vicariously something of the merits and defects of each other's points of view." This does not guarantee persuasion, "and, if it does, it need not be accompanied or followed by conversion . . . . For most people translation is a threatening process, and it is entirely foreign to normal science . . . . Nevertheless, as argument piles on argument and as challenge after challenge is successfully met," translation becomes a resource of persuasion and dialogue (Kuhn 1962, pp. 202–204).

I would suggest that late Bion's and Winnicott's theoretical and clinical thinking—and particularly the profound significance and implications of their thinking for the foundations of clinical psychoanalysis and for the analytic process—introduces a revolutionary change in psychoanalysis, stirring up a felt sense of ongoing transition, controversy, upheaval, struggle, and translation. This is especially true of late Bion's recondite conception of *transformation in O*, and of Winnicott's clinical-technical revision of analytic work, with its heavy emphasis on regression and primary communication in the treatment of more disturbed patients; both of these engender formative experiences of being and becoming in order to transform emotional experience from its initial inscription.

To contextualize this argument (and "translation"), let us return to Vermote's (2013) integrative model of psychic functioning for dealing with the unknown or the unthought, presented earlier in chapter 2. Vermote identifies three distinct *zones* or *modes* of psychic functioning to describe the scope of psychoanalytic work and the range of possible psychic changes, each characterized by varying degrees of differentiation, different major psychoanalytic models, and distinct clinical implications for the analyst:

1 The mode of reason—oedipal, understanding Ucs. system (Freud, Klein).
2 Transformation in Knowledge—container-contained, reverie, dream-work, alpha function (Bion, Marty, de M'Uzan, Bollas, Botella and Botella, Ogden, Ferro).
3 Transformation in O, when dealing with the most unthought, unknown, undifferentiated mode of psychic functioning (Winnicott, Milner, late Bion, late Lacan). Real psychic change occurs at the level of *radical experience*, unrepresented and unknowable-O (called O by Bion for Origin),[2] while the *epistemological exploration* of the traumatic unknown, in mode 2 of transformation in Knowledge or dream-thought, remains at the level of representations. Thus, the difference between *transformation in Knowledge* and *transformation in O* is that T(K) is a thought for something that has not been thought yet, and T(O) is a new experience that happens, that can only "be 'become,' but it cannot be 'known'" (Bion 1970, p. 26). "It can only be experienced" (Vermote 2013).

In my view, Vermote's mode 2, transformation in Knowledge, is an *extension* of the existing paradigm, while mode 3, transformation in O, introduces a *revolutionary ontological change* that is taking place in psychoanalysis, reflecting a fundamental commitment to the principle of being and becoming in the experience rather than an epistemological exploration; this extends the reach of psychoanalytic treatment to more disturbed patients and difficult treatment situations.

My own rendering (and synergism) of transformation in O in Winnicott's and late Bion's thinking (as distinct from Brown 2012, Lopez-Corvo 2014,

Ogden 2005b, Reiner 2012, Vermote 2011, and others) clinically underscores the radical, undifferentiated experience of patient-and-analyst being-in-oneness at a primordial point of origin: according to Bion, it is the primacy of the analyst becoming and being-at-one with the patient's unknown and unknowable, ultimate emotional reality-O. According to Winnicott, patient and analyst become merged in primary relatedness within deep therapeutic regressions, akin to the early two-in-one of mother–baby; and the object has to be the first, subjective object[3] of the early phases of emotional development and communication, when reaching in analysis to the deepest non-communicating layers of the patient's personality.

In addition, to my way of thinking, the unknown and unknowable emotional reality-O has become connected mainly with unthinkable breakdown (Winnicott) and catastrophe (Bion). I will discuss this later, after more fully exploring late Bion's and Winnicott's revolutionary ideas, and after briefly relating the "crisis" that triggered these ideas and the complex reactions they have evoked.

Bion

From extension to revolutionary change

The influential concepts of *alpha function*, *container-contained*, and *reverie* constitute the major phase of Bion's work. They have become a fundamental feature in the writings of many psychoanalysts, both Kleinian and non-Kleinian. For me (as I have written in Eshel 2004a), the most inspiring expression of the idea of containing was, and still remains, Bion's (1959) groundbreaking description in "Attacks on linking" (1959, pp. 103–104), in which he carved out a new dimension of normal emotional communication within the pathological nature of Melanie Klein's conceptualization of projective identification. The patient projects his or her unbearable, split-off parts and inner experiences into the analyst's psyche, and it is crucial that the analyst—like the mother for her infant—takes in, processes, and modifies them, thus enabling the patient to reintroject them safely. Hence, it can be said that the existence of containing ultimately depends upon what the recipient is able to bear (this is also vividly described by Bion, 2013, second seminar, of April 14, 1967). Successful containment enables both emotional growth and development of the capacity for thinking.

Thus, Bion's description of containing and reverie marked a divide in the evolution of the Kleinian approach to the transformative function of the real, external other. The availability and capacity of the object—via reverie and alpha function—to take in, experience, modify and contain unbearable projected parts are of vital importance.

Sandler (1988), in response to Bion's descriptions of containing, writes in his comprehensive study of the concept of projective identification:

> By no stretch of the imagination can this [Bion's containing] be understood as occurring in fantasy[4] only, nor is this what Bion intended to imply. What he describes here is a concrete "putting into the object." He [Bion] says: "An evacuation of the bad breast takes place through a realistic projective identification. The mother, with her capacity for reverie, transforms the unpleasant sensations linked to the 'bad breast' and provides relief for the infant who then reintrojects the mitigated and modified emotional experience, i.e., reintrojects . . . a non-sensual aspect of the mother's love."
>
> (p. 19)

Sandler therefore views Bion's containing as the most extreme stage—"third-stage projective identification"—in which "the externalization of parts of the self or of the internal object occurs directly into the external object" (1988, p. 18), whereas Klein's formulation of projective identification into the phantasy object is "first-stage projective identification."

In a similar vein, Spillius (1992), in distinguishing Klein and Bion, coined the term *evocatory* projective identification to describe the sort of projective identification that produces emotional effects on the recipient—as opposed to *nonevocatory*, which has no real effect on the other person (Britton 1998, Spillius 1988). But Sandler goes further and argues for separating the concept of projective identification from the "container" model:

> What I find unacceptable is the notion that this process [containing] is one of projective identification, unless the concept is stretched to extreme limits . . . . The "container" model can, I believe, be fruitfully separated from the developmental theory . . . as well as from the concept of projective identification . . . and has value in its own right.
>
> (1988, pp. 24–25)

However, for Bion, these were extensions. He introduces the concept of *extension* in *Elements of Psychoanalysis* (1963) as follows:

> Psychoanalytic elements and the objects derived from them have the following dimensions:
>
> 1 Extension in the domain of the senses.
> 2 Extension in the domain of myth.
> 3 Extension in the domain of passion.
>
> An interpretation cannot be regarded as satisfactory unless it illuminates a psychoanalytic object, and that object must, at the time of interpretation, possess these dimensions.
>
> (1963, p. 11)

Bion goes on to explain these extensions:

> Extension in the domain of senses . . . means that what is interpreted must amongst other qualities be an object of sense. It must, for example, be visible or audible, certainly to the analyst and presumably to the analysand.
>
> (p. 11)

> It is more difficult to give a satisfactory explanation of what I mean by extension in the domain of myth . . . . They are not statements of observed fact or formulations of theory intended to represent a realization: they are statements of a [the patient's] personal myth.
>
> (p. 12)

He then beautifully explains the last extension in the domain of passion:

> I mean the term [passion] to represent emotion experienced with intensity and warmth though without any suggestion of violence . . . . For senses to be active only one mind is necessary: passion is evidence that two minds are linked and that there cannot possibly be fewer than two minds if passion is present.
>
> (pp. 12–13)

Grotstein (2007) emphasizes that Bion's conception of alpha function and of container-contained "represented a *needed extension of Kleinian theory* into external reality" (p. 116, my italics), and "*modifications and extension of Kleinian technique* . . . [that are] subtle, profound, and far-ranging" (p. 93, italics in original). The major part of Bion's work (and that of his followers) consists of a further elaboration of these ideas into a theory of *transformation in Knowledge*, which is summarized in his grid, delineating the elements of the process and their relations and transition (Vermote 2013).

The emergence of a new be(com)ing

It was only a few years later that Bion radically transformed his psychoanalytic theory and technique with the creation of the concept of O—beginning at the end of his book *Transformations* (1965a), continuing on through his article "Notes on Memory and Desire" (1967a) and *Bion in Buenos Aires*, Third seminar (2018/1968), and particularly in his book *Attention and Interpretation* (1970). This abrupt, radical change was accompanied by his move in 1967–1968 from London to Los Angeles, for the last twelve years of his life.

It was "a transformational moment in Bion's life and thinking . . . on the very nature of psychoanalysis itself" (Grotstein 2013, p. xi). Bion's concept of O necessitated a complete revision of what analysis is; it represented an awareness of the limits of knowledge gained through the senses (Green 1973; Hinshelwood 2010, quoted in Reiner 2012 and Brown 2012) and the limits of analytic thinking (Vermote 2011). Rather than epistemological exploration (knowing), Bion focused on the unknown and unknowable ultimate emotional reality-O, the primacy of the analyst's being "at-one with the reality of the patient" (1970, p. 28),[5] and of lived, new experience. Bion's enigmatic words acquire their full meaning here:

> The psycho-analytic vertex is O. With this the analyst cannot be identified: he must *be* it . . . . No psycho-analytic discovery is possible without at-one-ment with it and evolution . . . . The interpretation is an actual event in the evolution of O that is common to analyst and analysand.
>
> (1970, pp. 27, 30, italics in original)

Bion subsequently offers important guiding words for the practical work of psychoanalysis: "To my belief, K has much to do with understanding, knowing. Basically, I do not consider it to be of great importance for the analyst because he is not interested in knowing O, but in becoming O" (2018/1968, p. 43). "K depends on the evolution of O → K. At-one-ment with O would seem to be possible through K → O, but it is not so" (1970, p. 30). "In practice this means *not* that the analyst recalls some relevant memory but that a relevant constellation will *be evoked during the process of at-one-ment with O*, the process denoted by transformation O → K" (p. 33, my italics).

Furthermore, "the transformation O → K depends on ridding K of memory and desire" (1970, p, 30). The analyst is required to discipline himself with the suspension of memory, desire, and even understanding, in order to preclude any "hindrance to the psychoanalyst's intuition of the reality with which he must be at one" (Bion 1967a, p. 272); to *be in-tu-it* (intuit). To this Bion (1970) added "attention" and "'patience' and 'security'" (p. 124) and called the ability to be at one with O an "act of faith" (p. 32), faith in O. Borrowing the words "dark night of/to the soul" from St. John of the Cross, he took them further to a "'dark night' to K [knowledge]" in analytic work (Bion 1965a, p. 159) and thus to the need for an ontological-intuitive psychoanalytic approach of being in the experience, rather than an epistemological (K) one: "The intuitive approach is obstructed because the 'faith' involved is associated with absence of inquiry, or 'dark night' to K" (p. 159). It can be exerted only when the analyst allows him/herself to experience the "dark night" of the soul (p. 159).

Bion thus "recommend[s] a complete change of the analyst's attitude . . . . In fact, psychoanalysis rests on an act of faith" (Green 1973, p. 117). Eigen (2014) terms this "faith-work" (p. 123).

These unique and radical ideas were a profound ontological change after Bion's long epistemological odyssey (Eigen 2012; Vermote 2013). What was the "crisis" (Kuhn 1962) that triggered his revolutionary exploration and ideas? It seems to me to be deeply connected to *Bion's struggling with psychotic terrors*, both in working clinically with his psychotic patients and, as has been suggested in recent years, with his own severely traumatic experiences as a child and his deathly World War I experience, which have been increasingly explored (Williams 1985; Souter 2009; Szykierski 2010; Brown 2012).

Clinically, I can almost hear this imminent fundamental change lurking in Bion's questioning, poignant words regarding his analytic work with two psychotic patients in the entry entitled: "The Attack on the Analyst's a-Function: The Analyst's Odyssey" (1992):

> "Oh shut up." He [the patient] whispered, "Shut up: shut up."
>
> There are many interpretations I could give, and have given in the past. They are apparently quite ineffectual, there seems to be no particular point in repeating them. What, I wonder, can have happened to them? Years of analytic interpretations, and patience and knowledge that go with them, have been swallowed up by him, or poured into him by me, without apparently leaving the slightest trace. He might simply be a gaping hole or mouth, with nothing beyond it . . . . What in fact links us is endurance, fortitude, patience, anger, sympathy, love. Is the task in hand, the analysis itself, a link? It seems hardly possible because it rarely comes to a point where it might be called analysis . . . .
>
> Take now a different patient. Out it pours—masses of semi-whispered, disjointed stuff, name after name, some of which I know, some I may be supposed to know, some presumably I cannot be expected to know. They are mostly doing something that the patient sees: "It didn't occur to him . . ."; "I ask him, he did realize . . . ." It does not require interpretation so much as loud cries of, "Help! Help! I'm drowning, not waving."[6]
>
> What is it all? Can anyone stem the flood? What interpretation, when there must be many millions? . . . The overburdened mind just deposits it in the lap of the analyst and says, "Here, *you* do it!" . . .
>
> The essential thing is that nothing can be made of it—there is no selected fact, nothing to make it all cohere. If it is so, then perhaps the essential thing is an emotional situation . . . .
>
> . . . It can be content *and* . . . [breaks off here.]
>
> (1992, pp. 219–221, italics in original)

This entry is broken off in mid-sentence.

Bion's own early "horrors of psychic abandonment" (Souter, 2009, p. 795), and especially his traumatic World War I horrors, where he "died—on August 8th 1918" (Bion, 1982, p. 265), were related by Szykierski (2010) to Bion's ending the "Amiens" war diary in mid-sentence:

> Bion's attempt in "Amiens" (published in 1997, though written in 1958) to revisit his war experiences was aborted in order to write what can be regarded as the three books of his metapsychology (1962, 1963, 1965)[7]. Bion abandoned the writing of "Amiens" in

> mid-sentence . . . . it reads as though Bion were about to formulate the great unknown of mental catastrophe, but could not find the words, and went on an intellectual journey to find the elements and factors determining the transformations that determine whether a mind will *learn from experience* or "crack up."
>
> (p. 959, italics in original)

I would like to offer my further impression, that Bion's "intellectual journey" and his theory of containment and dream-work-alpha failed to encompass, contain, or dream a horror that could not be dreamed in the sense of turning it into an emotional experience, memory, or dream-thought (Vermote's mode 2—transformation in Knowledge).

Thus, the "great unknown of mental catastrophe" had to further develop into the radical conception of the unknown and unknowable-O and of being and becoming at-one with it. "The transformation in K must be replaced by the transformation in O, and K must be replaced by F [faith]" (Bion 1970, p. 46). Indeed, Bion's fourth and last metapsychological book, *Attention and Interpretation* (1970), opens with a "catastrophic emotional explosion . . . felt as an immensity so great that it cannot be represented even by astronomical space because it cannot be represented at all," with debris, remnants, and scraps of personality floating in space, going farther and farther away from the point of explosion and farther from each other. In this vast horrid space in analysis, the "I scream" of Bion's patient was unmet and aborted after two-and-a-half years and became "no—I scream" (1970, pp. 12–14).

Bion (1991) further conveys his unabated struggle with this immensity of mental pain "from the past" and the loss of meaning in a very different way, in his dramatic and enigmatic last book, *A Memoir of the Future*:

> *Mind:* You are borrowing [words] from me; do you get them through the diaphragm?
>
> *Body:* *They* penetrate *it*. But the meaning does not get through. Where did you get your pains from?
>
> *Mind:* Borrowed from the past. The meaning does not get through the barrier though. Funny—the meaning does not get through whether it is from you to me, or from me to you.
>
> *Body:* It is the meaning of pain that I am sending to you; the words get through—which I have not sent—but the meaning is lost.
>
> (pp. 433–434, italics in original)

In my view, Bionian faith and at-one-ment are needed so that—despite the breakdown of alpha function—new, different experiences will continue to be generated in the psychic reality of patient–analyst, beyond the great destruction of catastrophic trauma.

"An analyst should leave room for the growth of ideas that are being germinated in the analytic experience, even though the germ of an idea is going to displace him and his theories," said Bion (2005b, p. 49) at age 81, one year before his death, in a Tavistock seminar held on July 3, 1978. I believe that this profound change regarding the analyst's being and becoming the experience of O was crucially important to Bion and came from a very deep inner conviction.

In April 1990, Leon Grinberg, a leading pioneer of Bion's ideas, appeared before the Israel Psychoanalytic Society and presented Bion's paper "Notes on Memory and Desire" (1967a). I was a very young analyst at the time and I did not understand it (this was the general reaction to the presentation), but something about these ideas intrigued me. Therefore, after the presentation, I approached Dr. Grinberg and said that I would like to read the paper. He responded enthusiastically, and upon his return to Spain, sent me by express mail two copies of *The Psychoanalytic Forum*, in which Bion's paper was published, along with five commentaries by respected psychoanalysts (from Chicago, Los Angeles, Mexico, England, and Pennsylvania), and Bion's response.

I was alarmed to read the first commentary, by Thomas French. It was brief and most dismissive:

> I am completely unable to understand W. R. Bion's paper, "Notes on Memory and Desire." Dr. Bion starts by reminding us that memory is often distorted by desire. This is self-evident, but Dr. Bion advises us to eschew memory and desire entirely, even to the point of the analyst's not remembering the preceding session. On the other hand, he makes a great point of "intuiting" the evolution of the patient's emotional experience.
>
> But what is evolution unless it occurs in time? And is emotional experience a mere succession of moods, each forgotten before the next emerges, and without relation to any external reality?
>
> (1967a, p. 274)

The other discussants also objected to and were confused by Bion's injunction to abandon memory and desire, past and future, and thus to be in contact only with a present "evolution." One of them, Gonzales, emphasized the obvious contradictions with what Bion had written in *Elements of Psycho-Analysis* (1963). To this argument, Bion responded directly and frankly:

> Dr. Gonzales draws attention to a defect of which I am very conscious. My own feeling is that my views have "evolved" . . . . I think that the expressions he rightly quotes from *Elements of Psycho-Analysis* are wrongly framed, but wrong though the formulations now seem to be, they were good enough to lead me to my present formulations which I think are better.
>
> (1967a, p. 280)

Another discussant, Herskovitz, wrote, "Dr. Bion's thesis is, at best, illogical" (1967a, p. 278). Only Lindon, the editor of *The Psychoanalytic Forum*, expressed a more favorable viewpoint; although finding the paper "provocatively nihilistic of all that we have learned as psychoanalysts" (1967a, p. 274), he recounted that it helped him considerably in a difficult analysis that had been bogged down for months.

Six years later, Green (1973) in his review of Bion's *Attention and Interpretation* also related strongly to the contradictions with what Bion had written in *Elements of Psychoanalysis*:

> One can also wonder whether, since the publication of *Elements of Psycho-Analysis* (the emphasis in this book was mostly on the elements in as much as they constituted an extension to the realms of the senses, of myth and of passion), the development of the author's thought has led him to support a point of view further and further away from these propositions, as, for example, when he now states that "the central phenomena of psychoanalysis have no background in sense data" (1970, p. 57).
>
> (Green 1973, p. 118)

Bion's injunction to abandon memory, desire, and understanding as essential to analytic technique, and his "struggling to present something really new" (Hinshelwood, 2013), finds strong expression in the choice of powerful words he uses with regard to this injunction in much of his writing in those years (Bion 1965b, 1967a, 2013/1967; see also Bernat, 2018) and later in 1970. Specific examples of such word are: "banishment" (1965b, p. 17), "get out" (1965b, p. 13), "avoidance" (1967a, p. 272), "exclusion" (1967a, p. 273; 1970, p. 57), "*suppress*" (2013, p. 5, italics in original), "*forget*" (2013, p. 25, italics in original), "removed" (1970, p. 32), "discard" (1970, p. 33), "denial" (1970, p. 41), "avoid" (1970, p. 42), "suspension, suppression" (1970, p. 46), and "*divest*" (1970, p. 49, italics in original).

Later, I also read that:

> At the International Congress of Psycho-Analysis in 1975 in London, Leo Rangell, who was immediate past President, opposed this recommendation [that the analyst should approach the session without "memory and desire"] by saying that if he were to approach an analytic session in this vein he would not feel justified in charging a fee.
>
> (Symington and Symington 1996, p. 166)

In view of these harsh reactions, I felt that great courage and unabated faith were required for Bion to go on struggling and further elaborating his revolutionary ideas, which forged a completely new approach to analytic work. He veritably "'*dare[d] to disturb the universe*' of psychoanalytic ideas and beyond" (Grotstein 2007, p. 329, italics in original) and introduced "perhaps the greatest paradigm shift in psychoanalysis to date" (p. 12) in traditional psychoanalytic thinking and technique. "Psychoanalysis seen through Bion's eyes is a radical departure from all conceptualizations which preceded him" (Symington and Symington 1996, p. xii).

I will conclude this section with Grotstein's (2007) powerful words on the "Bionic revolution" for psychoanalysis:

> Bion crossed the Rubicon of psychoanalytic respectability in London and launched a metapsychological revolution whose echoes are still reverberating across the psychoanalytic landscape worldwide . . . .
>
> I believe that the concept of O transforms all existing psychoanalytic theories (e.g., the pleasure principle, the death instinct, and the paranoid-schizoid and depressive positions) into veritable psychoanalytic manic defences against the unknown, unknowable, ineffable, inscrutable, ontological experience of ultimate being.
>
> (pp. 114, 121)

Winnicott

Clinical psychoanalysis at its most formative edge

> I am asking for a kind of revolution in our work. Let us re-examine what we do.
>
> (Winnicott, "DWW's Notes for the Vienna Congress, 1971" [never presented because of his untimely death]; cited by Abram 2013, pp. 1, 312)

"In essence, from his early days as a psychoanalyst, Winnicott's quest is to address the stage of human development that precedes object relations," writes Abram (2008, p. 1189). I would suggest that from the outset, and over the years, Winnicott's way of exploring, experiencing, and practicing psychoanalysis consistently offered a revolutionary change in psychoanalysis, which is based on "essentially natural processes" (1989, p. 156). His core ideas of self-development and human subjectivity evolved out of very early infantile psychic processes and environmental mother–infant relatedness that precede object relationships, and these are powerfully applied to the treatment process and situation. His fundamental model of psychoanalytic treatment is the mother–infant, mother–child relationship.

Winnicott's important theoretical contributions have been thoroughly and comprehensively described (Abram 2007, 2008, 2013; Caldwell and Joyce 2011; Dethiville 2014; Dias 2016; Eigen 1981, 2009; Fulgencio 2007; Girard 2010; Goldman 2012; Loparic 2002, 2010; Ogden 1986, 2001a, 2005b; Phillips 1988; Spelman 2013; Spelman and Thomson-Salo 2015). In this context, Loparic (2002, 2010) claims that Winnicott's theoretical thinking with regard to mother–baby, two-body psychoanalysis constitutes a Kuhnian paradigm change in Freud's oedipal, triangular psychoanalysis—a claim subsequently referred to by Fulgencio (2007), Abram (2008, 2013), Eshel (2013c), Minhot (2015), and Dias (2016). Minhot (2015) extends it to the profound change in Winnicott's thinking regarding the core aspects of *feeling alive* or *feeling real* that were not considered by traditional psychoanalysis and to the shift from a language of instincts and wishes to a language of needs and environment.

I have chosen, rather, to focus on and re-examine the revolutionary vision of Winnicott's *clinical* thinking, which is profoundly linked to his theory of regression. This essentially means moving experientially *beyond the space-time confines of traditional clinical psychoanalysis* to work with primal processes in the treatment situation and setting, thus reaching and correcting basic self-processes and unthinkable early breakdown—and enlarging the scope of psychoanalytic practice. "There was no class of illness that he considered impossible to analyze, as Freud regarded narcissistic neuroses and psychoses" (Little 1985, p. 39).

In a previous paper (Eshel 2013c), I related in detail to Winnicott's unique clinical thinking as constituting a paradigm shift, drawing primarily on his revision of the foundations of clinical psychoanalysis, and I entitled it "Reading Winnicott into *Nano-Psychoanalysis*." The title refers to concepts and terminology borrowed from nanoscience and nanotechnology, and in particular to physicist Richard Feynman's (1959) visionary presentation hailing nanotechnology and its radical potential: "There's plenty of room at the bottom—An invitation to enter a new field in physics." I paraphrased this title and applied it to Winnicott and to psychoanalysis, as an invitation to enter and develop a new field of psychoanalysis. Indeed, Winnicott's psychoanalytic thinking, and particularly his clinical-technical theory, with its emphasis on regression in the treatment of more disturbed patients, share the fundamental principle proposed by Feynman and nanotechnology—that of going back to the "bottom," to the elemental early states and processes and to early mothering techniques, thereby enabling the initiation of formative developmental processes.

In my view, this is a psychoanalytic revolution that has been in process since the beginning of Winnicott's writing, although he tried to view his theory of regression in the analytic situation as an extension of Freud's work to areas Freud had not addressed (Winnicott 1954a, 1964a, 1969c). He did write in his last years: "Freud seems to me to be struggling to use what he knows to be true, because of his analytic experience, to cover what he does not know" (Winnicott, 1969c, p. 240). But only at the very end of his life did he venture "asking for a kind of revolution in our work" (cited in Abram 2013, pp. 1, 312).

Abram (2013), too, writes about this:

> Perhaps by now, so near to death, Winnicott was able to articulate something that he had been in the process of since 1945—a psychoanalytic revolution. Thomas Kuhn had only just published his book *The Structure of Scientific Revolutions* (1962), and although Winnicott never refers to this book, his use of this word at the beginning of these

> notes suggests that he intuited his formulations were moving psychoanalysis toward something new.
>
> (p. 313)

In this regard, Phillips (1988) writes that Winnicott introduced important "innovations in psychoanalytic practice and technique followed by explicit assertions of the continuity of his work with a more orthodox psychoanalytic tradition," which represent "in fact, a certain disingenuousness in the way Winnicott disguises his radical departures from Freud" (p. 5).

Similarly, Mitchell (1993) contends:

> Winnicott had a tendency to introduce his extremely innovative contributions with references to non-neurotic psychopathology and therefore outside psychoanalysis proper. Over time, the contributions broadened in their implications, and it became clear that Winnicott had introduced a novel vision of the analytic process itself. He came to see regression as a central feature of the therapeutic action of analysis, and regression has everything to do with hope.
>
> (pp. 206–207)

Home (1966) stated in a lecture at the British Psycho-Analytical Society that with regard to

> . . . the psycho-analytic theory of regression, in which there are two sorts of regression—ego regression and instinct regression, when Winnicott (1954) presented his clinical experiences of regression in analysis, . . . he found that it fell into neither category. This meant that, strictly speaking, it could not exist as regression so far as psychoanalytic theory was concerned.
>
> (p. 46)

In effect, over the years Winnicott explored, described, and struggled, theoretically and clinically, with "any degree" of regression to dependence, especially in the treatment of severely disturbed patients and also in difficult treatment situations with neurotic patients (1949a, 1949b, 1954a, 1954b, 1955–1956, 1963b, 1964a, 1967a, 1988a, 1988b; see also Little 1985). He "fully believe[d]" that regression must be allowed "absolutely full sway" (Winnicott 1954a, p. 279), even to the earliest stages of prenatal life and rebirth. For regression carries with it, within the analytic process, the hope and a new opportunity for reliving and correcting the original maternal failure and inadequate adaptation to need in the patient's infancy, and the early traumatic unthinkable breakdown that happened at the time of early environmental failure. According to Winnicott:

> All this can be very clearly demonstrated in psychoanalytic work provided one is able to follow the patient *right back in emotional development as far as he needs to go*, by regression to dependence, in order to get behind the period at which impingements became multiple and unmanageable.
>
> (1949a, pp. 192–193, my italics)

There, by providing the needed environmental essentials of holding, adaptation to need, and reliability, which should have been provided earlier but were not available, he creates for the first time in the patient's life a facilitating environment in which development can start anew.

Regression in the present tense

In Winnicott's revolutionary clinical model of regression and its healing quality, "the self cannot make new progress unless and until the [frozen] environment failure situation is [unfrozen and] corrected" (1954a, p. 291) through the analytic setting and process. Unless and until the deeply traumatic origins of the unthinkable, not-yet-experienced breakdown—which is therefore "past and future," never and forever—are relived and experienced "for the first time in the present" with the analyst (1974, p. 179). It is not a linear return to the past. The regression to dependence and early psychic processes in treatment calls forth *a radical possibility of actually influencing and altering the patient's "past and future" in the present*, by

> . . . allow[ing] the past to *be* the present. Whereas in the transference neurosis the past comes into the consulting-room, in this work it is more true to say that the present goes back into the past, and *is* the past. Thus the analyst finds himself confronted with the patient's primary process in the setting in which it had its original validity.
>
> (Winnicott 1955–1956, pp. 297–298, italics in original)

Furthermore, Winnicott posits:

> Let me add that for Freud there are three people, one of them excluded from the analytic room. If there are only two people involved then there has been a regression of the patient in the analytic setting, and the setting represents the mother with her technique, and the patient is an infant. There is a further state of regression in which there is only one present, namely the patient, and this is true even if in another sense, from the observer's angle, there are two.
>
> (1954a, p. 286)

This enables moving beyond the space-time confines of traditional clinical psychoanalysis and techniques to encompass and influence primal stages and processes of development, so that the treatment process actualizes a new experiential possibility within a new psychic environment.[8] The regression creates what has not existed and could not exist before. Winnicott writes:

> In a peculiar way we can actually alter the patient's past, so that a patient whose maternal environment was not good enough can change into a person who has had a good enough facilitating environment, and whose personal growth has therefore been able to take place, though late.
>
> (1988a, p. 102)

And through Winnicott's words that convey and describe this innovative clinical-technical thinking, there emerge his profound belief, hope, quest, and yearning for a psychoanalytic treatment that would enable a new opportunity for correcting past experiences and forward emotional development for all patients, especially severely disturbed patients. This "hope of getting at something here in the analysis which had never been before" (1986a, p. 32), can transpire if the analyst is willing to go back "in emotional development as far as . . . [the patient] needs to go" (Winnicott 1949a, p. 192); to meet and adapt to the very basic needs of the patient; to contend with the depth of the regression, the profound dependence, the "exacting," specialized early environmental provision that is needed within each treatment of regressed patients; and to cope with the terrors involved.

Winnicott particularly relates to the need for therapeutic regression in the psychoanalytic treatment of schizoid, false-self, borderline, and psychotic disorders, which constitute the third, most regressed group in Winnicott's 1954a classification. (From my clinical experience, I would add patients with severe sexual perversions to this list of the most regressed group [Eshel 2005, 2013a; now chapters 7 and 8 here].) Of the psychotic patient, he writes:

> The regression represents the psychotic individual's hope that certain aspects of the environment which failed originally may be relived, with the environment this time succeeding instead of failing in its function of facilitating the inherited tendency in the individual to develop and to mature.
>
> (1959–1964, p. 128)

Winnicott was very much aware of the great difficulties met in the course of psychoanalytic work with long, deep, or "total" regressions to dependence, which around the same time bothered two of his contemporaries—Balint in London and Nacht in Paris. Balint (1968, with regard to the *basic fault* psychopathology) and Nacht (1963) and Nacht and Viderman (1960) also dealt with the place of therapeutic regression in the psychoanalytic situation, but with rather restrained and cautious clinical-theoretical conclusions (Eshel 2013c). The last 20 years have given rise to several critical reflections on this way of working with more disturbed patients, and its utility and necessity have been questioned (Spurling 2008; Tyson and Tyson 1990) and criticized (Segal 2006). But Winnicott's clinical thinking insists on the fundamental transformative importance of such regressions for the patient, the analyst, and clinical psychoanalysis. He therefore emphasizes that the analyst must be experienced at meeting the dependence and managing the regressed patient during this stormy, primal, and needy state. Referring to a severely regressed analytic case that he has "all the time in mind," he writes:

> I cannot help being different from what I was before this analysis started . . . . This one experience that I have had has tested psychoanalysis in a special way and has taught me a great deal.
>
> The treatment and management of this case has called on everything that I possess as a human being, as a psycho-analyst, and as a paediatrician. I have had to make personal growth in the course of this

> treatment which was painful and which I would gladly have avoided. In particular I have had to learn to examine my own technique whenever difficulties arose, and it has always turned out in the dozen or so resistance phases that the cause was in a counter-transference phenomenon which necessitated further self-analysis in the analyst . . . .
>
> The main thing is that in this case, as in many others that have led up to it in my practice, I have needed to re-examine my technique, even that adapted to the more usual case.
>
> (Winnicott 1954a, p. 280)

Elsewhere, in a very different tone, Winnicott characteristically addresses this point through the baby:

> I am still referring to the very early stages. Certainly there is something that happens to people when they are confronted with the helplessness that is supposed to characterize a baby. It is a terrible thing to do to plant a baby on your doorstep, because your reactions to the baby's helplessness alter your life and perhaps cut across the plans you have made. This is fairly obvious but it needs some kind of restatement in terms of dependence . . . . We could almost say that those who are in the position of caring for a baby are as helpless in relation to the baby's helplessness as the baby can be said to be. Perhaps there can be a battle of helplessness.
>
> (1988b, pp. 102–103)

Thus, Winnicott's clinical theory of regression, with its invitation to go back and enter the most fundamental, elemental, and early states in order to enable new developmental processes (in Winnicott's theory, this relies heavily on mother–infant natural processes[9]), offers a living experiential possibility for broadening the reach of psychoanalytic practice. In my view, his thinking presents clinical psychoanalysis at its most formative edge.

Clinical illustrations

Vexed, Bion (1992) writes:

> There are many interpretations I could give and have given in the past. They are apparently quite ineffectual, there seems to be no particular point in repeating them. What, I wonder, can have happened to them?

> Years of analytic interpretations, and patience and knowledge that go with them, have been swallowed up by him, or poured into him by me, without apparently leaving the slightest trace.
>
> (pp. 219–220; quoted earlier in this chapter, p. 245)

It is difficult to convey through brief clinical illustrations the radical move from the analyst's epistemological position to the more fundamental and more enigmatic *experiencing-with*, *becoming*, and *being at-one with* the patient's unthinkable psychic reality. To this end, I will first demonstrate the kind of Kleinian-based interpretations that Bion gave during the epistemological period (to which he referred in the passage quoted above). I have chosen to quote the interpretations he presented in clinical example (vi) in his October 1957 lecture to the British Psychoanalytic Society on "Attacks on linking" (1959). This clinical example also allows me to introduce Winnicott's very different approach to similar symptoms and immense fear in the session, as described by Little (1985). Winnicott emphasized regression in the transference as his alternative way of understanding, experiencing, reliving, holding, and interpreting the session when working with regressed patients—an approach that had already characterized his mode of interpreting since 1949 and the early 1950s. I will then relate to Bion's clinical statements regarding the examples from his Los Angeles seminars (2013), at the critical point of the transformation in his clinical thinking as put forth in his controversial paper "Notes on Memory and Desire" (1967a), discussed earlier in this chapter. And finally, I will present a clinical example of my own.

Bion and Winnicott: attack on linking or deep regression to rebirth

In his lecture of October 20, 1957, Bion (1959) described six clinical examples showing the significance of destructive attacks on linking seen in some symptoms encountered in borderline psychosis, and the interpretations he gave the patient regarding his "conduct designed to destroy whatever it was that linked two objects together" (p. 308).

I will focus on clinical example (vi):

> Half the session passed in silence; the patient then announced that a piece of iron had fallen on the floor. Thereafter he made a series of

> convulsive movements in silence as if he felt he was being physically assaulted from within. I said he could not establish contact with me because of his fear of what was going on inside him. He confirmed this by saying that he felt he was being murdered. He did not know what he would do without the analysis as it made him better. I said that he felt so envious of himself and of me for being able to work together to make him feel better that he took the pair of us into him as a dead piece of iron and a dead floor that came together not to give him life but to murder him. He became very anxious and said he could not go on. I said that he felt he could not go on because he was either dead, or alive and so envious that he had to stop good analysis. There was a marked decrease of anxiety, but the remainder of the session was taken up by isolated statements of fact which again seemed to be an attempt to preserve contact with external reality as a method of denial of his phantasies.
>
> (1959, pp. 309–310)

Winnicott's very different approach to similar symptoms and immense fear in the session is described by Little (1985) in her "personal record" of "Winnicott working in areas where psychotic anxieties predominate," as she entitled her account. Since her analysis with him lasted from 1949 until 1955, and this was early in the analysis, we may assume that it was around 1950. She writes:

> Throughout a whole session I was seized with recurring spasms of terror. Again and again I felt a tension begin to build up in my whole body, reach a climax, and subside, only to come again a few seconds later. I grabbed his hands and clung tightly till the spasms passed. He said at the end that he thought I was reliving the experience of being born; he held my head for a few minutes, saying that immediately after birth an infant's head could ache and feel heavy for a time. All this seemed to fit, for it was birth into a relationship, via my spontaneous movement which was accepted by him. Those spasms never came again, and only rarely that degree of fear.
>
> (p. 20)

This is indeed a very different way of understanding, experiencing, reliving, holding, and interpreting convulsive symptoms and terror in the session.

For Winnicott, in *regression to dependence* the patient is not responding defensively, but:

> regresses because of a new environmental provision which allows of dependence. . . It is another thing if a patient breaks down into some new environment provision that offers reliable care . . . [and a] new opportunity for dependence.
>
> (1967a, p. 197)

> In [these] cases, I have found that the patient has needed phases of regression to dependence in the transference, these giving experience of the full effect of adaptation to need that is in fact based on the analyst's (mother's) ability to identify with the patient (her baby). In the course of this kind of *experience* there is a sufficient quantity of being merged in with the analyst (mother) to enable the patient to live and to relate without the need for projective and introjective identificatory mechanisms.
>
> (1971a, p. 160, italics in original)

Winnicott thus emphasizes regression in the treatment experience that "reaches the limit of the patient's need," even to the earliest stages and rebirth, until, "at the bottom of the regression, there came a new chance for the true self to start" (1949b, pp. 249, 252).

Is it not amazing, and perhaps even terrifying, to think that "spasms of terror" (Little 1985, p. 20) can become a rebirth in analysis with Winnicott, while Bion (1959) interprets them as an (inner) murder, a destructive attack on linking in which the patient "took the pair of us into him as a dead piece of iron and a dead floor that came together not to give him life but to murder him" (p. 310)?

Bion's different way of being and relating—1967

Ten years after presenting it in lecture form, Bion republished "Attacks on linking" (1959) in his book *Second Thoughts* (1967b). However, his controversial paper "Notes on Memory and Desire" (1967a) was also published that year in *The Psychoanalytic Forum*, and, as described earlier, it introduced a completely different mode of analytic work—of becoming at one with the psychic reality of the patient during the analytic session. The analyst is required to suspend memory, desire, and even understanding in order to prevent any "hindrance to the psychoanalyst's intuition of the reality with which he must be at one" (Bion, 1967a, p. 272) —to become all the more *intuit* (in-tu-it).[10] Bion's clinical illustrations from this critical year appeared only posthumously, in Bion's (2013) Los Angeles seminars from April 1967. Another clinical illustration from March 1967 (for presentation on 20 April in Los Angeles) was previously published under the entry "Reverence and awe" in *Cogitation* (1992). These are also cases of psychotic and severely disturbed patients, but in these illustrations Bion conveys a very different mode of "becoming" and not-becoming of understanding and interpreting that radically challenges the all-knowing imposing position of the analyst seen in his earlier examples. It seems that he has come a long way from the Bion who knows and decodes everything militantly.

He says in the Los Angeles third seminar of his "actual experience" in the treatment of a psychotic patient who told him a dreadful dream, in which he and his children were being swept down the weir:

> I had nothing to interpret to him. I did not know what to say about this. But it made the focusing point for a good deal of thought because one felt (as I felt about this) that I'd simply been handed it on a plate, and had failed to understand, and had failed to be able to make any contribution . . . . As far as I was concerned, it was simply a lost opportunity; I felt certain that it was very important.
>
> (2013, pp. 56–57; see also Eshel, 2017b)

At that time, when relating to his March 1967 clinical example Bion (1992) powerfully writes:

> While listening to the patient the analyst should dwell on those aspects of the patient's communication which come nearest to arousing feelings corresponding to persecution and depression. . . . I am fortified in this belief by the conviction that has been borne in on me by the analysis of psychotic or borderline patients. I do not think such a patient will ever accept an interpretation, however correct, unless he feels that the *analyst has passed through this emotional crisis as a part of the act of giving the interpretation.*
>
> (1992, p. 291, my italics)

Furthermore, he says at that year in Los Angeles:

> . . . especially if we are going to deal with patients which are not really like the sort of patient which is spoken of in classical psychoanalysis, then not only are we to treat these patients, but we have to invent the methods by which we are going to treat them.
>
> (2013, p. 66)

And later on, Bion returns to consider his patient (from the third Los Angeles seminar) with new, different thoughts, even coming close to some of Winnicott's terms of interpreting:

> I'm referring here to the association of the patient who says he's had a dream of being swept down the weir. To come back to that point, if I had an association of that kind today, I would try to interpret it much more in terms of this having been an *experience*; that what he was describing was not a dream at all. It was really his fear about emerging from his foetal state of mind; making this fact public by talking to me, using the language of the adult, that he does the counterpart in the actual session of something which in physical terms one could say was one of the *rebirth*—you emerge from one state of mind into another, you risk being caught at it . . . .
>
> it's an experiment in which he expects to be swept away, drowned, disposed of, if he dares to come out into the open as having the capacity to communicate and talk and so forth . . . I think that the actual experience as near as you can describe it—the description of that experience—has its own validity, I take it—a kind of wisdom after the event.
>
> (2013, p. 67, my italics)

Clinical example: a voice from a haunting dungeon of madness

I would now like to demonstrate my way of understanding this *becoming at-one* with the patient's unthinkable psychic reality with my own clinical example—also involving the treatment of a psychotic patient. This treatment took place a decade after Bion's 1967a paper, very early on in my therapeutic work as a clinical psychologist, when I was not yet familiar with these writings of Bion and Winnicott. However, for both Bion and Winnicott, the truest form of learning is *learning from experience* (Bion) and from *my clinical experiences* (Winnicott); and I was working deeply within the clinical experience.

Nir was referred to me for intensive psychotherapy in the state psychiatric hospital in which I was working, due to extraordinary circumstances. He was about 30 years old, the only son of elderly Holocaust survivors, and had been hospitalized for years in an open ward of the hospital with an indeterminate diagnosis of schizophrenia. Nir was extremely closed and cut-off, having no contact with anyone in the hospital—neither patients nor staff. As his intellectual functions were unimpaired and his thinking appeared logical, he served as the editor of the hospital newsletter. In fact, he could have been discharged were it not for his sudden and severe occasional suicide attempts that endangered him and his surroundings. After each of these attempts, he was transferred to a locked ward where he would remain for a week or two. However, due to his unimpaired intellectual state, there was no point in keeping him there for long, and thus he was transferred back to the open ward until he unexpectedly again made another severe suicide attempt, usually in the dead of night, when security was minimal.

Nir's suicide attempt prior to starting treatment with me was extremely serious. He hung himself from a rope above his bed and set his mattress on fire to burn himself to death. He was freed from the hanging rope at the last moment and the flames were extinguished; however, many patients had to be evacuated from the panic-stricken, smoke-filled ward, a particularly difficult undertaking as most of them were under the influence of sleeping drugs. Nir was again moved to a locked ward, but it was clear that things could not continue in this way, and that if no solution could be found, he would have to be transferred to a closed psychiatric facility for chronic patients.

Therefore, in a last-ditch effort, the hospital manager and the chief psychologist, came up with the idea that if someone could manage to establish therapeutic contact with Nir and to talk to him, it might be possible to pre-empt future suicide attempts. But since Nir was so cut-off, the ward psychologist did not see any possibility of establishing a therapeutic relationship with him, and I was asked to take the case, since I was dealing with severe cases in the hospital.

And so Nir and I began treatment. We met three times a week. The sessions were extremely difficult. Nir came to the sessions, but scarcely spoke; he was very detached and impenetrable, avoided eye contact, and was withdrawn somewhere into his own world; but he did reply when I asked him questions.

Regardless of the season, I would wipe drops of sweat from my brow at the end of each session. Yet, with time, a hidden sense of contact slowly began to be felt, though in the innermost psychic underground—unseen, and inaccessible to any questioning. After nine months, Nir unexpectedly told me his greatest secret. He said that he did not want to commit suicide, he did not wish to die, but the secret service was sending men to capture and torture him and then execute him in unbearable suffering. Therefore, when he saw them coming, he would rather kill himself than be caught, tortured and executed by them.

When Nir finished speaking, I knew he had told me his deepest, most precious secret, the inner sanctum of his psychic reality. At that moment, starkly gripped by feelings of the screaming voice of dread and crucial urgency that filled the room, I found myself saying: "Nir, next time they come, come to me and I'll protect you." Nir stared at me with a direct, intent look. It was the first time that I had seen his eyes, which were an extraordinarily light blue, almost water-like, as though they had not been designed for seeing. It was hard to know what he was thinking.

After a long pause he asked, "Will you?" "Yes," I replied. Then he asked, "And if you're with another patient?" "Then knock on my door, and I'll come out to protect you," I replied." "All right," he said.

Nir never attempted another suicide. The hospital staff was overwhelmed. I continued to work with him for years; this great change allowed him to leave the hospital and live with his parents.

Writing now in current terms that I did not know back then, I think that this vignette illustrates my *becoming-at-one* with the dread of the patient's psychic reality. I had completely *been-with* his dread and profound need to be rescued, and this enabled him to risk accepting my promise to protect him without questioning just how a young female psychologist, slender, rather pale and delicate-looking, would be able to protect him from a terrifying gang of secret service assassins. I might also point out that he did not ask how I would protect him if they showed up at the hospital at 3 a.m.—the time he usually made his suicide attempts—while I was at home. He only asked that I could make myself totally available to him when he called me, and that I not leave him to battle all alone through a "dark night of the soul."

I have recounted what being *in-tu-it*, within the patient's innermost, mad psychic reality enabled me to experience and to be in the case of Nir. In Eigen (2004) words "It [became] clear to me that no amount of defensive imposition on deep madness would win the day. Something had to happen on the level of the madness itself" (p. 171). In the many years that have passed since then, I have come to realize that transformation in the most cut-off, blocked, deadening, empty, desperate and despairing psychic zones—zones of psychic breakdown, madness, annihilation and catastrophe—may become possible only when the analyst/therapist is willing and able to *be-within* (and *with-in*) the patient's experiential world and within the grip of the analytic process, with the ensuing patient–analyst deep-level interconnectedness or "withnessing," psyche-with-psyche (Eshel, 2004a, 2005, 2006, 2010, 2012, 2013b, 2016a, 2016b, 2017b, 2017c; now chapters 1 to 9 here). This interconnectedness, which becomes at-one-ment when the analyst puts him-/herself entirely within the patient's emotional reality, is difficult and demanding, an unyielding, ongoing struggle with the underlying catastrophe to reach a new and formative deep experiencing, beyond epistemological exploration-K. "The analyst apprehends that reality because he has *become it in the depth of his being*" (Symington and Symington, 1996, p. 166, my italics).

Concluding thoughts

Reading late Bion and Winnicott into "quantum psychoanalysis"

Having reviewed the main radical clinical ideas in late Bion's and Winnicott's psychoanalytic thinking and presented some clinical illustrations, I would now like to put forth my own rendering of these ideas, and the meaning and implications of the psychoanalytic revolutionary change that they introduced.

Toward this aim, I will refer again to Vermote's (2013) integrative model of psychic functioning for dealing with the unknown in psychoanalytic work, which identifies three distinct zones or modes of psychic functioning with varying degrees of differentiation, different psychoanalytic models, and clinical implications for the analyst: 1—reason (Freud, Klein); 2—transformation in Knowledge (Bion, Marty, de M'Uzan, Bollas, Botella and Botella, Ogden, Ferro); and 3—transformation in O, when dealing with the most unthought, unknown, undifferentiated mode of psychic functioning (Winnicott, Milner, late Bion, late Lacan). I argued earlier in this chapter, using Kuhnian terminology, that Vermote's mode 2—*transformation in Knowledge* constitutes an extension of the existing psychoanalytic paradigm, while mode 3—*transformation in O* introduces a revolutionary shift.

Continuing with this framework, I wish to suggest a further categorization of varying states of the unknown or unthought with different experiences associated with them in the analytic work:

> Unconscious-conscious: mode 1, consisting of psychic material that could have been repressed.
>
> The unrepressed unknown: modes 2 and 3—neither of which could be repressed—ranging from traumatically dissociative processes–mode 2, to primordial, unknown and unknowable unrepresented processes–mode 3 (cf. Bergstein, 2014, "the unrepressed unconscious"; Levine, Reed, and Scarfone, 2013, "Unrepresented states").

The strength of the words "the *unthinkable* states of affairs" of early breakdown (Winnicott) and "*catastrophic* emotional explosion" (Bion) captures the difference in intensity between mode 2 and mode 3. This intensity is related to the extent of the traumatization and of the failure of not being held and contained at the time, as well as to how early on it occurred, since early trauma breaks the personality that forms at the beginning of the individual's life. According to Winnicott (1967a), the varieties of experience of "unthinkable" or "psychotic" anxiety can be classified "in terms of the amount of integration that survived the disaster" of early environmental failures (p. 198).

Thus, mode 2 is the mode of the "traumatic" unknown that remains at the level of representations or that can be transformed by analytic representations, while mode 3 is the mode of the primordial unknowable and unthinkable realm of experience, in particular, the great unknown of mental catastrophe, early breakdown and madness. In Bion, this mode is the "domain of the non-existent" (Bion,1970, p. 20), "a nameless dread" (Bion, 1962b), "a breakdown of dream-work-a" (1992, p. 59), "the complete dissociation" (2013, p. 68), "complete meaninglessness" (1965a, p. 101), and the "dark night of/to the soul," which is the "'dark night' to K" in analytic work (1965a, p. 159); "it is off the ends of the spectrum" (2013, p. 63; see also p. 60).

In Winnicott, mode 3 is the agonizing, unthinkable early breakdown or madness that has already happened but could not be experienced (Winnicott, 1974, 1965a), and therefore is "unlived" (Ogden, 2014) and "undreamt" (Ogden, 2005c); it is x + y + z degree of mother deprivation in which the baby has experienced a break in life's continuity (Winnicott, 1971a); an "annihilation" before the person even existed (Little, 1985). It is also "a-void—to avoid the void of the 'domain of the nonexistent' or nothingness" (Emanuel, 2001); and I would add here Lopez-Corvo's description of "early or pre-conceptual traumas" that represent "living fossils" left in the mind by psychic traumas that took place at a time when a mind capable of digesting and containing the impact of such psychic facts did not exist, and also, and very significantly, when the mother's alpha function had also failed (2014, pp. xxvii, 44).

It is interesting to note that Winnicott and Bion even use similar words to describe this unrepresented unknown zone of early breakdown and catastrophe. Winnicott writes: ". . . it is not possible to remember something that has not yet happened, and this thing of the past has not happened yet because the patient was not there for it to happen to" (1974, p. 105). Bion describes "something that is unconscious and unknown because it has not happened" (1970, p. 35).

Rather than an epistemological exploration for recovering repressed material (mode 1) and the need for the analyst's reverie, dream-thought and containing capacity for further epistemological exploration and transformation of the unbearable traumatic unknown (TK, mode 2), the depths of the unknown and unknowable mode 3, which is unrepresented, unthinkable, and unexperienced, are beyond the limits of the level of representations and analytic thinking. *The unthinkable cannot be thought, but only relived and gone through with the analyst.*

Thus, "Real psychic change" happens in mode 3 (Vermote, 2013) at the level of the radical ontological experience of patient-and-analyst's being-in-oneness at a primordial point of origin: For Bion, it is the primacy of the analyst becoming at-one with the patient's unknown and unknowable, ultimate reality-O. For Winnicott, patient and analyst become merged in primary relatedness within deep therapeutic regression, akin to the early two-in-one of mother–baby, and the object is the first, subjective object when reaching to the deepest non-communicating layers of the patient's personality; this offers a crucially new opportunity for correcting past experiences and for forward emotional development and true communication (Winnicott, 1954a, 1963c), which is life-giving. It is therefore essential to the practical work of psychoanalysis. For only the great intensity of being and becoming at-one-with the patient's unknown and unknowable ultimate emotional reality can reach the innermost *annihilated-annihilating states of ultimate trauma, and create a new experience* within the depths of core catastrophe, unthinkable breakdown and madness.

I believe that this radical and profound importance of essential *being* is conveyed in Bion's much criticized mystical statement that O is "represented by terms such as ultimate reality, absolute truth, the godhead, the infinite, the thing in-itself . . . it can be 'become', but it cannot be 'known'" (Bion, 1970, p. 26). The most criticized of these daring terms, "godhead," (which Grotstein, 2007, suggests reading as "godhood") becomes much more understandable if we consider the closeness of the association between unknown infinite, ultimate *being*, and the Biblical Hebrew name for God אהיה אשר אהיה (Exodus, 3:14). This name for God, which is derived from a verb that means "to be," "to become," is most commonly translated as "I AM THAT I AM" or "I shall be what I shall be" (In Hellenistic Greek of Jewish literature this phrase was rendered in Greek as "*ego eimi ho on*"—"I am the BEING".) It is God's response when Moses asks for his name. And it appears in a chapter that is impregnated with a call for being: with Moses answering God's call out of the midst of the burning bush: "Here am I" (3:4); and God promising him: "Certainly I will be with thee" (3:12), "Thus shalt thou say unto the children of Israel: I AM hath sent me unto you" (3:14).

Winnicott similarly refers to this essential state of being in his paper "*Sum*, I AM" (1986). With regard to the early Hebrew name for God, he writes:

> Monotheism seems to be closely linked to the name I AM. I am that I am. (*Cogito, ergo sum* is different: *sum* here means I have a sense of existing as a person, that in my mind I feel my existence has been proved. But we are concerned here with an unselfconscious state of being, apart from intellectual exercises in self-awareness.)
>
> (p. 57)

I would now like to elaborate further on the meaning of my contention that late Bion's and Winnicott's radical clinical ideas introduce a revolutionary change in traditional clinical psychoanalysis. The essential unity of being at the heart of late Bion's and Winnicott's revolutionary ideas regarding working with the patient's primordial, unknown psychic reality summons to my mind the quantum mechanics revolution in 20th-century physics; for with the quantum revolution, we move into a probabilistic, entangled realm of unity rather than division; of profound interconnectedness rather than separateness,[11] that operates at primary, deep, invisible levels. This is underscored by Grotstein's (2007) radical choice of words when he states that late Bion, in his concept of O,

> . . . turned to Heisenberg's concept of uncertainty[12]. . . . His psychoanalytic precision changed to a stoic acceptance of uncertainty, the ultimate result being his psychoanalytic metatheory, arguably the most far-reaching paradigm shift in psychoanalytic history and the most suitable one to date to anticipate the newer era of relativism, probabilism, and uncertainty . . .
>
> Bion's metapsychological revolution . . . perforated the flat world of Freud's and Klein's positivism (the instinctual drives as first cause) and introduced inner and outer cosmic uncertainty, infinity, relativism, and numinousness as its successor.
>
> (pp. 16, 114)

This view is in sharp contrast to Blass's concern ("Psychoanalytical Controversies," 2011, 2012) over whether late Bion's and especially Winnicott's clinical innovations can actually co-exist with traditional concepts and practices in psychoanalysis, or whether they go "beyond the limits of psychoanalysis" (2012, p. 1441). But are there limits to psychoanalysis and to its quest to reach the suffering human psyche? Should clinical psychoanalysis shy away from following the more radical possibilities that the revolutionary ideas of Winnicott and late Bion provide?

In modern physics, different paradigms—classical physics and quantum mechanics—do co-exist (Kuhn, 1962). Whereas classical physics is based on assumptions of linear causality, determinism, and a sharp separation between observer and observed, quantum mechanics introduced into scientific thinking enigmatic principles of uncertainty and inseparability of observer and observed, the crucial formative effect of the process of observation, and the fundamental organization of unbroken wholeness that underlies our perceived world of separateness at the particle level

(Bohm, 1980; Godwin, 1991; Sucharov, 1992; Field, 1996; Mayer, 1996; Kulka, 1997; Botella and Botella, 2005; Eshel, 2002a, 2005, 2006, 2010, 2013a,c, chapter 2 here; Gargiulo, 2016; Suchet, 2017). Physicist David Bohm (1980) describes "the quantum interconnectedness of distant systems" and the "implicate order" (or "enfolded" order) as a deeper and more fundamental order of reality, in contrast to the "explicate or unfolded" order that humans normally perceive. I believe that the fundamental claim of quantum physics finds its quantum-like psychoanalytic counterpart in the analytic oneness which is rooted in the revolutionary ideas of late Bion and Winnicott; and the elemental, unified counterpart in psychoanalysis may be described as the "implicate order" of psychoanalysis.

Thus, I would venture that the profound change introduced by late Bion's and Winnicott's revolutionary theoretical and clinical-technical thinking, and especially their revision of the foundations of clinical psychoanalysis, is to classical psychoanalysis what quantum physics is to classical physics.[13] Hence, I would term them "*quantum psychoanalysis*" (and more specifically, Winnicott's theoretical and clinical thinking—*nano-psychoanalysis*, with its quantum effects [2013]), and it may co-exist with classical psychoanalysis in the same way that classical physics co-exists with quantum physics.

Final notes on "quantum psychoanalysis"

In the context of the quantum revolution in physics, it is interesting to note the *practical meaning* of the assimilation and the co-existence of quantum theory with the older paradigm of classical physics.

Kuhn (1962) recounts that after Heisenberg's paper on matrix mechanics pointed the way to a new quantum theory, Wolfgang Pauli wrote, "Heisenberg's type of mechanics has again given me hope and joy in life. To be sure, it does not supply the solution to the riddle, but I believe it is again possible to march forward" (Pauli quoted by Kuhn 1962, p. 84).

But when Kuhn (1962) addresses the practical aspect of the assimilation of quantum theory into physics, it is in a far more pragmatic way than when he relates to the emergence of a new theory:

> The transition from Newtonian to quantum mechanics evoked many debates about both the nature and the standards of physics, some of which continue. . .

> How can a change of paradigm ever affect only a small subgroup? . . .
>
> Consider, for a single example, the quite large and diverse community constituted by all physical scientists. Each member of that group is taught the laws of quantum mechanics, and most of them employ these laws at some point in their research or teaching. But they do not all learn the same applications of these laws, and they are not therefore all affected in the same way by changes in quantum-mechanical practice . . . . What quantum mechanics means to each of them depends upon what courses he has had, what texts he had read, and which journals he studies. It follows that, though a change in quantum-mechanical law will be revolutionary for all these groups, a change that reflects only on one or another of the paradigm applications of quantum mechanics need be revolutionary only for the members of a particular professional subspecialty. For the rest of the profession and for those who practice other physical sciences, that change need not be revolutionary at all.
>
> (pp. 48–50)

I believe that it is the same with the new paradigm applications of "*quantum psychoanalysis*" (Eshel, 2013c, 2017a; Gargiulo, 2016; Suchet, 2017).

For me, the revolutionary ideas of late Bion and Winnicott are profoundly important, both theoretically and practically; they consist a rainbow's edge where patient–analyst "quantum interconnectedness" and at-one-ment comes into being to provide a formative matrix and a mode of transformation that relationships cannot offer at deeper levels of disturbance. This *ontological experience*, suspended, even if momentarily, from epistemological and relational discourse, becomes an experience and language of new possibility, especially within states of breakdown, devastation, core deadness and emptiness—off the spectrum. It is, in my view, the place wherein lies the very core of psychoanalysis, and, I would add, its wonder.

Therefore, I would like to end with the concluding lines of Dante's epic journey in the *Divine Comedy*:

> such was I at that new sight. I wished to see how the image was fitted to the circle and how it has its place there; *but my own wings were not*

sufficient for that, had not my mind been smitten by a flash wherein came its wish.

(*Paradiso*, Canto 33, pp. 136–141, my italics)

For me, this is the flash, the inspiration, that the radical ideas of Winnicott and late Bion confer.

Notes

1 Over the years, several authors have used Kuhn's terminology to relate to the history of psychoanalytic thinking (Britton 1998; Govrin 2016; Hughes 1989; Levenson 1972; Lifton 1976; McDougall 1995; Modell 1986, 1993), or to study Winnicott's paradigm change (Abram 2008, 2013; Eshel 2013c; Loparic 2002, 2010) and that of Bion (Brown 2013).

2 See footnote 6, chapter 2.

3 The term *subjective object* is used in Winnicott's writing "in describing the first object, the object *not yet repudiated as a not-me phenomenon*" (1971a, p. 93, italics in original).

4 Sandler refers to *f*antasy, whereas Kleinians refer to *ph*antasy.

5 Years later, I also read Francesca Bion's description that Bion "would sometimes emerge from his study, where he had been deep in thought, struggling with these seemingly intractable problems, looking pale and what I can only describe as 'absented.' It was alarming until I realized that he had been digging so deep into the nature of the psychotic mind that he had become 'at-one' with the patient experience" (1995, p. 96).

6 I think of Stevie Smith's poignant poem, "Not Waving but Drowning" (1957).

7 The three books are: *Learning from Experience*, 1962; *Elements of Psychoanalysis*, 1963; *Transformations*, 1965.

8 A*ctualize* is intended here in its two meanings: "In the present and in the process of actualization, that is, trying to bring into existence what didn't happen" (Pontalis 2003, p. 45).

9 In my opinion, Winnicott has introduced the most extreme theoretical and clinical-technical psychoanalytic thinking evolving out of earliest human infancy. However, the shift toward primal forms in clinical psychoanalysis does not have to be limited solely to mother–infant natural processes and states, as can be seen in the writings of Searles (1961, 1986) and Botella and Botella (2005).

10 It is interesting to note that Bion does mention this change in the lengthy "Commentary" he added at the end of *Second Thoughts* (1967b), where he writes about the importance of the "*experience*" of both psychoanalytic work and psychoanalytic reading, and "a *defensive* . . . substitute for experiencing . . .—what I have elsewhere called 'Transformation under K as contrasted with Transformation under O'" (1967b, p. 156, italics in original).

11 Wolfgang Pauli, one of the pioneers of quantum physics and Nobel laureate in physics In 1945, describes in his classical book on quantum mechanics, "This solution (to the long-sought wave–particle duality problem) is obtained at the cost of abandoning the possibility of treating physical phenomena objectively, i.e. by abandoning the classical space-time and causal description of nature which essentially rests upon our ability to separate uniquely the observer and the observed" (1958, p. 1).

12 I recently learned that in the 1970s Bion frequently talked about the uncertainty principle (Reiner, 2015, personal communication).

13 For a further explanation of what I view as the quantum-like psychoanalytic counterpart, see Eshel, 2002b, 2010.

References

Abram, J. (2007) *The Language of Winnicott: A Dictionary of Winnicott's Use of Words*. Second edition. London: Karnac Books.

Abram, J. (2008) Donald Woods Winnicott (1896–1971): A brief introduction. *International Journal of Psychoanalysis*, 89:1189–1217.

Abram, J. (2013) Introduction and Notes for the Vienna Congress 1971: A consideration of Winnicott's theory of aggression and an interpretation of the clinical implication (2012). In J. Abram (ed.), *Donald Winnicott Today* (pp. 1–25, 302–330). London & New York: Routledge/The New Library of Psychoanalysis.

Akhtar, S. (2009) *Comprehensive Dictionary of Psychoanalysis*. London: Karnac.

Alexander, R. (1981) On the analyst's "sleep" during the psychoanalytic session. In J.S. Grotstein (ed.), *Do I Dare Disturb the Universe: A Memorial to Wilfred R. Bion* (pp. 46–57). London: Maresfield.

Alvarez, A. (2012) *The Thinking Heart: Three Levels of Psychoanalytic Therapy with Disturbed Children*. London & New York: Routledge.

Amichai, Y. (1962) God full of mercy. In B. & B. Harshav (trans.), *Shirim [Poems], 1948–1962*. Jerusalem, Israel: Schocken, 1977.

Amir, D. (2012) The inner witness. *International Journal of Psychoanalysis*, 93:879–896.

Amir, I. (2000) Telepathic dreams in psychotherapy. Paper presented at the Conference of the Israel Psychoanalytic Institute, May 27.

Ansky, S. (1914) The Dybbuk, or between two worlds: A dramatic legend in four acts. In D.G. Roskies (ed.), G. Werman (trans.), *The Dybbuk and Other Writings*. New Haven, CT/London: Yale University Press, 2002.

Anzieu, D. (1989) *The Skin Ego*. New Haven/London: Yale University Press.

Arendt, H. (1965) *On Revolution*. London: Penguin.

Aron, L. (1996) *A Meeting of Minds: Mutuality in Psychoanalysis*. Hillsdale, NJ: The Analytic Press.

Aron, L. & Harris, A. (1993) Sandor Ferenczi: Discovery and rediscovery. In L. Aron & A. Harris (eds.), *The Legacy of Sandor Ferenczi* (pp. 1–35). Hillsdale, NJ: The Analytic Press.

Bach, S. (2011) Chimeras: Immunity, interpenetration, and the true self. *Psychoanalytic Review*, 98:39–56.

Baird, K., & Kracen, A.C. (2006) Vicarious traumatization and secondary traumatic stress: A research synthesis. *Counselling Psychology Quarterly*, 19:181–188.

Balint, M. (1955) Notes on parapsychology and parapsychological healing. *International Journal of Psycho-Analysis*, 36:31–35.

Balint, M. (1968) *The Basic Fault: Therapeutic Aspects of Regression*. London: Tavistock/Routledge.

Balter, L., Lothane, Z. & Spencer, J.H. (1980) On the analyzing instrument. *Psychoanalytic Quarterly*, 49:474–504.

Banai, E. (1996) 'Please hurry.' [Audio] On *Soon*. All Rights Reserved to Ehud Banai and ACUM.

Baranger, M. & W. (2009) *The Work of Confluence: Listening and Interpreting in the Psychoanalytic Field*. H. Breyter & D. Alcorn (trans.). London: Karnac.

Bass, A. (2001) It takes one to know one; or, whose unconscious is it anyway? *Psychoanalytic Dialogues*, 11:683–702.

Benjamin, J. (1988). *The Bonds of Love*. New York: Pantheon Books.

Benyamini, I. & Zivoni, I. (eds.) (2002) Introduction. In *Slave, Enjoyment, Master: On Sadism and Masochism in Psychoanalysis and in Cultural Studies* (pp. 9–14). Tel-Aviv: Resling Publishing.

Bergstein, A. (2008) On the capacity to bear the patient's love. *Sihot—Dialogue, Israel Journal of Psychotherapy*, 22:118–125.

Bergstein, A. (2014) Beyond the spectrum: Fear of breakdown, catastrophic change and the unrepressed unconscious. *Rivista di Psicoanalisi*, 60:847–868.

Berman, E. (1998) Arthur Penn's *Night Moves*: A film which interprets us. *International Journal of Psychoanalysis*, 79:175–178.

Berman, E. (2004) *Impossible Training: A Relational View of Psychoanalytic Education*. Hillsdale, NJ: The Analytic Press.

Berman, E. & Rolnik, E.J. (2002) In E.J. Rolnik (trans.), Introduction and Epilogue in E.J. Rolnik (trans.), *Sigmund Freud, Psychoanalytic Treatment: Essays, 1890–1938* (pp. 7–47, 244–278). Tel-Aviv: Am Oved Publishers.

Bernat, I. (2018) Negation as a method for psychoanalytic discoveries: Bion's turning-point in "Notes on memory and desire" and beyond. *Sihot—Dialogue, Israel Journal of Psychotherapy*, 33:11–22.

Bernstein, A. (2001) The fear of compassion. *Modern Psychoanalysis*, 26:209–219.

Bion, F. (1995) The days of our years. In C. Mawson (ed.), *The Complete Works of W. R. Bion, Vol. XV* (pp. 91–111). London: Karnac, 2014.

Bion W.R. (1959) Attacks on linking. *Int. J. Psychoanal.*, 40:308–315. Also in *Second Thoughts* (pp. 93–109). London: Maresfield Library/Karnac, 1967.

Bion, W.R. (1962a) A theory of thinking. In *Second Thoughts* (pp. 110–119). London: Maresfield Library/Karnac, 1967.

Bion, W.R. (1962b) *Learning from Experience*. London: Maresfield Library/ Karnac.

Bion, W.R. (1963) *Elements of Psychoanalysis*. London: Maresfield Library/ Karnac.

Bion W.R. (1965a) *Transformations*. London: Maresfield Library/Karnac.

Bion, W.R. (1965b) Memory and desire. In C. Mawson (ed.), *The Complete Works of W.R. Bion*. Vol. VI. London: Karnac Books, 2014.

Bion, W.R. (1967a) Notes on memory and desire. *The Psychoanalytic Forum*, 2:272–273.

Bion, W.R. (1967b) *Second Thoughts*. London: Maresfield.

Bion W.R. (1970) *Attention and Interpretation*. London: Maresfield Library/ Karnac.

Bion, W.R. (1975). *Bion's Brazilian Lectures, 2:* Rio/Sao Paulo, 1974. Rio de Janeiro, Brazil: Image Editora.

Bion, W.R. (1982) *The Long Week-End, 1897–1919: Part of a Life*. Abingdon, UK: Fleetwood Press.

Bion, W.R. (1985) *All My Sins Remembered: Another Part of a Life & The Other Side of Genius: Family Letters*. F. Bion (ed.). London: Karnac, 1991.

Bion, W.R. (1987) Clinical Seminars. In *Clinical Seminars and Other Works* (pp. 1–240). London: Karnac.

Bion, W.R. (1991) *A Memoir of the Future*. London: Karnac.

Bion W.R. (1992) *Cogitations*. London: Karnac.

Bion, W.R. (2005a) *The Italian Seminars*. P. Slotkin (trans.). London: Karnac.

Bion, W.R. (2005b) *The Tavistock Seminars*. London: Karnac.

Bion, W.R. (2013/1967) *Los Angeles Seminars and Supervisions*. J. Aguayo & B. Malin (eds.). London: Karnac.

Bion, W.R. (2018/1968). *Bion in Buenos Aires: Seminars, Case Presentation and Supervision*. Joseph Aguayo, Lia Pistiner de Cortinas, & Agnes Regeczkey (eds.). London: Karnac.

Blass, R.B. (2011) Introduction to On the value of "late Bion" to analytic theory and practice. *International Journal of Psychoanalysis*, 92:1081–1088.

Blass, R.B. (2012) On Winnicott's clinical innovations in the analysis of adults: Introduction to a controversy. *International Journal of Psychoanalysis*, 92:1439–1448.

Bohm, D. (1980) *Wholeness and the Implicate Order*. London: Routledge/Kegan Paul.

Bollas, C. (1987) *The Shadow of the Object: Psychoanalysis of the Unthought Known*. New York: Columbia University Press.

Bollas, C. (1990) Regression in the countertransference. In L.B. Boyer & P.L. Giovacchini (eds.), *Master Clinicians on Treating the Regressed Patient* (pp. 339–352). Northvale, NJ: Aronson.

Bollas, C. (1995) *Cracking Up: The Work of Unconscious Experience*. London: Routledge.

Bollas, C. (1999) *The Mystery of Things*. London & New York: Routledge.

Bollas, C. (2011) Introduction. In J. Sklar, *Landscapes of the Dark: History, Trauma, Psychoanalysis* (pp. xv–xxiii). London: Karnac.

Boris, H.N. (1987) Tolerating nothing. *Contemporary Psychoanalysis*, 23:351–366.

Botella, C. & Botella, S. (2005) *The Work of Psychic Figurability: Mental States without Representation*. Hove and New York: Brunner-Routledge/The New Library of Psychoanalysis.

Boyer, L.B. (1979) Countertransference with severely regressed patients. In L. Epstein & A. H. Feiner (eds.), *Countertransference* (pp. 347–374). Northvale, NJ/London: Aronson.

Brabant, E., Falzeder, E., & Giampieri-Deutsch P. (eds.) (1993) In P.T. Hoffer (trans.), *The Correspondence of Sigmund Freud and Sandor Ferenczi, Vol 1: 1908–1914*. Cambridge, MA: Harvard University Press.

Branfman, T.G. & Bunker, H.A. (1952) Three "extrasensory perception" dreams. *Psychoanalytic Quarterly*, 21:190–195.

Brenman Pick, I. (1988) Working through in the counter-transference. In E. Bott Spillius (ed.), *Melanie Klein Today, Vol. 2, Mainly Practice* (pp. 34–47). London: Routledge.

Brenner, I. (1994) The dissociative character: A reconsideration of "multiple personality." *Journal of the American Psychoanalytic Association*, 42:819–846.

Brenner, I. (2001) Intersubjectivity and beyond. In *Dissociation of Trauma: Theory, Phenomenology, and Technique* (pp. 177–200). Madison, CT: International University Press.

Britten, T. & Lyle, G. (1984) What's love got to do with it? [Audio recorded by Tina Turner.] On *Private Dancer*. England: Capitol Records.

Britton, R. (1998) *Belief and Imagination: Explorations in Psychoanalysis*. London & New York: Routledge.

Bromberg, P.M. (1998) *Standing in the Spaces: Essays on Clinical Process, Trauma, and Dissociation*. Hillsdale, NJ: Analytic Press.

Bromberg, P.M. (2006) *Awakening the Dreamer: Clinical Journeys*. Mahwah, NJ: Analytic Press.

Bromberg, P.M. (2011) *The Shadow of the Tsunami and the Growth of the Relational Mind*. New York: Routledge.

Brown, D.G. (1977) Drowsiness in the countertransference. *International Review of Psychoanalysis*, 4:481–492.

Brown, L.J. (2012) Bion's discovery of Alpha Function: Thinking under fire on the battlefield and in the consulting room. *International Journal of Psychoanalysis*, 93:1191–1214.

Brown, L.J. (2013) Bion at a threshold: Discussion of papers by Britton, Cassorla, Ferro & Foresti, & Zimmer. *Psychoanalytic Quarterly*, 82:413–433.

Brunswick, D. (1957) A comment on E. Servadio's A presumptively telepathic-precognitive dream during analysis. *International Journal of Psycho-Analysis*, 38:56.

Burlingham, D. (1935) Child analysis and the mother. *Psychoanalytic Quarterly*, 4:69–92.

Caldwell, L. & Joyce, A. (eds.) (2011) *Reading Winnicott*. London & New York: Routledge/The New Library of Psychoanalysis.

Carson, A. (1995) The truth about God. In *Glass, Irony and God*. New York: A New Directions Book.

Caruth, C. (1995) Introduction. In C. Caruth (ed.), *Trauma: Explorations in Memory* (pp. 3–12). Baltimore, MD: Johns Hopkins University Press.

Caruth C. (1996) *Unclaimed Experience: Trauma, Narrative, and History*. Baltimore, MD & London: The Johns Hopkins University Press.

Coen, S.J. (2000) Why we need to write openly about our clinical cases. *Journal of the American Psychoanalytic Association*, 48:449–470.

Cohen, L. (1967) Suzanne. On *Songs of Leonard Cohen*. [Audio] Sony/ATV Music Publishing LLC.

Crastnopol, M. (1997) Incognito or not? The patient's subjective experience of the analyst's private life. *Psychoanalytic Dialogues*, 7:257–280.

Dante Alighieri ((1320)) *Inferno*. In *Divine Comedy*. Trans. C. H. Sisson. Oxford: Oxford University Press/Oxford World's Classics, 2008..

Davies, J.M. (1996) Linking the pre-analytic with the postclassical: Integration, dissociation, and the multiplicity of unconscious processes. *Contemporary Psychoanalysis*, 32:553–576.

Davies, J.M. & Frawley, M.G. (1991) Dissociative processes and transference-countertransference paradigms in the psychoanalytically oriented treatment of adult survivors of childhood sexual abuse. *Psychoanalytic Dialogues*, 2:5–36.

Davies, J.M. & Frawley, M.G. (1992) Reply to Gabbard, Shengold, and Grotstein. *Psychoanalytic Dialogues*, 2:77–96.

Davies, J.M., & Frawley, M.G. (1994) *Treating the Adult Survivor of Childhood Sexual Abuse: A Psychoanalytic Perspective*. New York: Basic Books.

Davoine, F. & Gaudillière, J-M. (2004) *History Beyond Trauma*. S. Fairfield (trans.). New York: Other Press.

Dean, E.S. (1957) Drowsiness as a symptom of countertransference. *Psychoanalytic Quarterly*, 26:246–247.

De Masi, F. (2003) *The Sadomasochistic Perversion: The Entity and the Theories*. London: Karnac.

de M'Uzan, M. (1973) A case of masochistic perversion and an outline of a theory. *International Journal of Psycho-Analysis*, 54:455–467.

de M'Uzan, M. (1984/2003) Slaves of quantity. *Psychoanalytic Quarterly*, 72:711–725.

de M'Uzan, M. (2006) Invitation to frequent the shadows. *European Psychoanalytical Federation Bulletin*, 60:14–28.

de Peyer, J. (2016). Uncanny communication and the porous mind. *Psychoanalytic Dialogues*, 26:156–174.

Derrida, J. (1988) Telepathy. N. Royle (trans.), *Oxford Literary Review*, 10:3–41.

Dethiville, L. (2014) *Donald W. Winnicott: A New Approach*. S.G. L'evy (trans.). London: Karnac.

Devereux, G. (ed.) (1953) *Psychoanalysis and the Occult*. New York: International University Press.

Dias, E.O. (2016) *Winnicott's Theory of the Maturational Processes*. London: Karnac.

Dickes, R. (1965) The defence function of an altered state of consciousness: A hypnoid state. *Journal of the American Psychoanalytic Association*, 13:356–403.

Dickes, R. & Papernik, D.S. (1977) Defensive alternations of consciousness: Hypnoid states, sleep and the dream. *Journal of the American Psychoanalytic Association*, 25:635–654.

Dimen, M. (2001) Perversion is us? Eight notes. *Psychoanalytic Dialogues*, 11:825–860.

Dupont, M.A. (1984) On primary communication. *International Review of Psycho-Analysis*, 11:303–311.

Eaton, J.F. (2013) Discussion of Eshel's Tustin's "diabolon" and "metabolon" revisited: Further clinical explorations. The 18th Annual Frances Tustin Memorial Lecture, Los Angeles, California, November 16, 2013.

Eaton, J.L. (2011) *A Fruitful Harvest: Essays after Bion*. Seattle, WA: The Alliance Press.

Ehrenwald, H.J. (1942) Telepathy in dreams. *British Journal of Medical Psychology*, 19:313–323.

Ehrenwald, H.J. (1944) Telepathy in the psychoanalytic situation. *British Journal of Medical Psychology*, 20:51–62.

Ehrenwald, H.J. (1950a) Psychotherapy and the telepathic hypothesis. *American Journal of Psychotherapy*, 4:51–79.

Ehrenwald, H.J. (1950b) Presumptively telepathic incidents during analysis. *Psychoanalytic Quarterly*, 24:726–743.

Ehrenwald, H.J. (1956) Telepathy: Concepts, criteria and consequences. *Psychoanalytic Quarterly*, 30:425–444.

Ehrenwald, H.J. (1957) The telepathy hypothesis and doctrinal compliance in psychotherapy. *American Journal of Psychotherapy*, 11:359–379.

Ehrenwald, H.J. (1960) Schizophrenia, neurotic compliance, and the psi hypothesis. *Psychoanalytic Review*, 47:43–54.

Ehrenwald, H.J. (1971) Mother–child symbiosis: Cradle of ESP. *Psychoanalytic Review*, 58:455–466.

Ehrenwald, H.J. (1972) A neurophysiological model of psi phenomenon. *The Journal of Nervous and Mental Disease*, 54:406–418.

Eigen, M. (1981) The area of faith in Winnicott, Lacan, and Bion. *International Journal of Psychoanalysis*, 62:413–433.

Eigen, M. (1985) Towards Bion's starting point: Between catastrophe and faith. *International Journal of Psychoanalysis*, 66:321–330.

Eigen, M. (1993) *The Electrified Tightrope*. A. Phillips (ed.). Northvale, NJ/London: Jason Aronson.

Eigen, M. (1996) *Psychic Deadness*. Northvale, NJ: Aronson.

Eigen, M. (1999) *Toxic Nourishment*. London: Karnac.

Eigen, M. (2001) *Damaged Bonds*. London & New York: Karnac.

Eigen, M. (2002) *Rage*. Middletown, CT: Wesleyan University Press.

Eigen, M. (2004) *The Sensitive Self*. Middletown, CT: Wesleyan University Press.

Eigen, M. (2005) Interview with Micha Odenheimer. *Another Country (Eretz Acheret)*, 26:36–42.

Eigen, M. (2006) The annihilated self. *Psychoanalytic Review*, 93:25–38.

Eigen, M. (2009) *Flames from the Unconscious: Trauma, Madness, and Faith*. London: Karnac.

Eigen, M. (2010) *Eigen in Seoul: Volume 1: Madness and Murder*. London: Karnac.

Eigen, M. (2012) *Kabbalah and Psychoanalysis*. London: Karnac.

Eigen, M. (2014) *Faith*. London: Karnac.

Eisenbud, J. (1946) Telepathy and problems of psychoanalysis. *Psychoanalytic Quarterly*, 15:32–87.

Eisenbud, J. (1947) The dreams of two patients in analysis interpreted as a telepathicrève à deux. *Psychoanalytic Quarterly*, 16:39–60.

Eisenbud, J. (1948) Analysis of a presumptively telepathic dream. *Psychoanalytic Quarterly*, 22:103–135.

Eliot, T.S. (1940) Four Quartets, East Coker. In *Collected Poems: 1909–1962* (pp. 196–204). London: Faber and Faber, 1974.

Eliot T.S. (1942) Four Quartets, Little Gidding. In *Collected Poems: 1909–1962* (pp. 214–223). London: Faber and Faber, 1974.

Ellis, A. (1947) Telepathy and psychoanalysis: A critique of recent "findings" (with discussions by J. Eisenbud, G. Pederson-Krag, and N. Fodor). *Psychoanalytic Quarterly*, 21:607–659.

Ellis, A. (1949) Re-analysis of an alleged telepathic dream. *Psychoanalytic Quarterly*, 23:116–126.

Emanuel, R. (2001) A-void—An exploration of defences against sensing nothingness. *International Journal of Psychoanalysis*, 82:1069–1084.

Eshel, O. (1987) The silent patient (diploma thesis, Tel Aviv University, Sackler Faculty of Medicine). *Moshe Wulff Award*, 1987.

Eshel, O. (1996) Story-telling in the analytic situation. *Sihot—Dialogue, Israel Journal of Psychotherapy*, 10:182–193.

Eshel, O. (1998a) "Black Holes," deadness and existing analytically. *International Journal of Psychoanalysis*, 79:1115–1130.

Eshel, O. (1998b) Meeting acting out, acting in and enactment in psychoanalytic treatment, or: Going into the eye of the storm. *Sihot—Dialogue, Israel Journal of Psychotherapy*, 13:4–16.

Eshel, O. (2001) Whose sleep is it, anyway? Or "Night Moves." *International Journal of Psychoanalysis*, 82:545–562.

Eshel, O. (2002a) Let it be and become me: Notes on containing, identification, and the possibility of being [Hebrew]. *Sihot—Dialogue, Israel Journal of Psychotherapy*, 16:137–147.

Eshel, O. (2002b) My use of concepts from modern physics in psychoanalysis. In J. Raphael-Leff (ed.), *Between Sessions and Beyond the Couch* (pp. 173–176). University of Essex, Colchester UK: CPS Psychoanalytic Publications.

Eshel, O. (2004a). Let it be and become me: Notes on containing, identification, and the possibility of being. *Contemporary Psychoanal*ysis, 40:323–351.

Eshel, O. (2004b) From the "Green Woman" to "Scheherazade": The becoming of a fundamentally new experience in psychoanalytic treatment. *Contemporary Psychoanalysis*, 40:527–556.

Eshel, O. (2005) Pentheus rather than Oedipus: On perversion, survival and analytic "presencing." *International Journal of Psychoanalysis*, 86: 1071–1097.

Eshel, O. (2006) Where are you, my beloved? On absence, loss, and the enigma of telepathic dreams. *International Journal of Psychoanalysis*, 87: 1603–1627.

Eshel, O. (2007a) Do I dare be an analyst of a severely perverse patient? On being there ("presencing"), daring (passion), and caring (compassion). Manuscript prepared for a panel on perversion, IPA Berlin.

Eshel, O. (2007b) Facing three gates—The psyche's yearning for a new opportunity for becoming: Thoughts following Margaret Little and Winnicott. *Sihot—Dialogue, Israel Journal of Psychotherapy*, 22:1–31.

Eshel, O. (2009) To be "included" in the silence: On the silent patient and the analyst's "presencing." *Sihot—Dialogue, Israel Journal of Psychotherapy*, 23:221–235.

Eshel, O. (2010) Patient-analyst Interconnectedness: Personal notes on close encounters of a new dimension. *Psychoanalytic Inquiry*, 30:146–154.

Eshel, O. (2012a) In the dark depths "Beyond the pleasure principle": On facing the unbearable traumatic experience in psychoanalytic work. *Sihot—Dialogue, Israel Journal of Psychotherapy*, 27:5–15.

Eshel, O. (2012b) A beam of "chimeric" darkness: Presence, interconnectedness and transformation in the psychoanalytic treatment of a patient convicted of sex offences. *Psychoanalytic Review*, 99:149–178.

Eshel, O. (2013a) Patient–analyst "withness": On analytic "presencing," passion, and compassion in states of breakdown, despair, and deadness. *Psychoanalytic Quarterly*, 82:925–963.

Eshel, O. (2013b) Tustin's "diabolon" and "metabolon" revisited: Further clinical explorations. The Frances Tustin Memorial Prize, the 18th Annual Frances Tustin Memorial Lectureship in Los Angeles, California.

Eshel, O. (2013c) Reading Winnicott into nano-psychoanalysis: "There's plenty of room at the bottom." *Psychoanalytic Inquiry*, 33:36–49.

Eshel, O. (2014) On Intersubjectivity and beyond. *Sihot—Dialogue, Israel Journal of Psychotherapy*, 28:260–269.

Eshel, O. (2015a) The "hearing heart" and the "voice" of breakdown. In L. Aron & L. Henik (eds.), *Answering a Question with a Question: Contemporary Psychoanalysis and Jewish Thought, Vol. II: A Tradition of Inquiry* (pp. 133–152). Boston, MA: Academic Studies Press.

Eshel, O. (2015b) From extension to paradigm shift in clinical psychoanalysis: The revolutionary influence of Winnicott. Presentation at the 1st Congress of the International Winnicott Association (IWA), Sao Paulo, Brazil, May.

Eshel, O. (2015c) From extension to paradigm shift in clinical psychoanalysis: The revolutionary influence of Bion. Presentation at the International Psychoanalytic Summer Institute (PSI), Tuscany, Italy, August.

Eshel, O. (2016a) The "voice" of breakdown: On facing the unbearable traumatic experience in psychoanalytic work. *Contemporary Psychoanalysis*, 52:76–110.

Eshel, O. (2016b) Into the depths of a "black hole" and deadness. In A. Reiner (ed.), *Of Things Invisible to Mortal Sight: Celebrating the Work of James S. Grotstein* (pp. 39–68). London: Karnac, 2017.

Eshel, O. (2016c) In search of the absent analyst: Commentary on janine de peyer's "uncanny communication." *Psychoanalytic Dialogues*, 26:185–197.

Eshel, O. (2016d) Psychoanalysis in trauma: On trauma and its traumatic history in psychoanalysis. *Psychoanalytic Review*, 103:619–642.

Eshel O. (2017a) From extension to revolutionary change in clinical psychoanalysis: The radical influence of Bion and Winnicott. *Psychoanalytic Quarterly*, 86:753–794.

Eshel, O. (2017b) The vanished last scream. *Sihot—Dialogue, Israel Journal of Psychotherapy*, 31:116–125.

Eshel, O. (2017c) Beyond sexuality, beyond perversion: The annihilated last scream. *Studies in Gender and Sexuality*, 18:154–166.

Ettinger, B.L. (2006a) Fascinance: The woman-to-woman (girl-to-m/other) matrixial feminine difference. In G. Pollock (ed.), *Psychoanalysis and the Image* (pp. 60–93). Oxford: Blackwell.

Ettinger, B.L. (2006b) *The Matrixial Borderspace*. Minneapolis, MN: University of Minnesota Press.

Ettinger, B.L. (2010) (M)Other re-spect: Maternal subjectivity, the ready-made mother-monster and the ethics of respecting. *Studies in the Maternal*. Retrieved from: www.mamsic.bbk.ac.uk/mother_respect.html.

Fairbairn, W.R.D. (1952) *Psycho-analytic Studies of the Personality*. London: Routledge & Kegan Paul.

Falzeder, E. (1994) My grand-patient, my chief tormentor: A hitherto unnoticed case of Freud's and the consequences. *Psychoanalytic Quarterly*, 63:297–331.

Farrell, D. (1983) Freud's "thought-transference," repression, and the future of psychoanalysis. *International Journal of Psycho-Analysis*, 64:71–81.

Federn, P. (1952) *Ego Psychology and the Psychoses*. New York: Basic Books.

Feiner, A.H. (1993) Compassion and standards. *Contemporary Psychoanalysis*, 29:180–188.

Ferenczi, S. (1926) On the technique of psychoanalysis. In *Further Contributions to the Theory and Technique of Psycho-Analysis* (pp. 132–177). New York: Brunner-Mazel.

Ferenczi, S. (1932) *The Clinical Diary of Sandor Ferenczi*. J. Dupont (ed.), M. Balint & N.Z. Jackson (trans.). Cambridge, MA & London: Harvard University Press, 1988.

Ferenczi, S. (1933) Confusion of tongues between adults and the child: The language of tenderness and passion. In M. Balint (ed.), *Final Contributions to the Problems and Methods of Psycho-Analysis* (pp. 156–167). London: Karnac Books, 1980.

Ferro, A. (1999) *The Bi-Personal Field*. New York: Routledge.

Ferro, A. (2005) Some reflections on interpretation. *EPF Bulletin, Psychoanalysis in Europe*, 59:44–45.

Ferro, A. (2009) Who saw it? The spectre of the oneiric. *EPF Bulletin, Psychoanalysis in Europe*, 63:63–74.

Ferro, A. (2010) Book review essay: *The Work of Confluence*, by Madeline and Willy Baranger. *International Journal of Psychoanalysis*, 91:415–429.

Ferro, A. & Basile, R. (2009) The universe of the field and its inhabitants. In A. Ferro and R. Basile (eds.), *The Analytic Field: A Clinical Concept* (pp. 5–29). London: Karnac for EFPP.

Field, N. (1996) *Breakdown and Breakthrough: Psychotherapy in a New Dimension.* New York: Routledge.

Fiorini, L.G. (2011) Psychoanalytic ideas and applications series. In A. Green, *Illusions and Disillusions of Psychoanalytic Work* (pp. ix–x). London: Karnac.

Fodor, N. (1947) Telepathy in analysis: A discussion of five dreams. *Psychoanalytic Quarterly*, 21:171–189.

French, T.M. (1967) Discussant: Notes on memory and desire. *The Psychoanalytic Forum*, 2:274.

Freud, S. (1890) Psychical (or mental) treatment. *SE* 7:283–230 (1905).

Freud, S. (1895) (with J. Breuer). Studies on hysteria. *SE* 2:1–306.

Freud, S. (1896) The aetiology of hysteria. *SE* 3:189–221.

Freud, S. (1897) Letter to Wilhelm Fliess. *SE* 1:173–280.

Freud, S. (1900a) The interpretation of dreams (part 2). *SE* 5:339–621

Freud, S. (1900b) A premonitory dream fulfilled (appendix A). *SE* 5:623–625.

Freud, S. (1905) Three essays on the theory of sexuality. *SE* 7:125–245.

Freud, S. (1910) "Wild" psycho-analysis. *SE* 11:291–227.

Freud, S. (1912) Recommendations to physicians practising psycho-analysis. *SE* 12:109–120.

Freud, S. (1915a) Observations on transference-love. *SE* 12:159–171.

Freud, S. (1915b) The unconscious. *SE* 14:159–216.

Freud, S. (1917) Mourning and melancholia. *SE* 14:238–253.

Freud, S. (1919a) "A child is being beaten": A contribution to the study of the origin of sexual perversions. *SE* 17:177–204.

Freud, S. (1919b) The "uncanny." *SE* 17:217–253.

Freud, S. (1920) Beyond the pleasure principle. *SE* 18:1–64.

Freud, S. (1921) [1941] Psycho-analysis and telepathy. *SE* 18:177–193.

Freud, S. (1922) Dreams and telepathy. *SE* 18:197–220.

Freud, S. (1924) The economic problem of masochism. *SE* 19:157–170.

Freud, S. (1925) Some additional notes upon dream-interpretation as a whole. *SE* 19:127–138.

Freud, S. (1927) Fetishism. *SE* 21:149–157.

Freud, S. (1931) Female sexuality. *SE* 21:223–243.

Freud, S. (1933) Lecture XXX: Dreams and occultism. In New introductory lectures on psychoanalysis, *SE* 22:31–56.

Freud, S. (1937a) Analysis terminable and interminable. *SE* 23:216–253.

Freud, S. (1937b) Constructions in analysis. *SE* 23:255–269.

Freud, S. (1938) Splitting of the ego in the process of defence. *SE* 23:273–278.

Fulgencio, L. (2007) Winnicott's rejection of the basic concepts of Freud's metapsychology. *International Journal of Psychoanalysis*, 88:443–461.

Gampel, Y. (1996) The interminable uncanniness. In L. Rangell & R. Moses Hrushovski (eds.), *Psychoanalysis at the Political Border: Essays in Honor of Rafael Moses* (pp. 85–132). Madison, CT: International University Press.

Gargiulo, G.J. (2016) *Quantum Psychoanalysis: Essays on Physics, Mind, and Analysis Today*. New York: IPBooks.

Gartner, R.B. (2014) Trauma and countertrauma, resilience and counterresilience. *Contemporary Psychoanalysis*, 50:609–626.

Gay, P. (1988) *Freud: A Life for Our Time*. New York: Norton.

Ghent, E. (1990) Masochism, submission, surrender: Masochism as a perversion of surrender. In S.A. Mitchell & L. Aron (eds.), *Relational Psychoanalysis: The Emergence of a Tradition* (pp. 211–242). Hillsdale, NJ & London: The Analytic Press.

Gillespie, W.H. (1953) Extrasensory elements in dream interpretation. In *Life, Sex and Death: Selected Writings of William H. Gillespie* (pp. 151–161.) London: Routledge (New Library of Psychoanalysis,Vol. 23).

Gillespie, W.H. (1995) *Life, Sex and Death: Selected Writings of William H. Gillespie*. New York: Routledge.

Girard, M. (2010) Winnicott's foundation for the basic concepts of Freud's Metapsychology? *International Journal of Psychoanalysis*, 91:305–324.

Glasser, M. (1986) Identification and its vicissitudes as observed in the perversions. *International Journal of Psychoanalysis*, 67:9–16.

Glatzer, H.T. & Evans, W.N. (1977) On Guntrip's analysis with Fairbairn and Winnicott. *International Journal of Psychoanalytic Psychotherapy*, 6:81–98.

Glover, E. (1933) The relation of perversion formation to the development of reality sense. *International Journal of Psychoanalysis*, 14:486–503.

Godwin R.W. (1991) Wilfred Bion and David Bohm: Toward a quantum metapsychology. *Psychoanalytic Contemporary Thought*, 14(4):625–654.

Goldberg, A. (1975) A fresh look at perverse behaviour. *International Journal of Psychoanalysis*, 56:335–342.

Goldberg, A. (1999) *Being of Two Minds: The Vertical Split in Psychoanalysis and Psychotherapy*. Hillsdale, NJ & London: The Analytic Press.

Goldman, D. (2012) Vital sparks and the form of things unknown. In J. Abram (ed.), *Donald Winnicott Today* (pp. 331–357). New York: Routledge.

Govrin, A. (2016) *Conservative and Radical Perspectives on Psychoanalytic Knowledge: The Fascinated and the Disenchanted*. New York: Routledge/The Relational Perspectives Book Series.

Gonzalez, F. (2010) Nothing comes from nothing: Failed births, dead babies. In J.V. Buren & S. Alhanati (eds.), *Primitive Mental States* (pp. 122–134). New York: Routledge.

Grand, S. (2000) *The Reproduction of Evil*. Hillsdale, NJ: Analytic Press.
Green, A. (1973) On negative capability—A critical review of W.R. Bion's "Attention and Interpretation." *International Journal of Psychoanalysis*, 54:115–119.
Green, A. (1986) The dead mother. In *On Private Madness* (pp. 142–173). London: The Hogarth Press & The Institute of Psychoanalysis.
Green, A. (2010) Sources and vicissitudes of *being* in D.W. Winnicott's work. *Psychoanalytic Quarterly*, 79:11–35.
Green, A. (2011) *Illusions and Disillusions of Psychoanalytic Work*. London: Karnac.
Gribbin, J. (1992) *In Search of the Edge of Time: Black Holes, White Holes, Wormholes*. London: Penguin.
Grinberg, L. (1962) On a specific aspect of countertransference due to the patient's projective identification. *International Journal of Psychoanalysis*, 43:436–440.
Grinberg, L. (1991) Countertransference and projective counter-identification in non-verbal communication. *European Psychoanalytic Federation Bulletin*, 36:11–24.
Grinberg, L. (1997) Is the transference feared by the psychoanalyst? *International Journal of Psychoanalysis*, 78:1–14.
Grotstein, J.S. (1986) The psychology of powerlessness: disorders of self-regulation as a newer paradigm for psychopathology. *Psychoanalytic Inquiry*, 6:93–118.
Grotstein, J.S. (1989) A revised psychoanalytic conception of schizophrenia. *Psychoanalytic Psychology*, 6:253–275.
Grotstein, J.S. (1990a) "Black hole" as the basic psychotic experience: some newer psychoanalytic and neuroscience perspectives on psychosis. *Journal of the American Academy of Psychoanalysis*, 18:29–46.
Grotstein, J.S. (1990b) Nothingness, meaninglessness, chaos and "black hole" I. *Contemporary Psychoanalysis*, 26:257–291.
Grotstein, J.S. (1990c) Nothingness, meaninglessness, chaos and "black hole" II. *Contemporary Psychoanalysis*, 26:377–407.
Grotstein, J.S. (1993) Boundary difficulties in borderline patients. In L.B. Boyer & P.L. Giovacchini (eds.), *Master Clinicians on Treating the Regressed Patient, Vol. II* (pp. 107–142). Northvale, NJ: Aronson.
Grotstein, J.S. (2000) *Who Is the Dreamer Who Dreams the Dream? A Study of Psychic Presences*. Hillsdale, NJ & London: Analytic Press.
Grotstein, J.S. (2007) *A Beam of Intense Darkness: Wilfred Bion's Legacy to Psychoanalysis*. London: Karnac.
Grotstein, J.S. (2009) Dreaming as a "curtain of illusion": Revisiting the "Royal Road" with Bion as our guide. *International Journal of Psychoanalysis*, 90:733–752.

Grotstein, J.S. (2010) "Orphans of O": The negative therapeutic reaction and the longing for the childhood that never was. In J.V. Buren & S. Alhanati (eds.), *Primitive Mental States* (pp. 8–30). London & New York: Routledge.

Grotstein, J.S. (2013) Foreword. In J. Aguayo & B. Malin (eds.), Wilfred Bion: Los Angeles Seminars and Supervisions (p. xi). London: Karnac.

Guntrip, H. (1968) *Schizoid Phenomena, Object Relations and the Self.* London: The Hogarth Press.

Guntrip, H. (1975) My experience of analysis with Fairbairn and Winnicott: (How complete a result does psychoanalytic therapy achieve?) *International Review of Psychoanalysis*, 2:145–156.

Harding, C. (ed.) (2001) *Sexuality: Psychoanalytic Perspectives.* Hove, East Sussex: Brunner-Routledge.

Hawking, S. (1988) *A Brief History of Time: From the Big Bang to Black Holes.* London: Bantam.

Hawking, S. (1993) *Black Holes and Baby Universes, and Other Essays.* London: Bantam.

Haynal, A. (1998) *The Technique at Issue: Controversies in Psychoanalysis from Freud and Ferenczi to Michael Balint.* London: Karnac.

Hazan, Y. (2008) Thoughts on listening. Lecture at the Israel Psychoanalytic Society, October, Jerusalem, Israel.

Herman, J.L. (1992) *Trauma and Recovery.* New York: Basic Books.

Hermann, I. (1976/1936) Clinging-going-in-search—A contrasting pair of instincts and their relation to sadism and masochism. *Psychoanalytic Quarterly*, 12, 45:5–36.

Hernandez, M. (1998) Winnicott's "Fear of breakdown": On and beyond trauma. *Diacritics*, 28:134–143.

Herskovitz, H.H. (1967) Discussant: Notes on memory and desire. *The Psychoanalytic Forum*, 2:278–279.

Hinshelwood, R.D. (2010) Making sense: Bion's nomadic journey. Unpublished paper presented at PCC Bion Conference, Los Angeles.

Hinshelwood, R.D. (2013) Endorsement. In J. Aguayo & B. Malin (eds.), *Wilfred Bion: Los Angeles Seminars and Supervisions.* London: Karnac.

Hinshelwood, R.D. (2018 (2018)) Forward. In J. Aguayo, L. Pistiner de Cortinas, & A. Regeczkey (eds.), *Bion in Buenos Aires: Seminars, Case Presentation and Supervision* (pp. xviii–xx). London: Karnac.

Hitschmann, E. (1924) Telepathy and psycho-analysis. *International Journal of Psycho-Analysis*, 5:425–439.

Hitschmann, E. (1953) Telepathy during psychoanalysis. In G. Devereux (ed.), *Psychoanalysis and the Occult* (pp. 128–132). New York: International University Press.

Home, H.J. (1966) The concept of mind. *International Journal of Psychoanalysis*, 47:42–49.

Homer (800 BCE) The Odyssey. In S. Butler (trans.), The Project Gutenberg eBook of *The Odyssey*.

Howell, E. (2005) *The Dissociative Mind*. New York: Routledge.

Hughes, J.M. (1989) *Reshaping the Psychoanalytic Domain: The Work of Melanie Klein, W.R.D. Fairbairn, and D.W. Winnicott*. Berkeley, CA: University of California Press.

Ithier, B. (2016) The arms of the chimeras. *International Journal of Psycho-Analysis*, 97:451–478.

Jones, E. (1957) *The Life and Work of Sigmund Freud, Vol. 3: The Last Phase*. New York: Basic Books.

Kantrowitz, J.L. (2001) The analysis of preconscious phenomena and its communication. *Psychoanalytic Inquiry*, 21:24–39.

Kaplan, L.J. (1993) *Female Perversions*. London: Penguin.

Kelman, H. (1987) On resonant cognition. *International Review of Psychoanalysis*, 14:111–123.

Khan, M.M.R. (1963) The concept of cumulative trauma. In *The Privacy of the Self* (pp. 42–58). London: The Hogarth Press, 1986.

Khan, M.M.R. (1964) Ego-distortion, cumulative trauma and the role of reconstruction in the analytic situation. In *The Privacy of the Self* (pp. 59–68). London: The Hogarth Press, 1986.

Khan, M.M.R. (1971) To hear with eyes: Clinical notes on body as subject and object. In *The Privacy of the Self* (pp. 234–250). London: The Hogarth Press, 1986.

Khan, M.M.R. (1972) The use and abuse of dream in psychic experience. In *The Privacy of the Self* (pp. 306–315). London: The Hogarth Press.

Khan, M.M.R. (1979) *Alienation in Perversion*. London: The Hogarth Press and the Institute of Psychoanalysis.

Kohut, H. (1972) Lecture 1 (January 7, 1972) Perversions. In P. Tolpin & M. Tolpin (eds.), *The Chicago Institute Lectures* (pp. 1–11). Hillsdale, NJ & London: The Analytic Press, 1996.

Kohut, H. (1977) *The Restoration of the Self*. New York: International Universities Press.

Kohut, H. (1978) Reflections on advances in self-psychology. In P. Orenstein (ed.), *The Search for the Self* (Vol. 13, pp. 261–357). Madison, CT: International Universities Press.

Kohut, H. (1984) *How Does Analysis Cure?* A. Goldberg & P. Stepansky (eds.). Chicago: University of Chicago Press.

Kristof, N.D. (July 7, 1999) Alien abduction? Science calls it sleep paralysis. *The New York Times*, 6.

Kuhn, T.S. (1962) *The Structure of Scientific Revolutions*. Chicago & London: The University of Chicago Press.

Kulka, R. (1997) Quantum selfhood: Commentary on paper by Beebe, Lachman, and Jaffe. *Psychoanalytic Dialogues*, 7:183–187.

Kulka, R. (2008a) From civilization and its discontents to culture of compassion: Optimistic contemplation on Freud's pessimism. In G. Shefler (ed.), *Freud: Civilization and Psychoanalysis* [Hebrew] (pp. 98–121). Or-Yehuda, Israel: Kinneret, Zmora-Bitan, Dvir & Magnes Press.

Kulka, R. (2008b) Irony and compassion: The cessation of duality. Lecture, Israel Association for Self Psychology and the Study of Subjectivity.

Lamott, A. (1994) *Bird by Bird: Some Instructions on Writing and Life*. New York: Anchor Books, Doubleday.

Laplanche, J. (1999) Masochism and the general theory of seduction. In *Essays on Otherness* (pp. 197–213). London & New York: Routledge.

Lazar, R. (2003) Knowing hatred. *International Journal of Psychoanalysis*, 84:405–425.

Lazar, S.G. (2001) Knowing, influencing, and healing: Paranormal phenomena and implications for psychoanalysis and psychotherapy. *Psychoanalytic Inquiry*, 21:113–131.

Levenson, E. (1972) *The Fallacy of Understanding*. Hillsdale, NJ: Analytic Press, 2005.

Levine, H.B. (1990a) Clinical issues in the analysis of adults who were sexually abused as children. In H. B. Levine (ed.), *Adult Analysis and Childhood Sexual Abuse* (pp. 197–218). Hillsdale, NJ: The Analytic Press.

Levine, H.B. (1990b) Introduction. In H. B. Levine (ed.), *Adult Analysis and Childhood Sexual Abuse* (pp. 3–19). Hillsdale, NJ: The Analytic Press.

Levine, H.B. (1997) Difficulties in maintaining an analytic stance in the treatment of adults who were sexually abused as children. *Psychoanalytic Inquiry*, 17:312–328.

Levine, H.B. (2014) Psychoanalysis and trauma. *Psychoanalytic Inquiry*, 34:214–224.

Levine, H., Reed, G.S. & Scarfone, D. (eds.) (2013) *Unrepresented States and the Construction of Meaning: Clinical and Theoretical Contribution*. London: Karnac.

Lichtenberg, J., Lachmann, F. & Fosshage J. (1992) *Self and Motivational Systems: Toward a Theory of Psychoanalytic Technique*. Hillsdale, NJ/London: Analytic Press.

Lifton, R.J. (1976) From analysis to formation: Towards a shift in psychological paradigm. *Journal of American Academy of Psychoanalysis*, 4:63–94.

Lindner, R. (1976) *The Fifty-Minute Hour: A Collection of True Psychoanalytic Tales*. New York: Bantam Books.

Lindon, J.A. (1967) Discussant: Notes on memory and desire. *The Psychoanalytic Forum*, 2:274–275.

Little, M. (1981) Transference in borderline states. In *Transference Neurosis and Transference Psychosis* (pp. 135–153). Northvale, NJ: Jason Aronson.

Little, M. (1985) Winnicott working in areas where psychotic anxieties predominate. *Free Associations*, 3:9–42.

Little, M. (1986) On basic unity (primary total undifferentiatedness). In G. Kohon (ed.), *The British School Of Psychoanalysis: The Independent Tradition* (pp. 136–153). London: Free Association.

Löfgren, L.B. (1968) Recent publications on parapsychology. *Journal of American Psychoanalytic Association*, 16:146–178.

Loparic, Z. (2002) Winnicott's paradigm outlined. Retrieved from: www.centrowinnicott.com.br

Loparic, Z. (2010) From Freud to Winnicott: Aspects of a paradigm change. In J. Abram (ed.), *Donald Winnicott Today* (pp. 113–156). New York: Routledge, 2013.

Lopez-Corvo, R.E. (2014) *Traumatised and Non-Traumatised States of the Personality: A Clinical Understanding Using Bion's Approach*. London: Karnac.

Major, R. & Miller, P. (1981) Empathy, antipathy and telepathy in the analytic process. *Psychoanalytic Inquiry*, 1:449–470.

Marcus, D.M. (1997) On knowing what one knows. *Psychoanalytic Quarterly*, *66*:219–241.

Marcus, D.M. (1999) Personal communication.

Markillie, R. (1996) Some personal recollections and impressions of Harry Guntrip. *International Journal of Psychoanalysis*, 77:763–771.

Maroda, K. (1994) *The Power of Countertransference: Innovation in Analytic Technique*. Northvale, NJ & London: Aronson.

Matte Blanco, I. (1975) *The Unconscious as Infinite Sets: An Essay in Bi-logic*. London: Maresfield Library.

Mayer, E.L. (1996a) Changes in science and changing ideas about knowledge and authority in psychoanalysis. *Psychoanalytic Quarterly*, 65:158–200.

Mayer, E.L. (1996b) Subjectivity and intersubjectivity of clinical facts. *International Journal of Psycho-Analysis*, 77:709–737.

Mayer, E.L. (2001) On "Telepathic dreams?" An unpublished paper by Robert J. Stoller. *Journal of American Psychoanalytic Association*, 49:629–657.

McCann, I.L. & Pearlman, L.A. (1990) Vicarious traumatization: A framework for understanding the psychological effects of working with victims. *Journal of Traumatic Stress*, 3:131–150.

McDougall, J. (1995) *The Many Faces of Eros*. London: Free Association Books.

McLaughlin, J.T. (1975) The sleepy analyst: Some observations on states of consciousness in the analyst at work. *Journal of the American Psychoanalytic Association*, 23:363–382.

McLuhan, M. (1994) *Understanding Media: The Extensions of Man*. Cambridge, MA: MIT Press.

Meerloo, A.M. (1949) Telepathy as a form of archaic communication. *Psychoanalytic Quarterly*, 23:691–704.

Melville, H. (1851) *Moby Dick*. New York: Norton, 1967.

Minhot, L. (2015) Over the shoulders of a giant. Presentation at the International Winnicott Association (IWA) Conference, Sao Paulo, Brazil, May 15.

Mitchell, S.A. (1993) *Hope and Dread in Psychoanalysis*. New York: Basic Books.

Mitchell, S.A. (1998) The emergence of features of the analyst's life. *Psychoanalytic Dialogues*, 8:187–194.

Mitrani, J.L. (1995) Towards an understanding of unmentalized experience. *Psychoanalytic Quarterly*, 64:68–112.

Mitrani, J.L. (2001) "Taking the transference:" Some technical implications in three papers by Bion. *International Journal of Psychoanalysis*, 82:1085–1104.

Mitrani, J.L. (2015) *Psychoanalytic Technique and Theory: Taking the Transference*. London: Karnac.

Modell, A.H. (1986) *Psychoanalysis in a New Context*. New York: International Universities Press.

Modell, A.H. (1990) *Other Times, Other Realities*. Cambridge, MA: Harvard University Press.

Modell, A.H. (1993) *The Private Self*. Cambridge, MA and London: Harvard University Press.

Modell, A.H. (2005) Emotional memory, metaphor and meaning. *Psychoanalytic Inquiry*, 25:555–568.

Modell, A.H. (2006) *Imagination and the Meaningful Brain*. Cambridge, MA: MIT Press.

Modell, A.H. (2009) Metaphor—The bridge between feelings and knowledge. *Psychoanalytic Inquiry*, 29:6–17.

Mollon, P. (1997) Who am I speaking to? The challenge of dissociative states. Unpublished paper, presented at the conference "Mind traps: Disclaimers of reality," Tavistock Society of Psychotherapists, 20 September, 1997, London.

Nacht, S. (1963) The non-verbal relationship in psycho-analysis treatment. *International Journal of Psychoanalysis*, 44:333–339.

Nacht, S. (1965) Criteria and technique for the termination of analysis. *International Journal of Psychoanalysis*, 46:107–116.

Nacht, S. & Viderman, S. (1960) The pre-object universe in the transference situation. *International Journal of Psychoanalysis*, 41:385–388.

Nietzsche, F. (1886) *Beyond Good and Evil*. W. Kaufmann (trans.). New York: Random House, 1968.

Ofarim, Y. (1998) Personal communication.

Ogden T.H. (1986) *The Matrix of the Mind*. Northvale, NJ & London: Jason Aronson.

Ogden, T.H. (1994) *Subjects of Analysis*. London: Karnac.

Ogden, T.H. (1995) Analyzing forms of aliveness and deadness in the transference-countertransference. *International Journal of Psychoanalysis*, 76: 695–709.

Ogden, T.H. (1996). The perverse subject of analysis. *Journal of the American Psychoanalytic Association*, 44:1121–1146.

Ogden, T.H. (1997) *Reverie and Interpretation: Sensing Something Human*. London: Karnac.

Ogden, T.H. (2001a) Reading Winnicott. In *Conversations at the Frontier of Dreaming* (pp. 203–235). London & New York: Karnac.

Ogden, T.H. (2001b) Re-minding the body. In *Conversations at the Frontiers of Dreaming* (pp. 153–174). London: Karnac.

Ogden, T.H. (2004) This art of psychoanalysis: Dreaming undreamt dreams and interrupted cries. *International Journal of Psychoanalysis*, 85:857–877.

Ogden T.H. (2005a) Reading Bion. In *This Art of Psychoanalysis: Dreaming Undreamt Dreams and Interrupted Cries* (pp. 77–92). London & New York: Routledge.

Ogden, T.H. (2005b) On holding and containing, being and dreaming. In *This Art of Psychoanalysis: Dreaming Undreamt Dreams and Interrupted Cries* (pp. 93–108). London & New York: Routledge.

Ogden, T.H. (2009) Bion's four principles of mental functioning. In *Rediscovering Psychoanalysis: Thinking and Dreaming, Learning and Forgetting* (pp. 90–113). London & New York: Routledge.

Ogden, T.H. (2014) Fear of breakdown and the unlived life. *International Journal of Psychoanalysis*, 95:205–223.

Orange, D.M. (2006) For whom the bell tolls: Context, complexity and compassion in psychoanalysis. *International Journal of Psychoanalytic Self-Psychology*, 1:5–21.

Ornstein, P.H. & Ornstein, A. (1985) Clinical understanding and explaining: The empathic vantage point. In A. Goldberg (ed.), *Progress in Self-Psychology* (pp. 43–61). Northvale, NJ: Guilford Press.

Oz, A. (1972) *My Michael*. N. de Lange (trans.). London: Chatto & Windus.

Pacheco, M.A. (1980) Neurotic and psychotic transference and projective identification. *International Review of Psychoanalysis*, 7:157–164.

Padel, J. (1996) The case of Harry Guntrip. *International Journal of Psychoanalysis*, 77:755–761.

Pajaczkowska, C. (2000) *Perversion*. Cambridge, UK: Icon Book/Ideas in Psychoanalysis.

Pauli, W. (1958) *General Principles of Quantum Mechanics*. Translated from German by P. Achuthan and K. Venkatesan. Berlin and New York: Springer-Verlag,1980.

Pederson-Krag, G. (1947) Telepathy and repression. *Psychoanalytic Quarterly*, 16:61–68.

Penn, A. (Director) & Sherman, R. (Producer) (1975) *Night Moves* [Film]. United States: Warner Bros.

Phillips, A. (1988) *Winnicott*. London: Fontana Press.

Phillips, A. (1997) Adam Phillips. In A. Molino (ed.), *Freely Associated* (pp. 127–164). London & New York: Free Association Books.

Plath, S. (1962) Poppies in October, in *Ariel*. London: Faber and Faber, 2001.

Pontalis, J.-B. (2003) *Windows*. A. Quinney (trans.). Lincoln, NE & London: University of Nebraska Press.

Quinodoz, D. (1996) An adopted analysand's transference of a "hole-object." *International Journal of Psychoanalysis*, 77:323–336.

Quinodoz, D. (2002) Termination of a fe/male transsexual patient's analysis: An example of general validity. *International Journal of Psychoanalysis*, 83:783–798.

Quinodoz, J-M. (2008) Listening to Hanna Segal. D. Alcorn (trans.). London/ New York: Routledge/The New Library of Psychoanalysis.

Racker, H. (1968) *Transference and Countertransference*. London: Maresfield Reprints.

Reiner, A. (2012) *Bion and Being: Passion and the Creative Mind*. London: Karnac.

Reiner, A. (2017) Ferenczi's "Astra" and Bion's "O": A Clinical Perspective. In A. Reiner (ed.), *Of Things Invisible to Mortal Sight: Celebrating the Work of James S. Grotstein* (pp. 131–148). London: Karnac.

Reis, B. (2009a) Performative and enactive features of psychoanalytic witnessing: The Transference as the scene of address. *International Journal of Psychoanalysis*, 90:1359–1372.

Reis, B. (2009b) We: Commentary on papers by Trevarthen, Ammaniti & Trentini, and Gallese. *Psychoanalytic Dialogues*, 19:565–579.

Renik, O. (1991) One kind of negative therapeutic response. *Journal of the American Psychoanalytic Association*, 39:87–105.

Rittenberg, S.M. (1987) On charm. *International Journal of Psychoanalysis*, 68:389–396.

Rodman, R.F. (ed.) (1987) To Wilfred R. Bion. In *The Spontaneous Gesture: Selected Letters of D.W. Winnicott*. Cambridge, MA: Harvard University Press.

Róheim, G. (1932) Telepathy in a dream. *Psychoanalytic Quarterly*, 1:277–291.

Rolnik, E. J. (2002) On the stigmata of psychoanalysis: Presentation at Tel-Aviv University, June 2002.

Roudinesco, E. (2001) *Why Psychoanalysis?* R. Bowlby (trans.). New York: Columbia University Press.

Rowling, J. K. (2007) *Harry Potter and the Deathly Hallows* (Harry Potter 7). London: Bloomsbury.

Royle, N. (1991) *Telepathy and Literature: Essays on the Leading Mind.* Oxford: Blackwell.

Sandler, J. (1988) The concept of projective identification. In J. Sandler (ed.), *Projection, Identification, Projective Identification* (pp. 13–26). London: Karnac Books.

Saul, L.J. (1938) Telepathic sensitiveness as a neurotic symptom. *Psychoanalytic Quarterly*, 7:329–335.

Schwarz, B.E. (1969) Synchronicity and telepathy. *Psychoanalytic Review*, 56:44–56.

Scott, W.C. (1975) Remembering sleep and dreams. *International Review of Psychoanalysis*, 2:253–354.

Searles, H.F. (1959) Oedipal love in the countertransference. In *Collected Papers on Schizophrenia and Related Subjects* (pp. 284–303). London: Maresfield Library.

Searles, H.F. (1961) Phases of patient–therapist interaction in the psychotherapy of chronic schizophrenia. In *Collected Papers on Schizophrenia and Related Subjects* (pp. 521–559). New York: International University Press, 1986.

Searles, H.F. (1965) *Collected Papers on Schizophrenia and Related Subjects.* London: Maresfield.

Searles, H.F. (1979) *Countertransference and Related Subjects.* New York: International University Press.

Searles, H.F. (1986) Introduction. In *Collected Papers on Schizophrenia and Related Subjects* (pp. 19–38). New York: International Universities Press.

Segal, H. (2006) Reflections on truth, tradition, and the psychoanalytic tradition of truth. *American Imago*, 63:283–292.

Servadio, E. (1955) A presumptively telepathic-precognitive dream during analysis. *International Journal of Psycho-Analysis*, 36:27–30.

Servadio, E. (1956) Transference and thought-transference. *International Journal of Psycho-Analysis*, 37:392–395.

Servadio, E. (1957) Reply to Dr. Brunswick's comment. *International Journal of Psycho-Analysis*, 38:57.

Shainberg, D. (1976) Telepathy in psychoanalysis: An instance. *American Journal of Psychotherapy*, 30:463–472.

Shengold, L. (1989) *Soul Murder: The Effects of Child Abuse and Deprivation.* New Haven, CT: Yale University Press.

Simpson, R.B. (2003) Introduction to Michel de M'Uzan's "Slaves of quantity." *Psychoanalytic Quarterly*, 72:699–709.

Simonov K. (1941) Wait for me and I'll come back! *Pravda*, January, 1942, A. Shlonsky (trans.), 1943.

Slavin, J. (2002) The innocence of sexuality. *Psychoanalytic Quarterly*, 71:51–80.

Slavin, J. & Pollock, L. (1996) Mommy, you're beautiful: Is there a place for the concept of reparenting in psychoanalytic treatment? Paper presented at the Spring Meeting Division of Psychoanalysis (39), American Psychological Association, New York.

Smith, H.F. (2010) Being and the death drive: The quality of Green's thinking. *Psychoanalytic Quarterly*, 79:1–10.

Sobol, J. (1982) *Soul of a Jew: Weininger's Last Night* [Hebrew]. Tel Aviv, Israel: Or-Am.

Socarides, C.W. (1959) Meaning and content of a pedophiliac perversion. *Journal of the American Psychoanalytic Association*, 7:84–94.

Socarides, C.W. (1974) The demonified mother: a study of voyeurism and sexual sadism. *International Review of Psycho-Analysis*, 1:187–195.

Souter, K.M. (2009) The war memoirs: Some origins of the thought of W.R. Bion. *International Journal of Psychoanalysis*, 90:795–808.

Spelman, M.B. (2013) *The Evolution of Winnicott's Thinking: Examining the Growth of Psychoanalytic Thought Over Three Generations*. London: Karnac.

Spelman, M.B. & Thomson-Salo, F. (eds.) (2015) *The Winnicott Tradition: Lines of Development—Evolution of Theory and Practice over the Decades*. London: Karnac.

Spensley, S. (1995) *Frances Tustin*. London: Routledge.

Spiegelman, J.M. (2003) Developments in the concept of synchronicity in the analytic relationship and in theory. In N. Totton (ed.), *Psychoanalysis and the Paranormal: Lands of Darkness* (pp. 143–160). London: Karnac.

Spillius, E.B. (1988) Introduction: Projective identification. In E.B Spillius (ed.), *Melanie Klein Today, Vol. 1: Mainly Theory* (pp. 81–86). London & New York: Tavistock/Routledge.

Spillius, E.B. (1992) Clinical experiences of projective identification. In R. Anderson (ed.), *Clinical Lectures on Klein and Bion* (pp. 59–73). London & New York: Tavistock/Routledge.

Spurling, L.S. (2008) Is there still a place for the concept of "Therapeutic Regression" in psychoanalysis? *International Journal of Psychoanalysis*, 89:523–540.

Stanton, M. (1990) *Sandor Ferenczi: Reconsidering Active Intervention*. London: Free Association Books.

Stark, M. (1999) *Modes of Therapeutic Action: Enhancement of Knowledge, Provision of Experience, and Engagement in Relationship*. Northvale, NJ & London: Jason Aronson.

Stav, A. (2007) The Comedy: Introduction. In Dante Alighieri, *The Divine Comedy: Inferno*. A. Stav (trans.). Tel Aviv: Hakkibutz Hameuchad.

Stein, R. (2003) Why perversion? Paper presented on the IARPP Online Colloquium, November 2003.

Stern, D.B. (1997) *Unformulated Experience: From Dissociation to Imagination in Psychoanalysis*. New York: Routledge.

Stern, D.B. (2002) Language and the nonverbal as a unity: Discussion of 'Where is the Action in the "Talking Cure"?' *Contemporary Psychoanalysis*, 38:515–25.

Stern, D.B. (2003) The fusion of horizons: Dissociation, enactment, and understanding. *Psychoanalytic Dialogues*, 13:843–875.

Stern, D.B. (2004) The eye sees itself: dissociation, enactment, and the achievement of conflict. *Contemporary Psychoanalysis*, 40:197–237.

Stern, D.B. (2009) Shall the twain meet? Dissociation, metaphor, and co-occurrence. *Psychoanalytic Inquiry*, 29:79–90.

Stern, D.B. (2010) *Partners in Thought: Working with Unformulated Experience, Dissociation, and Enactment*. New York: Routledge.

Stern, D.B. (2012) Witnessing across time: Accessing the present from the past and the past from the present. *Psychoanalytic Quarterly*, 81:53–81.

Stern, D.N. (1985) *The Interpersonal World of the Infant*. New York: Basic Books.

Stern, D.N. (1995) *The Motherhood Constellation*. New York: Basic Books.

Stern, D.N. (2004) *The Present Moment in Psychotherapy and Everyday Life*. New York: Norton.

Stern, D.N., Sander, L.W., Nahum, J.P., Harrison, A.M., Lyons-Ruth, K., Morgan, A.C., Bruschweilerstern, N., & Tronick, E.Z. (1998) Non-interpretive mechanisms in psychoanalytic therapy: the "something more" than interpretation. *International Journal of Psychoanalysis*, 79:903–921.

Stevens, A. (1994) Jung. In *Freud and Jung: A Dual Introduction*. New York: Barnes & Noble.

Stewart, H. (1992) Interpretation and other agents for psychic change. In *Psychic Experience and Problems of Technique* (pp. 127–140). London: Routledge.

Stoller, R.J. (1974) Hostility and mystery in perversion. *International Journal of Psychoanalysis*, 55:425–434.

Stoller, R.J. (1975) *Perversion: The Erotic Form of Hatred*. New York: Pantheon Books.

Stoller, R.J. (1991) *Pain and Passion: A Psychoanalyst Explores the World of S & M*. New York & London: Plenum Press.

Stolorow, R.D. (1975a) Addendum to a partial analysis of a perversion involving bugs: an illustration of the narcissistic function of perverse activity. *International Journal Psychoanalysis*, 56:361–364.

Stolorow, R.D. (1975b) The narcissistic function of masochism (and sadism). *International Journal of Psychoanalysis*, 56:441–448.

Stolorow, R., Atwood, G. & Branchaft, B. (1994) Masochism and its treatment. In R. Stolorow, G. Atwood & B. Brandchaft (eds.), *The Intersubjective Perspective* (pp. 121–126). Northvale, NJ & London: Jason Aronson.

Strachey, J. (1955a) Editor's note. In Psycho-analysis and telepathy, *SE* 18:175–176.

Strachey, J. (1955b) Editor's note. In Dreams and telepathy, *SE* 18:196.

Strachey, J. (1961) Editor's note. In Some additional notes on dream-interpretation as a whole, *SE* 19:125–126.

Strachey, J. (1964) Editor's note. In New introductory lectures on psycho-analysis, *SE* 22:3–4, 47–48.

Strean, H.S. & Nelson, M.C. (1962) A further clinical illustration of the paranormal triangle hypothesis. *Psychoanalytic Review*, 49:61–73.

Sucharov, M.S. (1992) Quantum physics and self-psychology: Towards a new epistemology. *Progressive Self Psychology*, 8:199–211.

Suchet, M. (2017) Surrender, transformation, and transcendence. *Psychoanalytic Dialogues*, 26:747–760.

Sullivan, H.S. (1954) *The Interpersonal Theory of Psychiatry*. New York: Norton.

Symington J. & Symington N. (1996) *The Clinical Thinking of Wilfred Bion*. New York: Routledge.

Symington, N. (1986) The analyst's act of freedom as agent of therapeutic change. In G. Kohon (ed.), *The British School of Psychoanalysis: The Independent Tradition* (pp. 253–270). London: Free Association.

Symington, N. (1996) *The Making of a Psychotherapist*. London: Karnac.

Szykierski, D. (2010) The traumatic roots of containment: The evolution of Bion's metapsychology. *Psychoanalytic Quarterly*, 79:935–68.

Szymborska, W. (1983) Autotomy. In: *Postwar Polish Poetry*. 3rd edition, ed. and trans. C. Milosz (pp. 115–116). Berkeley, CA: University of California Press.

Tennes, M. (2007) Beyond intersubjectivity: The transpersonal dimension of the psychoanalytic encounter. *Contemporary Psychoanalysis*, 43:505–525.

Terr, L.C. (1985) Remembered images and trauma—A psychology of the supernatural. *Psychoanalytic Study of the Child*, 40:493–533.

Thomas, D. (1933) And death shall have no dominion. In *The Poems of Dylan Thomas*. New York: New Directions, 2003.

Torok, M. (1986) Afterword: What is occult in occultism? Between Sigmund Freud and Sergei Pankeiev wolf man. In N. Rand (trans.), N. Abraham & M. Torok (eds.), *The Wolf Man's Magic Word: A Cryptonomy* (pp. 84–106). Minneapolis, MN: University Minnesota Press.

Turner T. (1984). What's love got to do with it? Britten, T. & Lyle, G. [Audio recorded by Tina Turner.] On *Private Dancer*. England: Capitol Records.

Tustin, F. (1972) *Autism and Childhood Psychosis*. London: The Hogarth Press.

Tustin, F. (1986) *Autistic Barriers in Neurotic Patients*. London: Tavistock.

Tustin, F. (1990) *The Protective Shell in Children and Adults*. London: Karnac Books.

Tustin, F. (1991) Revised understandings of psychogenic autism. *International Journal of Psychoanalysis*, 72:585–591.

Tustin, F. (1992/1981) *Autistic States in Children*. Revised edition. London: Routledge.

Tustin, F. (1994) The perpetuation of an error. *Journal of Child Psychotherapy*, 20:3–23.

Tyson, P. & Tyson, R.L. (1963) *Psychoanalytic Theories of Development: An Integration*. New Haven, CT: Yale University Press.

Ullman, M. (2003) Dream telepathy: Experimental and clinical findings. In N. Totten (ed.), *Psychoanalysis and the Paranormal: Lands of Darkness* (pp. 15–46). London: Karnac.

Verhaeghe, P. (1999) *Love in a Time of Loneliness*. London: Rebus Press.

Vermote, R. (2011) On the value of "late Bion" to analytic theory and practice. *International Journal of Psychoanalysis*, 92:1089–1092.

Vermote, R. (2013) The undifferentiated zone of psychic functioning: An integrative approach and clinical implications. Presentation at the European Psychoanalytical Federation (EPF) Conference, Basel, March 24. See also: Vermote, R. The undifferentiated zone of psychic functioning. European Psychoanalytical Federation, *Psychoanalysis in Europe Bulletin*, 2013, 67:16–27.

Weiner, J. (1995) *The Beach of the Finch: A Story of Evolution in Our Time*. New York: Vintage Books.

Welldon, E.V. (1998) *Mother, Madonna, Whore: The Idealization and Denigration of Motherhood*. London: Free Association Books.

Welldon, E.V. (2002) Sadomasochism. Cambridge, UK: Icon Books/Ideas in Psychoanalysis.

Whan, M. (2003) Mercurius, archetype, and 'transpsychic reality': C.G. Jung's parapsychology of spirit(s). In N. Totten (ed.), *Psychoanalysis and the Paranormal: Lands of Darkness* (pp. 105–127). London: Karnac.

Widlöcher, D. (2004) The third in mind. *Psychoanalytic Quarterly*, 73:197–213.

Winnicott, C. (1974) Editorial note. Fear of breakdown, D.W. Winnicott. *International Review of Psychoanalysis*, 1:102.

Winnicott, C. (1980) Fear of breakdown: A clinical example. *International Journal of Psychoanalysis*, 61:351–357.

Winnicott, D.W. (1935) The manic defence. In *Through Pediatrics to Psycho-Analysis: Collected Papers* (pp. 129–144). London: Karnac Books and The Institute of Psychoanalysis, 1992.

Winnicott, D.W. (1945) Primitive emotional development. In *Through Pediatrics to Psycho-Analysis: Collected Papers* (pp. 145–156). London: Karnac, 1992.

Winnicott, D.W. (1949a) Birth memories, birth trauma and anxiety. In *Through Pediatrics to Psycho-Analysis: Collected Papers* (pp. 174–193). London: Karnack Books, 1992.

Winnicott, D.W. (1949b) Mind and its relation to the psyche-soma. In *Through Pediatrics to Psycho-Analysis: Collected Papers* (pp. 243–254). London: Karnack Books, 1992.

Winnicott, D.W. (1954a). Metapsychological and clinical aspects of regression within the psycho-analytical set-up. In *Through Pediatrics to Psycho-Analysis: Collected Papers* (pp. 278–294). London: Karnac, 1992.

Winnicott, D.W. (1954b). Withdrawal and regression. In *Through Pediatrics to Psycho-Analysis: Collected Papers* (pp. 255–261). London: Karnac, 1992.

Winnicott, D.W. (1954–5) The depression position in normal emotional development. In *Through Pediatrics to Psycho-Analysis: Collected Papers* (pp. 262–277). London: Karnack Books, 1992.

Winnicott, D.W. (1955–6) Clinical varieties of transference. In *Through Paediatrics to Psycho-Analysis: Collected Papers* (pp. 295–299). London: Karnack Books, 1992.

Winnicott, D.W. (1959–1964). Classification: Is there a psycho-analytic contribution to psychiatric classification? In *The Maturational Processes and the Facilitating Environment* (pp. 124–139). London: The Hogarth Press and the Intitute of Psycho-analysis, 1965.

Winnicott, D.W. (1962) The aims of psycho-analytical treatment. In *The Maturational Processes and the Facilitating Environment* (pp. 166–170). London: The Hogarth Press and the Intitute of Psycho-analysis, 1979.

Winnicott, D.W. (1963a) Psychiatric disorders in terms of infantile maturational processes. In *The Maturational Processes and the Facilitating Environment* (pp. 230–241). London: The Hogarth Press and the Institute of Psycho-Analysis, 1979.

Winnicott, D.W. (1963b) Dependence in infant-care, in child-care, and in the psycho-analytic setting. In *The Maturational Processes and the Facilitating Environment* (pp. 249–259). London: The Hogarth Press and the Institute of Psycho-Analysis, 1979.

Winnicott, D.W. (1963c). Communicating and not communicating leading to a study of certain opposites. In: *The Maturational Processes and the Facilitating Environment* (pp. 179–192). London: The Hogarth Press and the Intitute of Psycho-analysis, 1979.

Winnicott, D.W. (1964a) The importance of the setting in meeting regression in psycho-analysis. In C. Winnicott, R. Shepherd, & M. Davis (eds.), *Psycho-Analytic Explorations* (pp. 96–102). London: Karnac Books, 1989.

Winnicott, D. W. (1964b). The baby as a going concern. In: *The Child, the Family, and the Outside World* (pp. 25–29). Harmondsworth: Penguin Books.

Winnicott, D.W. (1965a) The psychology of madness: A contribution from psychoanalysis. In C. Winnicott R. Shepherd, M. Davis (eds.), *Psycho-analytic Explorations* (pp. 119–129). London: Karnac Books, 1989.

Winnicott, D.W. (1965b) The concept of trauma in relation to the development of the individual within the family. In C. Winnicott, R. Shepherd, M. Davis (eds.), *Psycho-analytic Explorations* (pp. 130–148). Cambridge, MA: Harvard, 1989.

Winnicott, D.W. (1967a). The concept of clinical regression compared with that of defence organization. In C. Winnicott, R. Shepherd, & M. Davis (eds.), *Psycho-Analytic Explorations* (pp. 193–199). London: Karnac Books, 1989.

Winnicott, D.W. (1967b) Delinquency as a sign of hope. In C. Winnicott, R. Shepherd & M. Davis (eds.), *Home Is Where We Start From* (pp. 90–100). London: Penguin Books, 1986.

Winnicott, D.W. (1968?) Thinking and symbol-formation. In C. Winnicott, R. Shepherd, & M. Davis (eds.), *Psycho-Analytic Explorations* (pp. 213–216). London: Karnac Books, 1989.

Winnicott, D.W. (1969a) Additional note on psycho-somatic disorder. In C. Winnicott, R. Shepherd, M. Davis (eds.), *Psycho-Analytic Explorations* (pp. 115–118). Cambridge, MA: Harvard University Press, 1989.

Winnicott, D.W. (1969b) The mother–infant experience of mutuality. In C. Winnicott, R. Shepherd, & M. Davis (eds.), *Psycho-analytic Explorations* (pp. 251–261). London: Karnac Books, 1989.

Winnicott, D.W. (1969c) The use of an object in the context of Moses and Monotheism. In C. Winnicott, R. Shepherd, & M. Davis (eds.), *Psycho-Analytic Explorations* (pp. 240–246). London: Karnac Books, 1989.

Winnicott, D.W. (1971a) *Playing and Reality*. Harmondsworth, Middlesex: Penguin.

Winnicott, D.W. (1971b) *Therapeutic Consultations in Child Psychiatry*. London: The Hogarth Press.

Winnicott, D.W. (1974) Fear of breakdown. *International Review of Psycho-Analysis*, 1:103–107.

Winnicott, D.W. (1986a) *Holding and Interpretation: Fragment of an Analysis*. London: Karnac Books and the Institute of Psycho-Analysis.

Winnicott, D.W. (1986b) Sum, I am. In C. Winnicott, R. Shepherd, & M. Davis (eds.), *Home Is Where We Start From* (pp. 55–64). Penguin Books.

Winnicott, D.W. (1988a) *Babies and their Mothers*. London: Free Association Books.

Winnicott, D.W. (1988b) *Human Nature*. London: Free Association Books.

Winnicott, D.W. (1989) *The Family and Individual Development*. London & New York: Routledge.

Wolf, N.S., Gales M.E., Shane, E., & Shane, M. (2001) The developmental trajectory from amodal perception to empathy and communication: The role of mirror neurons in this process. *Psychoanalytic Inquiry*, 21:94–112.

Wolfenstein, E.V. (1985) Three principles of mental functioning in psychoanalytic.

Woolf, V. (1976) Sketch of the past. In *Moments of Being: Autobiographical Writings* (pp. 78–160). London: Pimlico, 2002.

Young-Eisendrath, P. (2001) When the fruit ripens: Alleviating suffering and increasing compassion as goals of clinical psychoanalysis. *Psychoanalytic Quarterly*, 70:265–285.

Zulueta de, F. (2012) Making sense of the symptoms and behavior of survivors of child abuse who suffer from complex PTSD and borderline personality disorders. AIMS (UK) Clinical Workshop Series, Tavistock, London, March.

Index

For Product Safety Concerns and Information please contact our EU
representative GPSR@taylorandfrancis.com
Taylor & Francis Verlag GmbH, Kaufingerstraße 24, 80331 München, Germany

www.ingramcontent.com/pod-product-compliance
Ingram Content Group UK Ltd.
Pitfield, Milton Keynes, MK11 3LW, UK
UKHW022216190926
475702UK00003B/385

* 9 7 8 1 1 3 8 1 8 6 3 3 0 *